T0200171

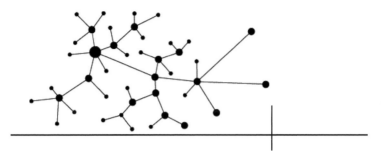

PRECISION PSYCHIATRY

Using Neuroscience Insights to Inform
Personally Tailored, Measurement-Based Care

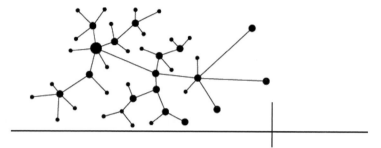

PRECISION PSYCHIATRY

Using Neuroscience Insights to Inform Personally Tailored, Measurement-Based Care

Edited by

Leanne M. Williams, Ph.D.
Laura M. Hack, M.D., Ph.D.

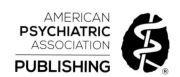

AMERICAN
PSYCHIATRIC
ASSOCIATION
PUBLISHING

If you wish to buy 50 or more copies of the same title, please go to www.appi.org/specialdiscounts for more information.

Copyright © 2022 American Psychiatric Association Publishing

ALL RIGHTS RESERVED

First Edition

Manufactured in the United States of America on acid-free paper
25   24   23   22   21   5   4   3   2   1

American Psychiatric Association Publishing
800 Maine Avenue SW
Suite 900
Washington, DC 20024-2812
www.appi.org

Library of Congress Cataloging-in-Publication Data
Names: Williams, Leanne M., editor. | Hack, Laura M., editor. | American Psychiatric Association Publishing, publisher.
Title: Precision psychiatry : using neuroscience insights to inform personally tailored, measurement-based care / edited by Leanne M. Williams, Laura M. Hack.
Description: First edition. | Washington, DC : American Psychiatric Association Publishing, [2022] | Includes bibliographical references and index.
Identifiers: LCCN 2021029289 (print) | LCCN 2021029290 (ebook) | ISBN 9781615371587 (paperback ; alk. paper) | ISBN 9781615374458 (ebook)
Subjects: MESH: Neuropsychiatry—methods | Precision Medicine—methods | Biomarkers—analysis
Classification: LCC RC341 (print) | LCC RC341 (ebook) | NLM WM 102 | DDC 616.8—dc23
LC record available at https://lccn.loc.gov/2021029289
LC ebook record available at https://lccn.loc.gov/2021029290

British Library Cataloguing in Publication Data
A CIP record is available from the British Library.

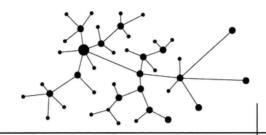

Contents

Part 1: Neuroimaging of Circuits

Part 2: Neurocognition, Neurophysiology, and Behavior

Part 3: Blood Markers

Part 4: Translational Neurobiological Approaches

Part 5: New Approaches and Computational Models That Bridge Neuroscience Insights and Clinical Application

Part 6: Developing the Academic Discipline of Precision Psychiatry

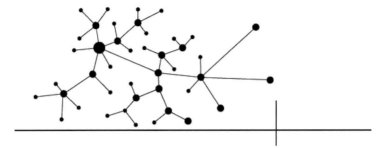

CONTRIBUTORS

Melissa R. Arbuckle, M.D., Ph.D.
Professor of Psychiatry, Columbia University Irving Medical Center; Vice Chair for Education and Director of Resident Education, Department of Psychiatry, Columbia University Irving Medical Center and the New York State Psychiatric Institute, New York

Tali M. Ball, Ph.D.
Instructor, Department of Psychiatry and Behavioral Sciences, Stanford University School of Medicine; Psychologist, Stanford Health Care, Stanford, California

Yosef A. Berlow, M.D., Ph.D.
Assistant Professor, Department of Psychiatry and Human Behavior, Alpert Medical School of Brown University and the VA RR&D Center for Neurorestoration and Neurotechnology, Providence VA Medical Center, Providence, Rhode Island

Isabel M. Berwian, Ph.D.
Postdoctoral Research Associate, Princeton Neuroscience Institute, Princeton University, Princeton, New Jersey

Chad A. Bousman, Ph.D.
Associate Professor, Departments of Medical Genetics, Psychiatry, Physiology, and Pharmacology, University of Calgary, Calgary, Alberta, Canada; Department of Psychiatry, University of Melbourne, Melbourne, Victoria, Australia

Joseph J. Cooper, M.D.
Associate Professor of Clinical Psychiatry, Director of Medical Student Education in Psychiatry, and Co-Director of Behavioral Neurology and Neuropsychiatry Fellowship, Department of Psychiatry, University of Illinois at Chicago, Chicago, Illinois

Docia L. Demmin, M.S.
Doctoral Student, Department of Psychology, and University Behavioral Health Care, Rutgers, The State University of New Jersey, Piscataway, New Jersey

Boadie W. Dunlop, M.D.
Professor and Director, Mood and Anxiety Disorders Program, Department of Psychiatry and Behavioral Sciences, Emory University School of Medicine, Atlanta, Georgia

Jennifer C. Felger, Ph.D.
Associate Professor and Laboratory Director, Behavioral Immunology Program, Department of Psychiatry and Behavioral Sciences, Emory University School of Medicine, Atlanta, Georgia

Malcolm P. Forbes, M.B.B.S.
Clinical Senior Fellow, Department of Psychiatry, University of Melbourne, Melbourne, Victoria, Australia

Samantha I. Fradkin, M.S.
Doctoral student, Department of Psychology, University of Rochester, Rochester, New York

David R. Goldsmith, M.D.
Assistant Professor; Faculty, Behavioral Immunology Program; Co-Director, Persistent Symptoms: Treatment, Assessment, and Recovery (PSTAR) Clinic, Department of Psychiatry and Behavioral Sciences, Emory University School of Medicine, Atlanta, Georgia

Laura M. Hack, M.D., Ph.D.
Postdoctoral Fellow, Advanced Fellowship in Mental Illness Research and Treatment, Palo Alto Veterans Affairs Health Care System, Sierra-Pacific MIRECC; Clinical Instructor and Director of the Translational Precision Mental Health Clinic, Department of Psychiatry and Behavioral Sciences, Stanford University School of Medicine, Stanford, California

Nathaniel G. Harnett, Ph.D.
Instructor, Neurobiology of Fear Laboratory, Division of Depression and Anxiety, McLean Hospital, Belmont, Massachusetts; Department of Psychiatry, Harvard Medical School, Boston, Massachusetts

Ebrahim Haroon, M.D.
Associate Professor and Medical Director, Behavioral Immunology Program, Department of Psychiatry and Behavioral Sciences, Emory University School of Medicine, Atlanta, Georgia

Peter Hitchcock, Ph.D.
Postdoctoral Research Associate, Laboratory of Neural Computation and Cognition, Department of Cognitive, Linguistic and Psychological Sciences, Brown University, Providence, Rhode Island

Quentin J.M. Huys, M.D., Ph.D.
Clinical Associate Professor, Division of Psychiatry and Max Planck UCL Centre for Computational Psychiatry and Ageing Research, University College London; Honorary Consultant Psychiatrist, Camden and Islington NHS Foundation Trust, London, United Kingdom

Carolina Medeiros Da Frota Ribeiro, M.D.
Assistant Professor, Department of Psychiatry and Behavioral Sciences, Emory University School of Medicine, Atlanta, Georgia

Andrew H. Miller, M.D.
William P. Timmie Professor, Vice Chair of Research, and Director, Behavioral Immunology Program, Department of Psychiatry and Behavioral Sciences, Emory University School of Medicine, Atlanta, Georgia

Jyoti Mishra, Ph.D.
Assistant Professor, Department of Psychiatry, University of California—San Diego, La Jolla, California

Mor Nahum, Ph.D.
Senior Lecturer, School of Occupational Therapy, Faculty of Medicine, Hebrew University, Jerusalem, Israel

Charles B. Nemeroff, M.D., Ph.D.
Chair and Professor, Department of Psychiatry; Director, Institute for Early Life Adversity Research, University of Texas Austin, Dell Medical School, Austin, Texas

Yael Niv, Ph.D.
Professor and Co-Director, Rutgers-Princeton Center for Computational Neuropsychiatry (CCNP), Princeton Neuroscience Institute and Psychology Department, Princeton University, Princeton, New Jersey

Martin P. Paulus, M.D.
Scientific Director and President, Laureate Institute for Brain Research, Tulsa, Oklahoma

Giampaolo Perna, M.D., Ph.D.
Professor, Department of Biological Sciences, Humanitas University, Milan, Italy; Chair, Department of Clinical Neurosciences, Villa San Benedetto Menni, Hermanas Hospitalarias, Como, Italy

Noah S. Philip, M.D.
Associate Professor, Department of Psychiatry and Human Behavior, Alpert Medical School of Brown University and the VA RR&D Center for Neurorestoration and Neurotechnology, Providence VA Medical Center, Providence, Rhode Island

Mary L. Phillips, M.D.
Pittsburgh Foundation—Emmerling Endowed Chair in Psychotic Disorders; Professor in Psychiatry and Clinical and Translational Science; Director of the Center for Research on Translational and Developmental Affective Neuroscience; Director of the Mood and Brain Laboratory, University of Pittsburgh, Pittsburgh, Pennsylvania

Daniel Pine, Ph.D.
Chief, Section on Developmental and Affective Neuroscience, and Co-Chief, Emotion and Development Branch, National Institute of Mental Health, Bethesda, Maryland

Diego A. Pizzagalli, Ph.D.
Professor of Psychiatry; Director, Center for Depression, Anxiety, and Stress Research; Director, McLean Imaging Center, McLean Hospital, Harvard Medical School, Belmont, Massachusetts

Ian S. Ramsay, Ph.D.
Assistant Professor, Department of Psychiatry and Behavioral Sciences, University of Minnesota Medical School, Minneapolis, Minnesota

Kerry J. Ressler, M.D., Ph.D.
Chief Scientific Officer; Chief, Center of Excellence in Depression and Anxiety Disorders; James and Patricia Poitras Chair in Psychiatry; and Director, Neurobiology of Fear Laboratory, McLean Hospital, Belmont, Massachusetts; Professor of Psychiatry, Department of Psychiatry, Harvard Medical School, Boston, Massachusetts

David A. Ross, M.D., Ph.D.
Associate Professor, Department of Psychiatry, Yale University School of Medicine, New Haven, Connecticut

Matthew D. Sacchet, Ph.D.
Instructor in Psychiatry and Assistant Neuroscientist, Center for Depression, Anxiety, and Stress Research, McLean Hospital, Harvard Medical School, Belmont, Massachusetts

Gila Schoen, M.D.
Psychiatrist, Child and Adolescent Division, Geha Mental Health Center, Petah Tikva, Israel

Antonia V. Seligowski, Ph.D.
Assistant Neuroscientist, Neurobiology of Fear Laboratory, Instructor in Psychology, Division of Depression and Anxiety, McLean Hospital, Belmont, Massachusetts; Department of Psychiatry, Harvard Medical School, Boston, Massachusetts

Steven M. Silverstein, Ph.D.
George L. Engel Professor of Psychosocial Medicine; Associate Chair of Research, Department of Psychiatry; Professor of Psychiatry, Neuroscience, and Ophthalmology; and Center for Visual Science, University of Rochester Medical Center, Rochester, New York

Michael J. Travis, M.D.
Associate Professor and Director of Residency Training, Department of Psychiatry, University of Pittsburgh School of Medicine, UPMC Western Psychiatric Hospital, Pittsburgh, Pennsylvania

Michael T. Treadway, Ph.D.
Associate Professor and Director, TReAD Lab, Department of Psychology, Emory University, Atlanta, Georgia

Sophia Vinogradov, M.D.
Donald W. Hastings Endowed Chair in Psychiatry and Department Head of Psychiatry and Behavioral Sciences, University of Minnesota Medical School, Minneapolis, Minnesota

Ashley E. Walker, M.D.
Associate Professor and Director of Residency Training, Department of Psychiatry, University of Oklahoma School of Community Medicine, Tulsa, Oklahoma

Christian A. Webb, Ph.D.
Assistant Professor of Psychiatry and Director, Treatment and Etiology of Depression in Youth (TEDY) Laboratory, Center for Depression, Anxiety, and Stress Research, McLean Hospital, Harvard Medical School, Belmont, Massachusetts

Leanne M. Williams, Ph.D.
Professor and Associate Chair of Translational Neuroscience and Director of the Precision Psychiatry and Translational Neuroscience Lab (PanLab), Stanford Department of Psychiatry and Behavioral Sciences; Director of the Stanford Center for Precision Mental Health and Wellness at Stanford University School of Medicine; and Director of Precision Medicine at the Department of Veterans Affairs, Sierra-Pacific MIRECC, California

Amin Zandvakili, M.D., Ph.D.
Assistant Professor, Department of Psychiatry and Human Behavior, Alpert Medical School of Brown University and the VA RR&D Center for Neurorestoration and Neurotechnology, Providence VA Medical Center, Providence, Rhode Island

DISCLOSURE OF COMPETING INTERESTS

The following contributors to this book have indicated a financial interest in or other affiliation with a commercial supporter, a manufacturer of a commercial product, a provider of a commercial service, a nongovernmental organization, and/or a government agency, as listed below:

Yosef A. Berlow, M.D., Ph.D.—Dr. Berlow's work is supported by grants from the National Institute of Mental Health (NIMH R25 MH101076) and the VA RR&D Center for Neurorestoration and Neurotechnology. The author reports no financial relationships with commercial interests.

Boadie W. Dunlop, M.D.—Dr. Dunlop has received honoraria for consulting services to Myriad Neuroscience, which markets the GeneSight Psychotropic Test.

Helen Mayberg, M.D.—Dr. Mayberg receives consulting and IP licensing fees from Abbott Neuromodulation.

Andrew H. Miller, M.D.—Dr. Miller is a paid consultant for Boehringer Ingelheim.

Charles B. Nemeroff, M.D., Ph.D.—Dr. Nemeroff reports the following: *Research/Grant:* National Institutes of Health (NIH); *Consulting (last three years):* Xhale, Takeda, Taisho Pharmaceutical, Signant Health, Sunovion Pharmaceuticals, Janssen Research & Development, Magstim, Navitor Pharmaceuticals, TC MSO, Intra-Cellular Therapies, EMA Wellness, Gerson Lehrman Group, Acadia Pharmaceuticals, Magnolia CNS, Compass Pathways, Epiodyne, Sophos, Axsome; *Stockholder:* Xhale, Celgene, Seattle Genetics, AbbVie, OPKO Health, Antares, BI Gen Holdings, Corcept Therapeutics Pharmaceuticals Company, TC MSO, Trends in Pharma Development, EMA Wellness; *Scientific Advisory Boards:* American Foundation for Suicide Prevention, Brain and Behavior Research Foundation, Xhale, Anxiety Disorders Association of America, Skyland Trail, Signant Health, Laureate Institute for Brain Research, Magnolia CNS; *Board of Directors:* Gratitude America, ADAA, Xhale Smart; *Income sources or equity of $10,000 or more:* American Psychiatric Association Publishing, Xhale, Signant Health, CME Outfitters, Intra-Cellular Therapies, Magstim, EMA Wellness; *Patents:* Method and devices for transdermal delivery of lithium (US 6,375,990B1), Method of assessing antidepressant drug therapy via transport inhibition of monoamine neurotransmitters by ex vivo assay (US 7,148,027B2), Compounds, compositions, methods of synthesis, and methods of treatment (CRF receptor binding ligand) (US 8,551, 996 B2).

Giampaolo Perna, M.D., Ph.D.—Dr. Perna is a consultant for Pfizer, Lundbeck, Menarini, and Mediobio Ldt.

Noah S. Philip, M.D.—Dr. Philip's work is supported by grants from the U.S. Department of Veterans Affairs (VA) (I01 RX002450), and the VA RR&D Center for Neurorestoration and Neurotechnology. In the past, Dr. Philip has received grant support from Janssen, Neosync, and Neuronetics through clinical trial contracts and has served as an unpaid scientific advisory board member for Neuronetics.

Diego A. Pizzagalli, Ph.D.—Dr. Pizzagalli has received consulting fees from Akili Interactive Labs, BlackThorn Therapeutics, Boehringer Ingelheim, Posit Science, and Takeda Pharmaceuticals, as well as an honorarium from Alkermes.

Kerry J. Ressler, M.D., Ph.D.—Dr. Ressler is on the Scientific Advisory Boards for Resilience Therapeutics, Sheppard Pratt–Lieber Research Institute, Laureate Institute for Brain Research, The Army STARRS Project, UCSD VA Center of Excellence for Stress and Mental Health—CES-AMH, and the Anxiety and Depression Association of America. He provides fee-for-service consultation for Alkermes and Resilience Therapeutics. He holds patents for use of D-cycloserine and psychotherapy, targeting PAC_1 receptor for extinction, targeting tachykinin-2 for prevention of fear, and targeting angiotensin to improve extinction of fear. He receives or has received research funding from NIMH, HHMI, Brainsway, Genomind, and NARSAD.

Matthew D. Sacchet, Ph.D.—Dr. Sacchet has received consulting fees from Vorso Corporation.

Michael T. Treadway, Ph.D.—Dr. Treadway has received consulting fees from Avanir Pharmaceuticals and BlackThorn Therapeutics. No funding or sponsorship was provided by these companies for the current work.

Sophia Vinogradov, M.D.—Dr. Vinogradov has received grant/research support from the Lynne and Andrew Redleaf Foundation and other financial or material support from Mindstrong Alkermes, Psyberguide, and Verily Life Sciences.

Leanne M. Williams, Ph.D.—U.S. Patent Applications 10/034,645 and 15/820,338: Systems and methods for detecting complex networks in MRI image data.

Amin Zandvakili, M.D., Ph.D.—Dr. Zandvakili's work is supported by grants from the National Institute of General Medical Sciences (NIGMS U54GM115677) and the VA RR&D Center for Neurorestoration and Neurotechnology. The author reports no financial relationships with commercial interests.

The following contributors have indicated that they have no financial interests or other affiliations that represent or could appear to represent a competing interferes with their contributions to this book:

Tali M. Ball, Ph.D.

Isabel M. Berwian, Ph.D.

Chad A. Bousman, Ph.D.

Docia L. Demmin, M.S.

Jennifer C. Felger, Ph.D.

Malcolm P. Forbes, M.B.B.S.

Samantha I. Fradkin, M.S.

David R. Goldsmith, M.D.

Laura M. Hack, M.D., Ph.D.

Nathaniel G. Harnett, Ph.D.

Ebrahim Haroon, M.D.

Peter Hitchcock, Ph.D.

Quentin J.M. Huys, M.D., Ph.D.

Carolina Medeiros Da Frota Ribeiro, M.D.

Jyoti Mishra, Ph.D.

Yael Niv, Ph.D.

Martin P. Paulus, M.D.

Mary L. Phillips, M.D.

Daniel Pine, Ph.D.

Ian S. Ramsay, Ph.D.

Gila Schoen, M.D.

Antonia V. Seligowski, Ph.D.

Steven M. Silverstein, Ph.D.

Michael J. Travis, M.D.

Christian A. Webb, Ph.D.

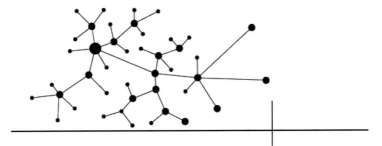

FOREWORD

While our strategies may vary, the vision of precision psychiatry is to optimize treatment for each and every patient. Toward this mission, dependable treatment selection algorithms, regardless of the indication, should not only match an individual to their best treatment option but also avoid an ineffective or potentially harmful one. Although this goal is seen by some as an impractical or, at best, naïve blue-sky goal, contemporary clinical neuroscience research speaks to the ultimate achievability of this holy grail quest. The contributors to this book provide clear evidence that the goal is indeed within sight.

The need has never seemed more urgent. Amplifying our impatience is the fact that current treatment selection continues to rely on experiential trial and error—the perennial stopgap. It is assumed that, while inefficient, this approach is generally effective, although the evidence is increasingly clear that the more treatments that are tried and failed, the less likely it is that any subsequent one will work, so getting the "right treatment" at the time of first intervention is paramount. More ominous is the hypothesis that exposure to the "wrong" treatment may itself contribute to the development of treatment resistance over time. Further underscoring this need is that patients are understandably suspect when told a treatment works well "on average," when what they really want to know is what treatment will work best for them. While frustration with this status quo serves as a useful scientific catalyst for many of us, despair, not frustration, is the upshot for many patients who have exhausted their available options. It is in this context that past ambivalence about the use of biomarkers to guide treatment is lessening, and development of biomarkers is now seen as a critical clinical need, complementing studies of disease pathophysiology and ultimately development of preventions and cures.

This book highlights the tremendous progress in the field toward these many important goals. Although the concept of "precision psychiatry" is not new, suitable tools to deconstruct and validate the multitude of putative moderators and mediators of illness risk, symptom severity, and phenotypical heterogeneity are relatively recent additions. Basic clinical and computational strategies are now routinely applied to address the complex interaction of molecular, developmental, chemical, structural, and environmental contributors to specific disorders and syndromes. As the precision psychiatry field has grown and matured, there are now means and methods to move beyond hypothesis-driven experiments in small prospective cohorts. Studies now include large-scale genetic, behavioral, and imaging phenotyping of increasingly larger cohorts of well-characterized patients and their families, informed by basic and translational studies in strategic animal models. The symbiosis of these multimodal strategies is at the core of precision psychiatry, with key examples highlighted in the various chapters of this book.

The tremendous progress of the field broadly provides the opportunity to reflect on just how far we have come since the 1980s toward actionable precision approaches for the treatment of major depression. My own studies, beginning in the mid-1980s, first examined brain metabolic patterns of depression in neurological patients. In those early days of functional neuroimaging using PET, the capacity to move beyond conducting static correlational analyses of postmortem or X-ray computed tomography lesions to mapping the living brain in action was a paradigm shift for the study of behavioral disorder when there were no pathognomonic markers. Resting-state studies of blood flow and metabolism identified a similar pattern of limbic-frontal abnormalities in depressed patients with stroke, Parkinson's disease, and Huntington's disease, a pattern also seen in unipolar depressed patients, suggesting a common depression signature, independent of etiology, and thus providing core elements for a putative depression circuit model (Mayberg 1994).

The simple-minded notion of a common depression pathway, while short-lived, did provide an anchor to interpret the variability revealed through studies of antidepressant treatment effects. In these early experiments, frontal abnormalities, common across all subjects at pretreatment baseline as previously noted, were accompanied by differential anterior cingulate metabolism that distinguished eventual medication responders from nonresponders. The concept of ongoing adaptive changes in patients prior to seeking care that might impact their ultimate response to treatment, although representing a shift from our initial hypothesis, was an important first clue to the notion of depression subtypes tied to treatment rather than symptom variability. We noted that the "presence of this metabolic signature in individual patients may prove useful in identifying those at risk for a difficult disease course" (Mayberg et al. 1997), a conclusion that unwittingly foretold the trajectory of our future work and defined what has become a cornerstone of the precision psychiatry mission—treatment selection biotyping.

These initial observations next led to a series of studies designed to characterize treatment mechanisms, starting with first-line antidepressant medications (Mayberg et al. 2000). In addition to identifying a nonlinear time course of brain changes over the course of 6 weeks of treatment, these studies also revealed distinct differences between responders and nonresponders (Mayberg 1997, 2000). Studies of single medications and placebo led to the natural next step—a complementary study of cognitive-behavioral therapy (CBT), an alternative first-line treatment. Interestingly, it was this experiment, designed to define a common response pathway independent of treatment type, that first demonstrated that different treatment classes target a common set of brain regions in complementary but non-overlapping patterns (Goldapple et al. 2004). These findings further enabled explicit testing of simple causal models and identification of putative treatment-specific "circuit" subtypes (Seminowicz et al. 2004). These preliminary studies also served to guide trial design and analytic strategies to define baseline imaging patterns that might differentially predict remission or failure to both medication and CBT (Mayberg 2003). Consecutive studies in distinct cohorts using fluorodeoxyglucose-PET and resting-state functional MRI to explore functional connectivity, respectively, independently defined two distinct imaging-based biotypes, both suitable for precision treatment selection in prospective trials (Dunlop et al. 2017; McGrath et al. 2013). In parallel, these data-driven depression models were also foundational to the development and testing of deep brain stimulation (DBS) of the subcallosal cingulate—a key node in our depression network—for treatment-resistant patients (Mayberg et al. 2005). Ongoing DBS studies continue to emphasize the importance of precision imaging, with surgical implantation of DBS leads now optimized using individualized tractography-guided methods (Riva-Posse et al. 2014), verified by predictable and reproducible intraoperative behavioral effects with therapeutic stimulation at predefined target locations (Riva-Posse et al. 2018).

Whether one uses a hypothesis-driven study in a small patient cohort or a model-free, "big data" approach, we share a common goal: to develop biomarkers and algorithms that will discriminate patient subgroups and optimize treatment selection in the management of individual patients across all stages of illness. Treatment selection is not a negotiation, but rather the best option given the current evidence. Ultimately, clinical use of such discoveries will require biomarkers that are not only robust but scalable. While the complexity of psychiatric disorders will always require a holistic approach, our evolving methodological toolkit now puts us in position to align our approaches with those in the fields of cardiology, oncology, and infectious disease, where treatment selection is routinely based not on preference or expediency but on explicit molecular, imaging, and biological markers. What is clear is that one size does not fit all; so the pursuit of a true precision approach, in all of its complexity, *is* our future.

Helen Mayberg, M.D.
Professor of Psychiatry, Neurology, Neuroscience, and Neurosurgery,
Icahn School of Medicine at Mount Sinai, New York, New York

References

Dunlop BW, Rajendra JK, Craighead WE, et al: Functional connectivity of the subcallosal cingulate cortex and differential outcomes to treatment with cognitive-behavioral therapy or antidepressant medication for major depressive disorder. Am J Psychiatry 174(6):533–545, 2017 28335622

Goldapple K, Segal Z, Garson C, et al: Modulation of cortical-limbic pathways in major depression: treatment-specific effects of cognitive behavior therapy. Arch Gen Psychiatry 61(1):34–41, 2004 14706942

Mayberg HS: Frontal lobe dysfunction in secondary depression. J Neuropsychiatry Clin Neurosci 6(4):428–442, 1994 7841814

Mayberg HS: Limbic-cortical dysregulation: a proposed model of depression. J Neuropsychiatry Clin Neurosci 9(3):471–481, 1997 9276848

Mayberg HS: Modulating dysfunctional limbic-cortical circuits in depression: towards development of brain-based algorithms for diagnosis and optimised treatment. Br Med Bull 65:193–207, 2003 12697626

Mayberg HS, Brannan SK, Mahurin RK, et al: Cingulate function in depression: a potential predictor of treatment response. Neuroreport 8(4):1057–1061, 1997 9141092

Mayberg HS, Brannan SK, Mahurin RK, et al: Regional metabolic effects of fluoxetine in major depression: serial changes and relationship to clinical response. Biol Psychiatry 48(8):830–843, 2000 11063978

Mayberg HS, Lozano AM, Voon V, et al: Deep brain stimulation for treatment-resistant depression. Neuron 45(5):651–660, 2005 15748841

McGrath CL, Kelley ME, Holtzheimer PE, et al: Toward a neuroimaging treatment selection biomarker for major depressive disorder. JAMA Psychiatry 70(8):821–829, 2013 23760393

Riva-Posse P, Choi KS, Holtzheimer PE, et al: Defining critical white matter pathways mediating successful subcallosal cingulate deep brain stimulation for treatment-resistant depression. Biol Psychiatry 76(12):963–969, 2014 24832866

Riva-Posse P, Choi KS, Holtzheimer PE, et al: A connectomic approach for sub-callosal cingulate deep brain stimulation surgery: prospective targeting in treatment-resistant depression. Mol Psychiatry 23(4):843–849, 2018 28397839

Seminowicz DA, Mayberg HS, McIntosh AR, et al: Limbic-frontal circuitry in major depression: a path modeling metanalysis. Neuroimage 22(1):409–418, 2004 15110034

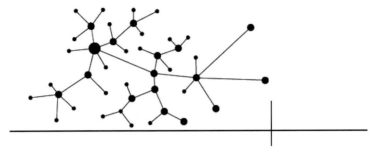

PREFACE

Precision Psychiatry: The Path Forward

Much of the world's health burden, measured in years lost to disability or premature mortality, is attributable to mental disorders. Every nation, every community, every family, and every person is affected, directly or indirectly, by these brain-based health conditions—conditions that are poorly understood, are often underrecognized, go untreated for years or for a lifetime, and are as yet incurable.

Psychiatry is the field of medicine that is dedicated to understanding mental disorders and helping people with these conditions to live fulfilling lives and to adapt to the unique challenges they face. In their clinical practice, psychiatrists work with courageous people who experience great distress and despair and also exhibit great resilience and dignity. Psychiatry also advances knowledge of the prevention, diagnosis, and treatment of mental disorders and awareness of how mental health and physical health go hand in hand.

Basic and clinical neuroscientists seek to discover the brain-based causes of different mental disorders and to discern patterns associated with mental disorders. Such discoveries will allow for better prevention, swifter treatment, and improved outcomes, benefiting people and populations today and in the future. This work has been hard going, however. The brain comprises nearly a hundred billion neurons, and these neurons connect in nearly a hundred trillion ways. These neurons adapt and change over the course of development, as do their many connections, and both are influenced by innumerable inherited and environmental factors. The phenomena that suggest or demonstrate the existence of an underlying mental disorder in people of different ages, genders, and across a continuum of cultures may be highly consistent or highly inconsistent. In this complexity one marvels that the brain works at all, rather than the fact that disorders may predictably arise.

Precision psychiatry represents a path forward, integrating findings from basic and clinical neuroscience, clinical practice, and population-level data. Precision psychiatry focuses on differentiating characteristics and patterns and, in an evidence-driven manner, developing therapeutic approaches that may be most helpful to specific individuals with a specific constellation of health issues, characteristics, strengths, and symptoms. In this book, the authors highlight progress in the treatment of common disorders such as depression, bipolar disorder, PTSD, and schizophrenia. Though treatment is remarkably effective in improving quality of life and reducing the burden of symptoms and impairments, finding the right treatment is too often a process of months or years. Moreover, mental disorders may complicate and worsen the risks associated with other health conditions. For example, depression increases the risk of cardiovascular-related deaths threefold. Addressing these challenges requires the very best, most cutting-edge approaches to prediction, prevention, and preemption that population science can possibly provide.

Harnessing advances in the fields of biomedical sciences, medicine, engineering, education, social sciences, and ethics will increasingly be the key to revolutionizing the diagnosis and treatment of mental illness with greater precision. With this book, we begin this new approach, advancing the care of our patients and advancing the field, which is dedicated to serving people living with mental disorders, and, ultimately, human health.

Laura Weiss Roberts, M.D., M.A.
Chairman and Katharine Dexter McCormick and Stanley McCormick Memorial Professor, Department of Psychiatry and Behavioral Sciences, Stanford University School of Medicine

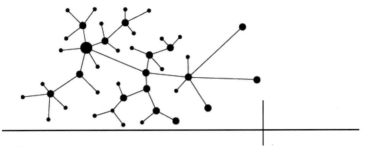

INTRODUCTION

A revolution is under way in psychiatry—one that integrates the scientific foundations of the discipline with recent advances in the neurosciences, data sciences, and technology in order to narrow the gap between discovery and clinical translation. This integration is motivated by the search for a model that connects a neurobiological understanding of mental disorder with clinical observation, in order to improve the precision of classification and treatment decisions. We feel the urgency to accelerate clinically applicable precision psychiatry and address the impact of major mental disorders on the very functions that enable us to live productive and satisfying lives. An estimated 970 million people worldwide experienced a mental or substance disorder in the past few years, and one in five people in the United States live with a mental disorder at some point in their lives.

Progress in precision medicine in disciplines outside of psychiatry, such as oncology and cardiology, has inspired progress reflected in the contributions in this book. In these disciplines, biomarkers are combined with clinical features to stratify patients into subtypes that are more coherent than are overarching diagnostic categories. This approach allows for identifying subtypes that are underserved by available therapies. It also allows for developing novel therapies aimed at targets that are based on specific mechanisms that affect measurable outcomes and that are closer to underlying disease processes than are traditional clinical endpoints.

We are gratified to offer this book to illustrate timely advances emerging in precision medicine in psychiatry. Contributors to this book have a common view that we require a neuroscience- and data-informed approach to advancing precision medicine in psychiatry. We believe that is it past time for mental health providers and educators to have ready access to the latest research in precise classification, treatment planning, and early identification across a spectrum of psychiatric disorders. While the scientific breakthroughs discussed in this book are exciting in their own right, they will only move our field forward if they are disseminated to trainees, clinicians, and, ultimately, our patients. Hence, throughout the chapters, our authors have included case examples of the applications of their topics, and the last chapter discusses the critical role of neuroscience education in precision psychiatry.

We are fortunate for the opportunity to bring together authors across a range of expertise who have played fundamental roles in the development of the discipline of precision psychiatry. They discuss biomarkers in neuroimaging, electrophysiology, and peripheral serum, as well as variations in genetic markers, neurocognition, and behavior. They examine the importance of computational approaches and machine learning. They take us on a journey through their topics from the history, sometimes dating back to the Middle Ages through the influential work of scholars like Gall and Kraepelin, through current knowledge, to what is needed to continue to progress the field. Our expert authors also review the precise application of multiple treatment modalities that include pharmacotherapy, cognitive-behavioral therapy, neurostimulation, and cognitive training programs on the individual level. Finally, throughout this book, they discuss issues of scalability and implementation, including the need for the tests we disseminate to our patients to have analytic and clinical validity as well as clinical utility.

We have elected to focus on mood and anxiety disorders as well as schizophrenia in adults given that the most robust evidence in precision psychiatry currently exists for these disorders and this age group. However, evidence is emerging in precision medicine for obsessive-compulsive, neurodevelopmental, and eating disorders and across the age range. We hope that future editions of this book will include chapters covering those disorders, a wider spectrum of age ranges, and the precise application of emerging therapies in mental health, including virtual reality, psychedelic medications, targeted delivery of drugs to specific regions of the brain, and digital therapies. While we are delighted with the topics covered in this book, we recognize that we were not able to include several emerging areas in precision psychiatry for which the evidence base is growing, such as epigenomics, proteomics, metabolomics, and induced pluripotent stem cells.

Our hope is that psychiatry will continue to follow the path of other fields that have advanced further in precision medicine, in its development of biological subtyping and tailored treatments in order to create a better future for our patients suffering from these devastating illnesses. We envision a future where providers will have access to mental health profiles that incorporate biological, clinical, and environmental information into an easily digestible format. Ideally, these profiles will be utilized collaboratively with our patients in conjunction with clinical expertise for the purpose of case formulation and treatment planning. These formulations and treatment plans will be updated through an iterative process that incorporates both active and passive information from mobile devices, wearables, and applications. In this way, we have the opportunity to merge technological advances with decades of research on the neurobiological, neurophysiological, genetic, and inflammatory mechanisms underlying mental illness and response to treatment into improved outcomes. Through this new understanding we also hope to help dissolve the stigma of mental disorders and the consequent discrimination and barriers to care. We hope that you will find this book engaging and enlightening and that it will serve as a stepping stone in your continual journey toward better care for your patients.

Laura M. Hack, M.D., Ph.D.
Leanne M. Williams, Ph.D.

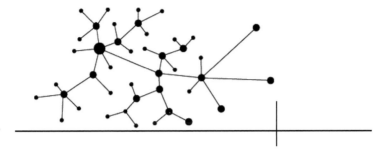

PART 1

Neuroimaging of Circuits

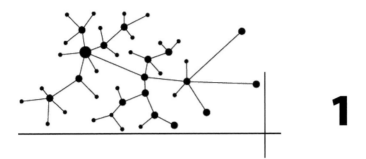

1

A Neural Circuit–Informed Taxonomy for Precision Psychiatry

Laura M. Hack, M.D., Ph.D.

Tali M. Ball, Ph.D.

Leanne M. Williams, Ph.D.

In this chapter, we make the case that precision psychiatry informed by neuroscience offers the opportunity to improve the precision of classification, treatment decisions, and prevention efforts. From this view, it is essential that advances in the neurobiological understanding of psychiatric disorders are mapped onto an understanding of clinical outcomes, and that clinical discoveries about treatment and disease progression can be interpreted relative to neural mechanisms. We focus on large-scale neural circuits of the human brain as assessed by functional MRI (fMRI) as a pertinent and proximal level of explanation for conceptualizing how a neurobiological understanding can offer more precise ways to classify psychiatric disorders and guide treatment choices. We use the term "large-scale neural circuit" or "network" to refer to the macroscale at which vast numbers of interconnected neurons constitute the anatomical and functional "connectome" of the brain.

We discuss emerging findings and case illustrations for major depressive disorder (MDD) and incorporate findings regarding anxiety, given the substantial overlap between features of depressive and anxiety disorders.

Incorporating Neural Circuit Dysfunction Into the Diagnostic Subtyping of Depressive and Anxiety Disorders: Biotyping Anchored in Neuroimaging

Researchers have identified circuits that are present intrinsically during task-free and at-rest states that are reproducible across studies and thought to underlie fundamental processes of self-reflection, salience perception and attention, and sensation (Buckner et al. 2013; Cole et al. 2014). Investigators have also identified circuits evoked by tasks that engage processes of emotional and cognitive function (Cole and Schneider 2007; Haber and Knutson 2010; Niendam et al. 2012). In illustrating a biotype approach to subtyping based on fMRI, we focus on six circuits: default mode, salience, negative affect, positive affect, attention, and cognitive control (Williams 2016, 2017). Knowledge about how disruptions of these circuits map onto clinical features and treatments is still emerging.

The *default mode circuit* (also known as the default mode network) has core connections between the anterior medial prefrontal cortex, posterior cingulate cortex, and angular gyrus (Greicius et al. 2003, 2009), and is typically assessed in task-free conditions. Disruptions in default connectivity are considered to reflect maladaptive self-referential processes expressed in rumination and worry. Distinct subtypes of depression have been distinguished by both hyperconnectivity (for meta-analysis, see Kaiser et al. 2016; for review, see Hamilton et al. 2015) and hypoconnectivity of the default mode (Price et al. 2017; Zhu et al. 2012; for meta-analysis, see Yan et al. 2019).

The *salience circuit* has core nodes in the anterior insula, anterior cingulate, and extended amygdala and is thought to detect salient interoceptive and exteroceptive changes. Salience circuit hypoconnectivity has been associated with greater symptom severity (Goldstein-Piekarski et al. 2020; Mulders et al. 2015) and may implicate generalized anxiety and anxious avoidance in particular (Mulders et al. 2015; Peterson et al. 2014; Williams 2016). Task-evoked insula hyperreactivity has been observed for sadness and disgust in MDD (Stuhrmann et al. 2011) and for anger, fear, and happiness in generalized anxiety disorder (Klumpp et al. 2013), suggesting in part a bias toward mood-congruent negative stimuli.

Affective circuits are robustly activated by stimuli that signal potential threats, negative events, or rewards. The *negative affect circuit* comprises the amygdala and connections with medial cortical regions, including ventral and dorsal medial prefrontal and anterior cingulate regions. Amygdala hyperreactivity occurs in depressive disorder, generalized anxiety disorder, social phobia/anxiety, and panic disorder elicited by threat-related stimuli (Fonzo et al. 2015; Jaworska et al. 2015; Killgore et al. 2014), and in depressive disorder elicited by sad stimuli (Williams 2016). Alterations in activation may also reflect a reduction in connectivity between the amygdala and regions of the anterior cingulate and medial prefrontal cortex (Matthews et al. 2008; Prater et al. 2013).

The *positive affect reward circuit* is defined by the nucleus accumbens (a key region of the ventral striatum) and ventral tegmental area, and their projections to the orbitofrontal cortex and medial prefrontal cortex. Hypoactivation of the ventral striatum characterizes at least a subgroup of individuals with depression, especially those with anhedonia (Greenberg et al. 2015) (for meta-analysis, see Hamilton et al. 2012; for reviews, see Der-Avakian and Markou 2012; Treadway and Zald 2011). In remitted depression, *hyper*activation of the frontal regions of this circuit has also been observed in response to happy faces (Keedwell et al. 2005; Mitterschiffthaler et al. 2003), reward outcomes (Dichter et al. 2012), and reward anticipation (Zhang et al. 2013).

Two additional circuits are relevant to the cognitive and concentration features of depression and anxiety, which are commonly given less emphasis than mood features. The frontoparietal *attention circuit* has been identified in the task-free state and is defined by core regions in the superior frontal cortex and anterior inferior parietal lobe, connecting with frontal eye fields. Relative hypoconnectivity within this circuit, and within constituent regions, has been implicated in the inattention and accompanying cognitive symptoms common across mood and anxiety disorders (Goldstein-Piekarski et al. 2020; Keller et al. 2020). The executive, or *cognitive control*, circuit involves the dorsal components of the lateral prefrontal cortex (dorsolateral prefrontal cortex [DLPFC]), anterior cingulate cortex (dACC), and parietal cortex engaged by tasks that require higher cognitive functions such as working memory and selective control of cognition (Niendam et al. 2012). In depression and social anxiety, DLPFC and dACC hypoactivation has been observed during cognitive tasks and in stress-induced situations (Korgaonkar et al. 2013; for review, see Williams 2016).

We anticipate that these circuit dysfunctions are modulated and refined as a result of other biological and environmental factors such as genetic variants and exposure to stress. As data accumulate, data-driven approaches will help define the optimal number of biotypes that account for the heterogeneity of mood and anxiety disorders (Figure 1–1). The utility of such pproaches has been demonstrated for subtypes of depression defined specifically by

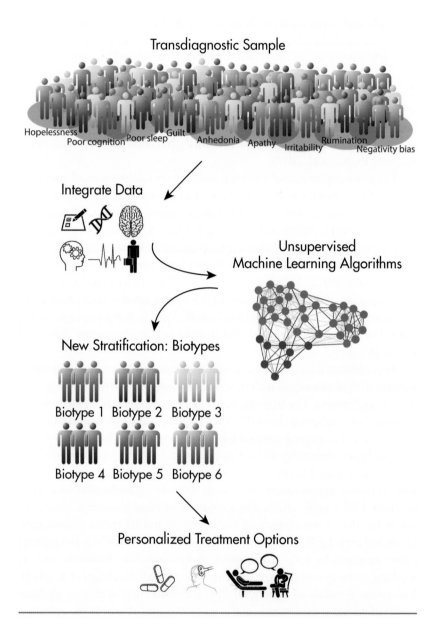

Figure 1–1. Example of how multimodal data and data-driven techniques may be used to help define the optimal number of biotypes accounting for the heterogeneity of mood and anxiety disorders.

To view this figure in color, see Plate 1 in Color Gallery.

The biotypes thus identified could then be utilized to guide patients to targeted treatments.

task-free circuit connectivity (Clementz et al. 2016; Drysdale et al. 2017; Goldstein-Piekarski et al. 2020; Maron-Katz et al. 2020).

Incorporating Neural Circuit Dysfunction Into Treatment Planning for Depressive and Anxiety Disorders

A goal of using neuroimaging to achieve more precise diagnosis of mood and anxiety disorder subtypes, based on underlying neural circuit function, is to provide clinicians with additional data to inform treatment choices (e.g., identifying which patients may benefit from pharmacotherapy, selecting a pharmacotherapy, limiting side effects). This goal has motivated large biomarker discovery trials that deploy neuroimaging along with other biomarker measures (Dunlop et al. 2012; Grieve et al. 2013; Trivedi et al. 2016).

In the International Study to Predict Optimized Treatment for Depression (iSPOT-D), for example, remission on typical first-line antidepressants depended on intact pretreatment connectivity of the default mode, whereas nonremission was predicted by hypoconnectivity (Goldstein-Piekarski et al. 2018; Korgaonkar et al. 2019). For the negative affect circuit evoked by emotion stimuli, pretreatment amygdala hyporeactivity to threat was a general predictor of subsequent response to a selective serotonin reuptake inhibitor (SSRI), whereas hyperreactivity to sadness was a specific predictor of nonresponse to the serotonin-norepinephrine reuptake inhibitor venlafaxine-XR (Williams et al. 2015). For the cognitive control circuit, intact activation and connectivity were predictive of response to SSRIs (Gyurak et al. 2016; Tozzi et al. 2020), while functional connectivity evoked by cognitive inhibition of task responses was shown to specifically differentiate responders to sertraline versus venlafaxine (Tozzi et al. 2020). In line with our earlier point about the modulation of these circuit dysfunctions, early life stress not only determines poor antidepressant responses overall (Williams et al. 2016a) but also, when combined with pretreatment negative affect circuit dysfunction, boosts the accuracy for identifying nonresponders (Goldstein-Piekarski et al. 2016).

Imaging biomarker studies that have formally evaluated sensitivity and specificity for first-line antidepressants have observed a predictive accuracy for response or remission of 70% or greater, which suggests these biomarkers have clinical utility. Although these figures may be reduced following external validation studies (i.e., when replications are attempted in independent samples), they still reflect great promise. Given that current treatment-matching approaches are essentially trial and error and a majority of patients do not respond to their first medication, even a small increase in predictive accuracy would be worthwhile. Furthermore, there is minimal risk in a novel strategy for selecting between FDA-approved treatments of comparable overall efficacy. Ultimately, the most valuable clinical predictions will be those that enable patients and providers to differentially select between treatment options.

The findings presented above also highlight the importance of identifying biomarkers that help guide the choice of alternative treatments for patients likely to be non-responders or who are already treatment resistant. Because of an arguably direct impact on large-scale neural circuits, transcranial magnetic stimulation (TMS), an FDA-cleared intervention for treatment-resistant depression, is of great interest in identifying circuit-based biotypes that discern patients who may not respond to pharmacotherapy but may benefit from TMS. Notably, default mode hypoconnectivity (predictive of pharmacotherapy nonremission in iSPOT-D) has been found to characterize responders to TMS (Philip et al. 2018). Hypoconnectivity of other circuits, such as the positive affect circuit, observed in the task-free state and implicated in pharmacotherapy nonresponse, also shows promise in identifying responders to TMS (Avissar et al. 2017; Downar et al. 2014). A disruption in the optimal anticorrelation between connectivity of the default mode (particularly the anterior portion) and the cognitive control circuit may characterize responders to TMS (Fox et al. 2012; Weigand et al. 2018). An accelerated form of TMS that targets this disruption may help regulate a more optimal anticorrelation between default mode and DLPFC connectivity and improve remission rates (Cole et al. 2020). See Chapter 2 ("The Future of Precision Transcranial Magnetic Stimulation in Psychiatry") for a more detailed discussion of baseline neuroimaging predictors of response and changes in functional connectivity as a result of TMS therapy.

Another promising avenue for neuroimaging biotypes and biomarkers is the rapid testing of new, alternative pharmacotherapies that have more targeted mechanisms of action. Reward circuit dysfunction and anhedonia do not appear to be modulated by typical antidepressants but offer candidates for novel therapies. For example, preclinical studies have found that the kappa opioid receptor (KOR) antagonist JNJ-67953964 is a promising candidate to modulate reward circuit dysfunction and anhedonia (Krystal et al. 2018). In a landmark study, Krystal and colleagues (2020) showed that targeting KOR antagonism with this drug in a transdiagnostic sample of patients with high anhedonia increased ventral striatal activation and concurrently improved anhedonia symptoms. A natural next step would be to assess whether KOR antagonism therapy preferentially improves outcomes when deployed in a stratified design in which individuals are preselected according to ventral striatal function (Williams and Hack 2020).

Accelerating the Clinical Translation of Neuroscience-Informed Precision Psychiatry

Precision psychiatry is not yet a clinical reality. Here, we outline three related initiatives we have launched at Stanford to accelerate progress in the clinical translation of precision psychiatry informed by neuroscience.

DISCOVERY CLINIC FOR NEUROSCIENCE-INFORMED PRECISION PSYCHIATRY

In 2013, LMW launched partnerships between her research lab at Stanford and two local area clinics: a community mental health center encompassing clinics for mood and anxiety issues with a combined focus on clinical training, and a technology-enabled health care company integrating mental health with primary care. These partnerships were centered around a project funded by the National Institute of Mental Health under the Research Domain Criteria (RDoC) initiative. This project recruited participants in 2013–2016 who were experiencing a range of palpable symptoms related to states of negative affect, unmedicated at the time of the study, and who completed functional neuroimaging as well as symptom, cognitive, daily function, and coping assessments (Williams et al. 2016b).

To initiate an understanding of the clinical utility of the RDoC approach, which is anchored in the neuroscience dimensions that underlie psychiatric disorders, LMW embedded a Discovery Clinic within the project flow. The Discovery Clinic consisted of several voluntary and confidential components included in the institutional review board–approved overall protocol: a feedback session after baseline assessments, a 12-week follow-up, quarterly meetings to discuss and refine the processes, and didactic sessions for clinic trainees. In feedback sessions involving LMW, the usual-care clinician, and the participating patient, LMW discussed a "beta" report that provided information about each patient's profile of symptoms, as well as cognitive and daily function data and information about fMRI. Clinician and patient could ask questions regarding the possible meaning of the information given the current state of scientific knowledge. Clinicians chose the extent to which they incorporated information into their ongoing case formulation process, then discussed the combined information and any implications for treatment choice to commence at their subsequent ongoing clinical sessions (at which LMW was not present). As the individualized fMRI data were refined as part of the ongoing parallel research project, they were also made available.

At the 12-week follow-up, symptom and daily function assessments were repeated, providing a naturalistic means to evaluate clinical outcomes. A debrief about the experience was also completed at this time via a brief survey and a video link with clinicians who provided qualitative feedback on each patient's experience. Fifty-one feedback sessions were completed, which identified two common themes: 1) the value to the clinician of having access to multiple sources of information perhaps not apparent in the clinical interview process (e.g., evidence of cognitive impairment, or evidence of extreme anhedonia even in the absence of overall severity of symptoms and knowledge about neural circuit dysfunction), and 2) the destigmatizing and demystifying experience of "seeing" individualized report information as described by participants. Indeed, having a shared tangible model of understanding for patients potentially provides a narrative that diminishes shame and self-blame, especially when the underlying biology is modifiable by interventions.

We present below two case illustrations of participants who received feedback from LMW and whose treatment plans were modified by the clinician after their sessions.

Clinical Case Illustrations

Mr. RT, a male engineer in his 50s with recurrent MDD, was unable to continue working due to the stress of his recent promotion. Six treatment trials (five SSRIs and electroconvulsive therapy) had failed. Mr. RT exhibited prominent anhedonia and hopelessness, while his cognitive testing revealed a slowed reaction to identifying happy faces. Increased time to identify happy emotions has been associated with symptoms of anhedonia (Vrijen et al. 2016). Mr. RT's biotype profile showed the greatest dysfunction in reward neurocircuitry. The ventral striatum, a key node in the reward circuitry, was shown to be hypoactive in neuroimaging studies of depressed patients who endorsed prominent anhedonia (Der-Avakian and Markou 2012; Greenberg et al. 2015). In developing a treatment plan in light of information from the feedback report, Mr. RT's mental health team considered prior evidence from a target engagement study that the selective D_3 dopamine receptor agonist pramipexole increased activation in a key region of the ventral striatum (Ye et al. 2011). Mr. RT tried pramipexole, and his anhedonia improved within 4 weeks. This improvement was maintained throughout a 16-week follow-up period.

Ms. B, a female college freshman, had a diagnosis of MDD at the time of her feedback session with LMW. Multiple SSRIs had failed to elicit a response, and she was not interested in trying another medication. Ms. B had a history of psychiatric hospitalization for active suicidality, and her symptom questionnaires indicated that she had prominent worry, rumination, self-blame, and poor sleep. Her imaging data revealed default mode disruptions implicating poor response to antidepressants (Goldstein-Piekarski et al.

2018). Given emerging evidence that default mode disruptions implicated in poor response to antidepressants may be associated with good response to TMS (Philip et al. 2018), and clinical information available to the patient's treatment team, this treatment team opted for an accelerated form of TMS. This treatment led to remission of MDD within 1 week, with the MDD still in remission during study follow-up and at a subsequent 10-month check-in.

INTEGRATING THE DISCOVERY CLINIC WITH RESIDENT TRAINING PROGRAMS

In 2017, building from the overall positive response of the initial Discovery Clinic process, LMW launched what is, to our knowledge, the first "Discovery Training Clinic" of its kind, a collaboration between researchers, educators, and clinicians in the Stanford Department of Psychiatry and Behavioral Sciences. The goal was to further inform the clinical translation of neuroscience-informed precision psychiatry by incorporating the principles of this approach directly into the clinical training of psychiatry residents. With the support of the Chief of Adult Psychiatry and Residency Training leadership (Director, Chris Haywood, M.D., and Assistant Director, Belinda Bandstra, M.D. [BB]), LMW designed and piloted a pragmatic clinical translational program that incorporated the feedback session principles from the initial Discovery Clinic process and the content of prior feedback sessions to develop structured case examples for teaching. TMB joined LMW to implement the program within the context of a yearlong third-year resident (PGY3) training rotation within the departmental Continuity Clinic. Over the year, researchers (TMB, LMW), residents, BB, and attendings met with two subgroups of approximately three residents each on alternating weeks. The program comprised three primary components: structured discussion of case examples based on prior cases, open discussion of case formulation issues (such as how to incorporate neuroscience measures into the clinical decision-making process), and discussion of new feedback session data from the residents' own consenting patients.

Participating patients (28 referred, 20 enrolled) undertook the same neuroimaging, cognitive, symptom, and function assessments as per the initial RDoC project–related Discovery Clinic. To facilitate learning about the impact of both residents and patients receiving neuroscience-related information, we randomized the feedback process so that half of the time residents (with attending) received the report prior to their first clinical appointment with the patient, and the other half of the time they received the report 12 weeks later. We evaluated the program after the first year. Residents indicated the experience was useful but expressed the need for the neuroscience information to be sequenced ahead of the direct clinical application, especially because they were new to the independent implementation of clinical decision making. Most patients agreed that the report information helped them understand how their brain functioned, provided new insights into their symptoms, and enabled them to feel more committed to treatment. Thus, in 2019, LMH joined the Discovery Clinic and with TMB further refined and expanded the program to include additional structured case studies and a didactic curriculum.

THE STANFORD TRANSLATIONAL PRECISION MENTAL HEALTH CLINIC

In 2018, LMW founded the Stanford Center for Precision Mental Health and Wellness, which has the translational goal of accelerating the insights of the Discovery Clinic into practice.

Then, in 2021, LMH and LMW launched the Stanford Translational Precision Mental Health Clinic; LMH is the director, and LMW serves as an expert advisor to the clinic regarding the imaging and biotype information. The goal of this translational consultation clinic is to offer a cutting-edge, multimodal assessment for treatment-resistant patients with mood and/or anxiety disorders in order to help better match their biological subtype to treatment. Any patient qualifying for one of our research studies has the opportunity to learn more about the clinic. Similar to our Discovery Clinic, participating patients undergo a comprehensive battery of evaluations assessing symptoms, neurocognition, pharmacogenetic variants, resting and task-based fMRI, and blood-based markers. All patients receive a report of the findings, along with a thorough explanation and their implications for treatment recommendations. This information is also discussed with their referring provider. Our hope is that, through this experimental approach, we may help relieve some of the tremendous suffering that is a consequence of our current trial-and-error approach to mental health treatment.

Conclusion and Future Directions

We envision a future that overcomes the gaps between research advances and their application in practice. New knowledge about neural circuits will be incorporated into models of assessment and care delivery, residency programs will prepare graduates with training in neuroscience, and clinicians will have access to neuroscience-based tools to inform their decision making as part of the routine, reimbursable workflow. We can foresee having a clinical toolkit that is the psychiatry equivalent of cardiology: multiple imaging modalities that help differentially diagnose the source of the underlying pathophysiology and guide choice of treatments accordingly, including lifestyle changes, medications, behavioral therapies, neuromodulation, and their combination. With such a precision approach that translates brain insights into clinically actionable tools, we have the opportunity to improve and save the lives of many.

KEY POINTS

- Precision psychiatry informed by neuroscience offers the opportunity to improve the precision of classification, treatment decisions, and prevention efforts.

- There is an urgent clinical need for this new approach because, although many effective treatments are available, finding the right treatment for the right patient remains largely a matter of trial and error, and we do not have a taxonomy for diagnosis and for guiding treatment choices that is based in an understanding of the underlying pathophysiology.

- Functional imaging of large-scale neural circuits of the human brain is one approach to developing such a taxonomy. Depression and anxiety may be conceptualized as disruptions to the neural circuits involved in the human functions of self-reflection, emotion processing, and cognitive control.

- Knowing about these disruptions can increase the accuracy of determining which patients are likely to benefit from an intervention. We have a rapidly increasing set of evidence for improvement in outcomes with pharmacotherapy and transcranial magnetic stimulation interventions utilizing knowledge of these disruptions.

- Multiple efforts are under way at Stanford to further neuroscience-informed precision psychiatry, including the creation of a Discovery Clinic, the Stanford Center for Precision Mental Health and Wellness, and the Stanford Translational Precision Mental Health Clinic.

References

Avissar M, Powell F, Ilieva I, et al: Functional connectivity of the left DLPFC to striatum predicts treatment response of depression to TMS. Brain Stimul 10(5):919–925, 2017 28747260

Buckner RL, Krienen FM, Yeo BT: Opportunities and limitations of intrinsic functional connectivity MRI. Nat Neurosci 16(7):832–837, 2013 23799476

Clementz BA, Sweeney JA, Hamm JP, et al: Identification of distinct psychosis biotypes using brain-based biomarkers. Am J Psychiatry 173(4):373–384, 2016 26651391

Cole EJ, Stimpson KH, Bentzley BS, et al: Stanford accelerated intelligent neuromodulation therapy for treatment-resistant depression. Am J Psychiatry 177(8):716–726, 2020 32252538

Cole MW, Schneider W: The cognitive control network: integrated cortical regions with dissociable functions. Neuroimage 37(1):343–360, 2007 17553704

Cole MW, Bassett DS, Power JD, et al: Intrinsic and task-evoked network architectures of the human brain. Neuron 83(1):238–251, 2014 24991964

Der-Avakian A, Markou A: The neurobiology of anhedonia and other reward-related deficits. Trends Neurosci 35(1):68–77, 2012 22177980

Dichter GS, Kozink RV, McClernon FJ, et al: Remitted major depression is characterized by reward network hyperactivation during reward anticipation and hypoactivation during reward outcomes. J Affect Disord 136(3):1126–1134, 2012 22036801

Downar J, Geraci J, Salomons TV, et al: Anhedonia and reward-circuit connectivity distinguish nonresponders from responders to dorsomedial prefrontal repetitive transcranial magnetic stimulation in major depression. Biol Psychiatry 76(3):176–185, 2014 24388670

Drysdale AT, Grosenick L, Downar J, et al: Resting-state connectivity biomarkers define neurophysiological subtypes of depression. Nat Med 23(1):28–38, 2017 27918562

Dunlop BW, Binder EB, Cubells JF, et al: Predictors of remission in depression to individual and combined treatments (PReDICT): study protocol for a randomized controlled trial. Trials 13:106, 2012 22776534

Fonzo GA, Ramsawh HJ, Flagan TM, et al: Common and disorder-specific neural responses to emotional faces in generalised anxiety, social anxiety and panic disorders. Br J Psychiatry 206(3):206–215, 2015 25573399

Fox MD, Buckner RL, White MP, et al: Efficacy of transcranial magnetic stimulation targets for depression is related to intrinsic functional connectivity with the subgenual cingulate. Biol Psychiatry 72(7):595–603, 2012 22658708

Goldstein-Piekarski AN, Korgaonkar MS, Green E, et al: Human amygdala engagement moderated by early life stress exposure is a biobehavioral target for predicting recovery on antidepressants. Proc Natl Acad Sci USA 113(42):11955–11960, 2016 27791054

Goldstein-Piekarski AN, Staveland BR, Ball TM, et al: Intrinsic functional connectivity predicts remission on antidepressants: a randomized controlled trial to identify clinically applicable imaging biomarkers. Transl Psychiatry 8(1):57, 2018 29507282

Goldstein-Piekarski AN, Ball TM, Samara Z, et al: Mapping neural circuit biotypes to symptoms and behavioral dimensions of depression and anxiety. SSRN Electronic Journal January 2020. Available at: www.researchgate.net/publication/343681272_Mapping_Neural_Circuit_Biotypes_to_Symptoms_and_Behavioral_Dimensions_of_Depression_and_Anxiety. Accessed February 9, 2021.

Greenberg T, Chase HW, Almeida JR, et al: Moderation of the relationship between reward expectancy and prediction error-related ventral striatal reactivity by anhedonia in unmedicated major depressive disorder: findings from the EMBARC study. Am J Psychiatry 172(9):881–891, 2015 26183698

Greicius MD, Krasnow B, Reiss AL, et al: Functional connectivity in the resting brain: a network analysis of the default mode hypothesis. Proc Natl Acad Sci USA 100(1):253–258, 2003 12506194

Greicius MD, Supekar K, Menon V, et al: Resting-state functional connectivity reflects structural connectivity in the default mode network. Cereb Cortex 19(1):72–78, 2009 18403396

Grieve SM, Korgaonkar MS, Etkin A, et al: Brain imaging predictors and the international study to predict optimized treatment for depression: study protocol for a randomized controlled trial. Trials 14:224, 2013 23866851

Gyurak A, Patenaude B, Korgaonkar MS, et al: Frontoparietal activation during response inhibition predicts remission to antidepressants in patients with major depression. Biol Psychiatry 79(4):274–281, 2016 25891220

Haber SN, Knutson B: The reward circuit: linking primate anatomy and human imaging. Neuropsychopharmacology 35(1):4–26, 2010 19812543

Hamilton JP, Etkin A, Furman DJ, et al: Functional neuroimaging of major depressive disorder: a meta-analysis and new integration of base line activation and neural response data. Am J Psychiatry 169(7):693–703, 2012 22535198

Hamilton JP, Farmer M, Fogelman P, Gotlib IH: Depressive rumination, the default-mode network, and the dark matter of clinical neuroscience. Biol Psychiatry 78(4):224–230, 2015 25861700

Jaworska N, Yang XR, Knott V, et al: A review of fMRI studies during visual emotive processing in major depressive disorder. World J Biol Psychiatry 16(7):448–471, 2015 24635551

Kaiser RH, Whitfield-Gabrieli S, Dillon DG, et al: Dynamic resting-state functional connectivity in major depression. Neuropsychopharmacology 41(7):1822–1830, 2016 26632990

Keedwell PA, Andrew C, Williams SC, et al: The neural correlates of anhedonia in major depressive disorder. Biol Psychiatry 58(11):843–853, 2005 16043128

Keller AS, Ball TM, Williams LM: Deep phenotyping of attention impairments and the "inattention biotype" in major depressive disorder. Psychol Med 50(13):2203–2212, 2020 31477195

Killgore WD, Britton JC, Schwab ZJ, et al: Cortico-limbic responses to masked affective faces across PTSD, panic disorder, and specific phobia. Depress Anxiety 31(2):150–159, 2014 DOI: 10.1002/da.22156 23861215

Klumpp H, Post D, Angstadt M, et al: Anterior cingulate cortex and insula response during indirect and direct processing of emotional faces in generalized social anxiety disorder. Biol Mood Anxiety Disord 3:7, 2013 23547713

Korgaonkar MS, Grieve SM, Etkin A, et al: Using standardized fMRI protocols to identify patterns of prefrontal circuit dysregulation that are common and specific to cognitive and emotional tasks in major depressive disorder: first wave results from the iSPOT-D study. Neuropsychopharmacology 38(5):863–871, 2013 23303059

Korgaonkar MS, Erlinger M, Breukelaar IA, et al: Amygdala activation and connectivity to emotional processing distinguishes asymptomatic patients with bipolar disorders and unipolar depression. Biol Psychiatry Cogn Neurosci Neuroimaging 4(4):361–370, 2019 30343134

Krystal AD, Pizzagalli DA, Mathew SJ, et al: The first implementation of the NIMH FAST-FAIL approach to psychiatric drug development. Nat Rev Drug Discov 18(1):82–84, 2018 30591715

Krystal AD, Pizzagalli DA, Smoski M, et al: A randomized proof-of-mechanism trial applying the "fast-fail" approach to evaluating kappa-opioid antagonism as a treatment for anhedonia. Nat Med 26(5):760–768, 2020 32231295

Maron-Katz A, Zhang Y, Narayan M, et al: Individual patterns of abnormality in resting-state functional connectivity reveal two data-driven PTSD subgroups. Am J Psychiatry 177(3):244–253, 2020 31838870

Matthews SC, Strigo IA, Simmons AN, et al: Decreased functional coupling of the amygdala and supragenual cingulate is related to increased depression in unmedicated individuals with current major depressive disorder. J Affect Disord 111(1):13–20, 2008 18603301

Mitterschiffthaler MT, Kumari V, Malhi GS, et al: Neural response to pleasant stimuli in anhedonia: an fMRI study. Neuroreport 14(2):177–182, 2003 12598724

Mulders PC, van Eijndhoven PF, Schene AH, et al: Resting-state functional connectivity in major depressive disorder: a review. Neurosci Biobehav Rev 56:330–344, 2015 26234819

Niendam TA, Laird AR, Ray KL, et al: Meta-analytic evidence for a superordinate cognitive control network subserving diverse executive functions. Cogn Affect Behav Neurosci 12(2):241–268, 2012 22282036

Peterson A, Thome J, Frewen P, et al: Resting-state neuroimaging studies: a new way of identifying differences and similarities among the anxiety disorders? Can J Psychiatry 59(6):294–300, 2014 25007403

Philip NS, Barredo J, van't Wout-Frank M, et al: Network mechanisms of clinical response to transcranial magnetic stimulation in posttraumatic stress disorder and major depressive disorder. Biol Psychiatry 83(3):263–272, 2018 28886760

Prater KE, Hosanagar A, Klumpp H, et al: Aberrant amygdala-frontal cortex connectivity during perception of fearful faces and at rest in generalized social anxiety disorder. Depress Anxiety 30(3):234–241, 2013 23184639

Price RB, Gates K, Kraynak TE, et al: Data-driven subgroups in depression derived from directed functional connectivity paths at rest. Neuropsychopharmacology 42(13):2623–2632, 2017 28497802

Stuhrmann A, Suslow T, Dannlowski U: Facial emotion processing in major depression: a systematic review of neuroimaging findings. Biol Mood Anxiety Disord 1(1):10, 2011 22738433

Tozzi L, Goldstein-Piekarski AN, Korgaonkar MS, et al: Connectivity of the cognitive control network during response inhibition as a predictive and response biomarker in major depression: evidence from a randomized clinical trial. Biol Psychiatry 87(5):462–472, 2020 31601424

Treadway MT, Zald DH: Reconsidering anhedonia in depression: lessons from translational neuroscience. Neurosci Biobehav Rev 35(3):537–555, 2011 20603146

Trivedi MH, McGrath PJ, Fava M, et al: Establishing Moderators and Biosignatures of Antidepressant Response in Clinical Care (EMBARC): rationale and design. J Psychiatr Res 78:11–23, 2016 27038550

Vrijen C, Hartman CA, Oldehinkel AJ: Slow identification of facial happiness in early adolescence predicts onset of depression during 8 years of follow-up. Eur Child Adolesc Psychiatry 25(11):1255–1266, 2016 27105995

Weigand A, Horn A, Caballero R, et al: Prospective validation that subgenual connectivity predicts antidepressant efficacy of transcranial magnetic stimulation sites. Biol Psychiatry 84(1):28–37, 2018 29274805

Williams LM: Precision psychiatry: a neural circuit taxonomy for depression and anxiety. Lancet Psychiatry 3(5):472–480, 2016 27150382

Williams LM: Defining biotypes for depression and anxiety based on large-scale circuit dysfunction: a theoretical review of the evidence and future directions for clinical translation. Depress Anxiety 34(1):9–24, 2017 27653321

Williams LM, Hack LM: A precision medicine-based, "fast-fail" approach for psychiatry. Nat Med 26(5):653–654, 2020 32405056

Williams LM, Korgaonkar MS, Song YC, et al: Amygdala reactivity to emotional faces in the prediction of general and medication-specific responses to antidepressant treatment in the randomized iSPOT-D trial. Neuropsychopharmacology 40(10):2398–2408, 2015 25824424

Williams LM, Debattista C, Duchemin AM, et al: Childhood trauma predicts antidepressant response in adults with major depression: data from the randomized international study to predict optimized treatment for depression. Transl Psychiatry 6:e799, 2016a 27138798

Williams LM, Goldstein-Piekarski AN, Chowdhry N, et al: Developing a clinical translational neuroscience taxonomy for anxiety and mood disorder: protocol for the baseline-follow up research domain criteria anxiety and depression ("RAD") project. BMC Psychiatry 16:68, 2016b 26980207

Yan CG, Chen X, Li L, et al: Reduced default mode network functional connectivity in patients with recurrent major depressive disorder. Proc Natl Acad Sci USA 116(18):9078–9083, 2019 30979801

Ye Z, Hammer A, Camara E, Münte TF: Pramipexole modulates the neural network of reward anticipation. Hum Brain Mapp 32(5):800–811, 2011 21484950

Zhang WN, Chang SH, Guo LY, et al: The neural correlates of reward-related processing in major depressive disorder: a meta-analysis of functional magnetic resonance imaging studies. J Affect Disord 151(2):531–539, 2013 23856280

Zhu X, Wang X, Xiao J, et al: Evidence of a dissociation pattern in resting-state default mode network connectivity in first-episode, treatment-naive major depression patients. Biol Psychiatry 71(7):611–617, 2012 22177602

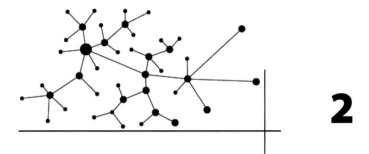

2

THE FUTURE OF PRECISION TRANSCRANIAL MAGNETIC STIMULATION IN PSYCHIATRY

Noah S. Philip, M.D.
Amin Zandvakili, M.D., Ph.D.
Yosef A. Berlow, M.D., Ph.D.

Drs. Berlow, Zandvakili, and Philip's work is supported by grants from the National Institute of Mental Health (NIMH R25 MH101076 [YAB]), the National Institute of General Medical Sciences (NIGMS U54GM115677 [AZ]), the U.S. Department of Veterans Affairs (VA) (I01 RX002450 (NSP), and the VA RR&D Center for Neurorestoration and Neurotechnology (YAB, AZ, NSP). In the past, Dr. Philip has received grant support from Janssen, Neosync, and Neuronetics through clinical trial contracts and has served as an unpaid scientific advisory board member for Neuronetics. The opinions herein represent those of the authors and not the National Institutes of Health or VA. The other authors report no financial relationships with commercial interests.

History

Since 2010, repetitive transcranial magnetic stimulation (TMS) has emerged as an evidence-based treatment in psychiatry. TMS has been clinically available since 2008, when it was cleared by the FDA for pharmacoresistant major depressive disorder (MDD) based on two multisite randomized controlled studies (George et al. 2010; O'Reardon et al. 2007). Recently, it received clearance for use in combination with symptom provocation to reduce symptoms of obsessive-compulsive disorder (Carmi et al. 2019). In addition to the registration studies, a number of groups have published studies on the efficacy of TMS for depression in naturalistic samples (Carpenter et al. 2012), its durability of effect (Philip et al. 2016), and its efficacy across the life span (Conelea et al. 2017; Sabesan et al. 2015; Wall et al. 2016). There is also emerging literature that supports the use of TMS for other psychiatric conditions, including PTSD (for review, see Koek et al. 2019) and schizophrenia (Hasan et al. 2016; Paillère-Martinot et al. 2017). A new form of TMS, called *theta-burst TMS*, has been developed. The burst pattern enables delivery of stimulation in much shorter periods for the same clinical benefit (see, e.g., Blumberger et al. 2018; Philip et al. 2019).

Current Knowledge and Approaches

TMS is particularly well suited for consideration from a precision psychiatry perspective, as described further below. The use of TMS requires an interdisciplinary understanding of electrical engineering and clinical research. Although the exact mechanisms of TMS remain unknown, it uses pulsed magnetic fields to induce depolarization in target brain regions, typically the dorsolateral prefrontal cortex (DLPFC) (described in more detail later in this section).

TMS starts with a precision medicine approach, in which the clinician calibrates the stimulation device to an individual's cortical excitability (typically described as a *motor threshold*, or MT). During MT determination, the clinician delivers single-pulse TMS over the motor cortex and records the amount of energy required to induce movement in the contralateral hand 50% of the time. Following this calibration, a course of TMS is delivered to the prefrontal cortex at 120% of MT daily for up to 30 (or more) sessions, often followed by a taper phase.

TMS parameters can vary and include the location of stimulation, its intensity and frequency, and other factors. Parameters have generally shifted over time, favoring higher intensity and greater exposure to a cumulative "dose" of stimulation. For example, initial work was done with a lower delivery of energy, and the intensity was increased up to 120% of MT once it was observed that increased stimulation intensity was required to overcome variability in coil-to-cortex distances that are associated with age and other factors (Kozel et al. 2000). Protocols have also evolved to incorporate more TMS sessions (i.e., increase from 10 sessions to >20); multiple sessions in a single day, which is termed *accelerated TMS* (for review, see Sonmez et al. 2019); and combination with symptom provocation (see, e.g., Carmi et al. 2019).

The location of stimulation is also germane to the discussion of precision medicine. For example, earlier TMS studies selected the DLPFC using an empirical "5 cm rule," in which the TMS device would be moved 5 cm anterior to the MT hotspot along the parasagittal line to be over the DLPFC. However, subsequent research convincingly demonstrated that this rule could reliably miss the DLPFC (Herbsman et al. 2009), a finding that led to the development of MRI-based neuronavigation or skull-based landmarks (Beam et al. 2009). To date, clinical evidence appears to show similar clinical outcomes using these modalities (Mir-Moghtadaei et al. 2015).

Despite the availability of TMS for over a decade, researchers continue the search to characterize its mechanism(s) of effect. For example, TMS for depression is typically delivered over the left DLPFC, yet as described above, evidence suggests that DLPFC stimulation can lead to improvement in symptoms in multiple other ailments, ranging from PTSD and other anxiety disorders to schizophrenia. This points to the fact that TMS treatment modulates networks of interest shared across psychiatric illnesses, and provides empirical evidence that current approaches to treatment parameter selection might not be accurate.

The selection of the left DLPFC as a TMS target was based on preliminary data that implicated hypoperfusion of the left prefrontal cortex as a potential mechanism for depression (Baxter et al. 1989; Martinot et al. 1990). Neuropsychiatric research since 2010 has made it clear that this mechanism is part of a larger element of broad-based dysfunction in depression and related disorders (e.g., Grisanzio et al. 2018). The choice of stimulation frequency (10 Hz) was based on studies on the motor cortex which showed that high stimulation frequencies yielded excitatory effects, whereas lower stimulation frequencies (typically ~1 Hz) appeared to suppress motor-evoked potentials (Chen et al. 1997). The results of stimulation delivered to the prefrontal cortex have some similarities to those of motor cortex stimulation. For example, early data suggested increased perfusion occurs after higher-intensity stimulation (Speer et al. 2000). However, these similarities become much less clear when assessing results from other neuroimaging methods such as functional connectivity (for review, see Philip et al. 2018a). Generally speaking, TMS follows the model of other conventional treatment modalities for mental illnesses; its parameters have been generally found through serendipity, and the initially speculated mechanisms of its action may not be accurate. One factor that makes TMS a complex treatment to study is the vast parameter space, which includes site of stimulation, frequency and temporal structure of TMS stimulations (bursts vs. single pulses), and duration of treatment.

TMS is thought to work through modulation of cortical connectivity and induction of neural plasticity (Hoogendam et al. 2010). Recent animal studies have shown that treatment with TMS leads to transient and large-scale remodeling of cortical connections via enhancing plasticity, which can last for hours posttreatment (Kozyrev et al. 2018). This means that stimulating over the DLPFC can lead to a cascade of changes in cortical networks, particularly in the sites to which TMS activity propagates (e.g., subgenual anterior cingulate cortex) (Vink et al. 2018). Indeed, such changes are apparent in the studies that tracked functional connectivity through a treatment course of TMS.

Depression is associated with enhanced connectivity between the frontoparietal network and the default mode network (DMN) and diminished functional connectivity between the frontoparietal and dorsal attention networks (Kaiser et al. 2015). Treatment with TMS appears to "normalize" some of these changes. In patients with depression, TMS treatment has led to a reduction in subgenual hyperconnectivity in the DMN and a modulation in the connectivity between the DLPFC and medial prefrontal DMN nodes (Liston et al. 2014). Similarly, in patients with comorbid PTSD and MDD, treatment with TMS is associated with reduced connectivity between the subgenual anterior cingulate cortex and the DMN, left DLPFC and insula, and reduced connectivity between the hippocampus and the salience network (Philip et al. 2018b).

Similar to functional imaging findings, TMS treatment also produces both transient and long-lasting changes in the electroencephalogram (EEG) signal. Combined TMS and electrographic studies have documented short-lived changes in both evoked potential and EEG power spectra after TMS treatment. Such changes were comparable in direction and magnitude to EEG changes associated with learning or fatigue. EEG changes have a short time course and usually last tens of minutes and up to 70 minutes (for review, see Thut and Pascual-Leone 2010). This time course could be related to the TMS-induced remodeling and cortical plasticity reported in animal studies (Kozyrev et al. 2018). Repeated TMS treatments, as are typically delivered in clinical treatment, have been shown to produce long-term modulation of functional connectivity metrics including coherence between the prefrontal site of stimulation and midline parieto-occipital regions, which lasts from days to weeks (Zandvakili et al. 2019), although findings in this domain require replication.

The functional connectivity patterns associated with depression are accompanied by structural and volumetric differences, most notably a reduction in the gray matter volume of the hippocampus and subgenual cingulate cortex (e.g., Botteron et al. 2002; Goodkind et al. 2015; Ongür et al. 2003). Interestingly, treatment with TMS leads to a volume increase in both the left subgenual cingulate cortex and hippocampus (Hayasaka et al. 2017; Lan et al. 2016). Beyond changes in functional connectivity, treatment with TMS is associated with partial normalization of anatomical connections. Additionally, multiple studies using diffusion tensor imaging have demonstrated that white matter integrity likely plays an important role in clinical improvement following TMS (for review, see Anderson et al. 2016). TMS has also been shown to induce changes in neurotransmitter levels that are detectable via magnetic resonance spectroscopy. These changes include elevation of glutamate levels in the DLPFC and anterior cingulate cortex (Croarkin et al. 2016; Yang et al. 2014), and GABA elevations in the medial prefrontal cortex. Although many of these findings still require replication, they present a nuanced picture of the multifactorial elements that likely compose the neurobiological mechanism of clinical TMS.

Clinical Illustration

As a clinical illustration, we describe current and future procedures at the Psychiatric Neuromodulation Clinic at the Providence VA Medical Center. Currently, patients with treatment-resistant psychiatric disorders are referred through standard clinical procedures. After an initial chart review for absolute contraindications to stimulation, patients receive a 1- to 2-hour clinical consultation visit with a TMS-credentialed attending physician in conjunction with resident trainees. This consultation includes a review of safety screening and a comprehensive review of the patient's experience with their illness, including their first episode of depression, their experience with antidepressant medications, and investigation of the pattern of their illness over the lifetime. Based on this information, a determination is made as to whether the patient is appropriate for stimulation, and whether the provider feels, in their opinion, a patient is likely to respond to stimulation. Assuming the patient is eligible for TMS and wants to pursue this option, they are also informed that rating scales—usually a series of self-rated scales and/or those related to psychiatric comorbidities—are administered every five TMS sessions. The patient is then offered the opportunity to participate in a series of research procedures that are affiliated with the clinic. These procedures often include MRI scans and EEGs throughout their course of TMS that are roughly timed to occur once per week. TMS then begins, often with a standard "one size fits all" initial approach that is then modified based on tolerability or other clinical factors that occur over the course of stimulation. Once TMS is completed, the TMS attending physician provides a detailed report to the referring physician.

Many aspects of this clinic lend themselves to the adoption of precision psychiatry. Currently, a great deal of biomarker data is obtained before stimulation and throughout the course of TMS. Therefore, if there were MRI or EEG biomarkers that could reasonably be used to assess whether a patient will respond to TMS or those that could inform on the possible length of treatment required, this information would be immediately actionable on multiple levels. Furthermore, as a thought experiment, a biomarker might also indicate whether TMS retreatment would work well for a patient over time and therefore provide information on diagnosis and longer-term prognosis. This would also provide an opportunity for trainees to obtain neuroscience exposure, during which they could receive hands-on experience utilizing neuroscience tools in clinical practice.

Conclusion and Future Directions

Researchers have been investigating various neuroimaging approaches to individualize TMS in order to match patients with the appropriate treatments and optimize efficacy. These efforts have included using structural and functional imaging to target stimulation sites, choose stimulation parameters, and more broadly predict treatment response. Although the use of neuroimaging to guide TMS treatment decisions has yet to be incorporated in clinical TMS centers, there are several practical and economic reasons to believe that TMS may be one of the first psychiatric treatments to translate neuroimaging approaches into clinical tools that guide psychiatric practice.

Several studies have used structural MRI combined with neuronavigation to identify individualized sites of stimulation for targeting the DLPFC. As described above, these methods overcame some of the variability of stimulation placement that was experienced when using the initially implemented "5 cm rule," which did not account for individual anatomy. However, other scalp-based approaches that adjust for head size, such as the "Beam F3" approach (Beam et al. 2009), have been shown to perform similarly to MRI-based neuronavigation with regard to locating a similar site of stimulation (Mir-Moghtadaei et al. 2015). MRI-based targeting has also been accompanied by individualized adjustments of the stimulation output to account for the depth of the DLPFC region (Stokes et al. 2005; Williams et al. 2018).

However, the use of higher intensities (i.e., 120% MT as applied in standard treatments) might overcome coil-to-cortex variability without the need for depth adjustments.

Other groups have used resting-state functional MRI to identify a region of the DLPFC that is most negatively correlated (i.e., "anticorrelated") with the subgenual anterior cingulate cortex to identify an optimized target for stimulation (Fox et al. 2012; Weigand et al. 2018). These approaches are based on the hypothesis that DLPFC stimulation indirectly modulates limbic regions that have connections to the DLPFC, resulting in decreased subgenual cingulate hyperactivity and antidepressant response. These groups have shown that the negative correlation in functional connectivity between the site of stimulation and the subgenual cingulate predicts antidepressant response. This work has been based on using normative group connectivity data and applying the coordinates to an individual (Weigand et al. 2018). It is still unknown whether targeting based on this approach yields stimulation sites that are substantially different compared with modern scalp-based approaches when considering the resolution of the TMS-induced electrical field (e.g., Deng et al. 2013), and whether this targeting represents a mechanism unique to TMS or a nonspecific antidepressant effect (e.g., Gärtner et al. 2019).

There is evidence that supports the use of alternative sites of stimulation, including the dorsomedial and orbitofrontal cortex, as therapeutic TMS targets to reduce depression (Downar and Daskalakis 2013; Downar et al. 2014; Feffer et al. 2018). Multiple TMS sites have been shown to be capable of producing an antidepressant response. It can be hypothesized that some individuals would respond to stimulation at any of these sites while others may only respond to one site over another, and some may not respond at all. An early case series demonstrated that 30% of patients who did not respond to dorsomedial stimulation did achieve remission with orbitofrontal stimulation (Feffer et al. 2018). Stimulation parameters, including frequency and stimulation patterns, may demonstrate a similar phenomenon requiring individualized adjustments to achieve an optimum response. Currently, some of these adjustments are made in the clinic to increase patient tolerance and comfort in completing treatment (e.g., Philip et al. 2015). However, early reports suggest that neuroimaging measures might provide additional information on treatment response to a given set of parameters before stimulation begins (Downar 2019). The pressing question is how to identify patients who are likely to respond to a given treatment.

Several studies have suggested that functional neuroimaging may provide patterns of connectivity that are predictive of TMS response (Philip et al. 2018a). For these approaches to be incorporated clinically, they will need to demonstrate reliability, cost-effectiveness, and a meaningful change in the likelihood of clinical response. While TMS has few side effects and is generally well tolerated, the cost and time commitment of a full treatment series can represent substantial factors to consider when choosing this modality. Remission rates for TMS are estimated to be 25%–35%, depending on treatment modality and method of defining remission (Blumberger et al. 2018; Carpenter et al. 2012), which implies that a majority of patients who complete a TMS treatment series do not achieve remission. TMS can also be considered a limited resource, given that only 60–80 patients can be treated on a single device per year. For these reasons, it is crucial that we develop predictive models that help guide individuals to treatments that are likely to succeed.

One potential approach, which is included here as a future direction for this field, is the use of decision curve analysis (DCA) (Vickers and Elkin 2006). DCA is a framework for evaluating the clinical utility of treatment strategies that could be used to provide information regarding what a clinically useful predictive neuroimaging model of TMS response would look like. DCA has been used to evaluate the predictive models in many fields of medicine, but it has yet to be widely adopted in psychiatry. DCA incorporates the concept of "threshold probability" (P_t), which is the probability above which the expected benefits of treatment outweigh the potential costs and harms of unnecessary treatment for a given individual. This threshold probability represents a significant clinical decision point at which additional information would be needed to inform a decision. While a precise threshold probability might be difficult for a clinician or patient to estimate, DCA does not require that a single threshold probability be determined. Instead, DCA plots the net benefit of a treatment strategy across a range of threshold probabilities, and this enables clinicians and patients to consider variations in their thresholds as part of the clinical decision-making process. The net benefit of the model is then compared with the net benefit of two alternative treatment strategies: treat everyone or treat no one. Net benefit is defined as the proportion of true positives minus a weighted proportion of false positives as determined by a ratio of the threshold probability over its complement ($1-P_t$), as shown in the equation below. Strategies with the highest net benefit at a given range of threshold probabilities are considered superior.

$$Net\ Benefit = \frac{True\ Positives}{n} - \frac{False\ Positives}{n} \left(\frac{P_t}{1 - P_t} \right)$$

Using this framework, we can apply DCA to a theoretical neuroimaging model that predicts TMS remission with a sensitivity of 70%, a specificity of 70%, and an accuracy of 70%. In this model, we assume an average baseline remission rate of 30%. The resulting DCA curves are shown in Figure 2–1, which demonstrates that the theoretical model with 70% accuracy achieves greater net benefit for all threshold probabilities above 15.5%. This higher net benefit means that a greater number of patients who are referred to undergo TMS treatment will achieve remission without increasing the number of patients who undergo treatment unsuccessfully. In 100 patients assessed, this theoretical treatment strategy would result in 42 patients being identified as likely to respond with a posttest probability of remission of 50%, and 58 patients being identified as unlikely to achieve remission with a posttest probability of 15.5% (compared with 30% pretest). If we assume the average cost and time of a TMS treatment series to be $15,000 and 36 clinical visits, the currently used treat-all strategy results in the cost and time for each remission being $50,000 and 120 clinical visits. Use of the theoretical predictive neuroimaging model described above would reduce the costs and time for each remission to $37,142 and 77 clinical visits, even after accounting for the addition of a clinical visit and a $1,500 MRI scan for each patient.

This example holds for more expensive neuroimaging and interventions; more inexpensive technologies, as well as improved and/or more reliable biological characterization of psychiatric illnesses, would reduce the threshold probability. Enthusiasm must also be tempered by the realities of acquiring single-participant functional MRI scans, although another approach would be the integration of clinical MRI scans into validated predictive models generated from representative research studies (e.g., Drysdale et al. 2017; Philip et al. 2018b).

In conclusion, there is a tremendous potential to develop precision psychiatry approaches by leveraging emerging knowledge about TMS mechanisms of action and incorporating novel tools and analytic approaches. Of the many fields in psychiatry, TMS already includes an element of precision (i.e., individualized MT determination), and as such provides an important venue for teaching and understanding the potential of precision psychiatry more broadly in the field.

KEY POINTS

- Repetitive transcranial magnetic stimulation (TMS), an FDA-cleared treatment for pharmacoresistant major depressive disorder (MDD), uses pulsed magnetic fields to induce depolarization in target brain regions.

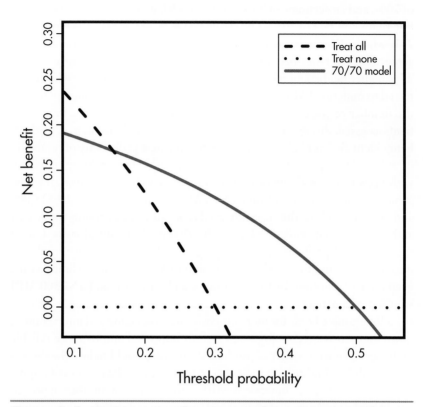

Figure 2–1. Decision curves for a theoretical neuroimaging model predictive of responsiveness to transcranial magnetic stimulation (TMS).

Threshold probability represents the point at which positive treatment response to TMS is valued equally to avoiding unnecessary treatment. Net benefit is defined as the percentage of individuals who receive TMS and achieve remission minus a weighted percentage of treated individuals who do not achieve remission. The solid line demonstrates the potential increase in net benefit that could be achieved with a predictive neuroimaging model with modest sensitivity (70%) and specificity (70%). When compared with the alternative strategies of "treat all" (dashed line) or "treat none" (dotted line) over a range of threshold probabilities above 15%, this theoretical model would be associated with greater net benefit and a higher proportion of successful TMS treatments.

- This treatment is well suited to a precision psychiatry approach in that the clinician calibrates the stimulation device to an individual's cortical excitability and multiple parameters can be modified, although standard parameters are typically used.
- Stimulating the dorsolateral prefrontal cortex, which is generally targeted in MDD because of evidence of dysfunction in this region in depression, appears to normalize aberrant functional

connectivity and produce both transient and long-lasting changes in the electroencephalogram (EEG) signal.

- TMS at the Psychiatric Neuromodulation Clinic at the Providence VA Medical Center begins with a "one size fits all" approach that is then modified based on tolerability or other clinical factors that occur over the course of stimulation.

- The clinic lends itself well to the precision psychiatry approach with the possibility of using neuroimaging-based targeting, customized stimulation parameters, and MRI or EEG biomarkers for prediction of treatment response and informing length of treatment.

References

Anderson RJ, Hoy KE, Daskalakis ZJ, et al: Repetitive transcranial magnetic stimulation for treatment resistant depression: Re-establishing connections. Clin Neurophysiol 127(11):3394–3405, 2016 27672727

Baxter LR Jr, Schwartz JM, Phelps ME, et al: Reduction of prefrontal cortex glucose metabolism common to three types of depression. Arch Gen Psychiatry 46(3):243–250, 1989 2784046

Beam W, Borckardt JJ, Reeves ST, et al: An efficient and accurate new method for locating the F3 position for prefrontal TMS applications. Brain Stimul 2(1):50–54, 2009 20539835

Blumberger DM, Vila-Rodriguez F, Thorpe KE, et al: Effectiveness of theta burst versus high-frequency repetitive transcranial magnetic stimulation in patients with depression (THREE-D): a randomised non-inferiority trial. Lancet 391(10131):1683–1692, 2018 29726344

Botteron KN, Raichle ME, Drevets WC, et al: Volumetric reduction in left subgenual prefrontal cortex in early onset depression. Biol Psychiatry 51(4):342–344, 2002 11958786

Carmi L, Tendler A, Bystritsky A, et al: Efficacy and safety of deep transcranial magnetic stimulation for obsessive-compulsive disorder: a prospective multicenter randomized double-blind placebo-controlled trial. Am J Psychiatry 176(11):931–938, 2019 31109199

Carpenter LL, Janicak PG, Aaronson ST, et al: Transcranial magnetic stimulation (TMS) for major depression: a multisite, naturalistic, observational study of acute treatment outcomes in clinical practice. Depress Anxiety 29(7):587–596, 2012 22689344

Chen R, Classen J, Gerloff C, et al: Depression of motor cortex excitability by low-frequency transcranial magnetic stimulation. Neurology 48(5):1398–1403, 1997 9153480

Conelea CA, Philip NS, Yip AG, et al: Transcranial magnetic stimulation for treatment-resistant depression: naturalistic treatment outcomes for younger versus older patients. J Affect Disord 217:42–47, 2017 28388464

Croarkin PE, Nakonezny PA, Wall CA, et al: Transcranial magnetic stimulation potentiates glutamatergic neurotransmission in depressed adolescents. Psychiatry Res Neuroimaging 247:25–33, 2016 26651598

Deng ZD, Lisanby SH, Peterchev AV: Electric field depth-focality tradeoff in transcranial magnetic stimulation: simulation comparison of 50 coil designs. Brain Stimul 6(1):1–13, 2013 22483681

Downar J: Theta-burst stimulation in major depression: clinical and neuroimaging results (should be attached to Symposium "Transdiagnostic Theta Burst Stimulation—the Future is Now" by Dr Noah Philip). Brain Stimul 12(2):524, 2019

Downar J, Daskalakis ZJ: New targets for rTMS in depression: a review of convergent evidence. Brain Stimul 6(3):231–240, 2013 22975030

Downar J, Geraci J, Salomons TV, et al: Anhedonia and reward-circuit connectivity distinguish nonresponders from responders to dorsomedial prefrontal repetitive transcranial magnetic stimulation in major depression. Biol Psychiatry 76(3):176–185, 2014 24388670

Drysdale AT, Grosenick L, Downar J, et al: Resting-state connectivity biomarkers define neurophysiological subtypes of depression. Nat Med 23(1):28–38, 2017 27918562

Feffer K, Fettes P, Giacobbe P, et al: 1Hz rTMS of the right orbitofrontal cortex for major depression: safety, tolerability and clinical outcomes. Eur Neuropsychopharmacol 28(1):109–117, 2018 29153927

Fox MD, Buckner RL, White MP, et al: Efficacy of transcranial magnetic stimulation targets for depression is related to intrinsic functional connectivity with the subgenual cingulate. Biol Psychiatry 72(7):595–603, 2012 22658708

Gärtner M, Aust S, Bajbouj M, et al: Functional connectivity between prefrontal cortex and subgenual cingulate predicts antidepressant effects of ketamine. Eur Neuropsychopharmacol 29(4):501–508, 2019 30819549

George MS, Lisanby SH, Avery D, et al: Daily left prefrontal transcranial magnetic stimulation therapy for major depressive disorder: a sham-controlled randomized trial. Arch Gen Psychiatry 67(5):507–516, 2010 20439832

Goodkind M, Eickhoff SB, Oathes DJ, et al: Identification of a common neurobiological substrate for mental illness. JAMA Psychiatry 72(4):305–315, 2015 25651064

Grisanzio KA, Goldstein-Piekarski AN, Wang MY, et al: Transdiagnostic symptom clusters and associations with brain, behavior, and daily function in mood, anxiety, and trauma disorders. JAMA Psychiatry 75(2):201–209, 2018 29197929

Hasan A, Guse B, Cordes J, et al: Cognitive effects of high-frequency rTMS in schizophrenia patients with predominant negative symptoms: results from a multicenter randomized sham-controlled trial. Schizophr Bull 42(3):608–618, 2016 26433217

Hayasaka S, Nakamura M, Noda Y, et al: Lateralized hippocampal volume increase following high-frequency left prefrontal repetitive transcranial magnetic stimulation in patients with major depression. Psychiatry Clin Neurosci 71(11):747–758, 2017 28631869

Herbsman T, Avery D, Ramsey D, et al: More lateral and anterior prefrontal coil location is associated with better repetitive transcranial magnetic stimulation antidepressant response. Biol Psychiatry 66(5):509–515, 2009 19545855

Hoogendam JM, Ramakers GM, Di Lazzaro V: Physiology of repetitive transcranial magnetic stimulation of the human brain. Brain Stimul 3(2):95–118, 2010 20633438

Kaiser RH, Andrews-Hanna JR, Wager TD, et al: Large-scale network dysfunction in major depressive disorder: a meta-analysis of resting-state functional connectivity. JAMA Psychiatry 72(6):603–611, 2015 25785575

Koek RJ, Roach J, Athanasiou N, et al: Neuromodulatory treatments for post-traumatic stress disorder (PTSD). Prog Neuropsychopharmacol Biol Psychiatry 92:148–160, 2019 30641094

Kozel FA, Nahas Z, deBrux C, et al: How coil-cortex distance relates to age, motor threshold, and antidepressant response to repetitive transcranial magnetic stimulation. J Neuropsychiatry Clin Neurosci 12(3):376–384, 2000 10956572

Kozyrev V, Staadt R, Eysel UT, et al: TMS-induced neuronal plasticity enables targeted remodeling of visual cortical maps. Proc Natl Acad Sci USA 115(25):6476–6481, 2018 29866856

Lan MJ, Chhetry BT, Liston C, et al: Transcranial magnetic stimulation of left dorsolateral prefrontal cortex induces brain morphological changes in regions associated with a treatment resistant major depressive episode: an exploratory analysis. Brain Stimul 9(4):577–583, 2016 27017072

Liston C, Chen AC, Zebley BD, et al: Default mode network mechanisms of transcranial magnetic stimulation in depression. Biol Psychiatry 76(7):517–526, 2014 24629537

Martinot JL, Hardy P, Feline A, et al: Left prefrontal glucose hypometabolism in the depressed state: a confirmation. Am J Psychiatry 147(10):1313–1317, 1990 2399999

Mir-Moghtadaei A, Caballero R, Fried P, et al: Concordance between BeamF3 and MRI-neuronavigated target sites for repetitive transcranial magnetic stimulation of the left dorsolateral prefrontal cortex. Brain Stimul 8(5):965–973, 2015 26115776

Ongür D, Ferry AT, Price JL: Architectonic subdivision of the human orbital and medial prefrontal cortex. J Comp Neurol 460(3):425–449, 2003 12692859

O'Reardon JP, Solvason HB, Janicak PG, et al: Efficacy and safety of transcranial magnetic stimulation in the acute treatment of major depression: a multisite randomized controlled trial. Biol Psychiatry 62(11):1208–1216, 2007 17573044

Paillère-Martinot ML, Galinowski A, Plaze M, et al: Active and placebo transcranial magnetic stimulation effects on external and internal auditory hallucinations of schizophrenia. Acta Psychiatr Scand 135(3):228–238, 2017 27987221

Philip NS, Carpenter SL, Ridout SJ, et al: 5Hz Repetitive transcranial magnetic stimulation to left prefrontal cortex for major depression. J Affect Disord 186:13–17, 2015 26210705

Philip NS, Dunner DL, Dowd SM, et al: Can medication free, treatment-resistant, depressed patients who initially respond to TMS be maintained off medications? A prospective, 12-month multisite randomized pilot study. Brain Stimul 9(2):251–257, 2016 26708778

Philip NS, Barredo J, Aiken E, et al: Neuroimaging mechanisms of therapeutic transcranial magnetic stimulation for major depressive disorder. Biol Psychiatry Cogn Neurosci Neuroimaging 3(3):211–222, 2018a 29486862

Philip NS, Barredo J, van't Wout-Frank M, et al: Network mechanisms of clinical response to transcranial magnetic stimulation in posttraumatic stress disorder and major depressive disorder. Biol Psychiatry 83(3):263–272, 2018b 28886760

Philip NS, Barredo J, Aiken E, et al: Theta-burst transcranial magnetic stimulation for posttraumatic stress disorder. Am J Psychiatry 176(11):939–948, 2019 31230462

Sabesan P, Lankappa S, Khalifa N, et al: Transcranial magnetic stimulation for geriatric depression: promises and pitfalls. World J Psychiatry 5(2):170–181, 2015 26110119

Sonmez AI, Camsari DD, Nandakumar AL, et al: Accelerated TMS for depression: a systematic review and meta-analysis. Psychiatry Res 273:770–781, 2019 31207865

Speer AM, Kimbrell TA, Wassermann EM, et al: Opposite effects of high and low frequency rTMS on regional brain activity in depressed patients. Biol Psychiatry 48(12):1133–1141, 2000 11137053

Stokes MG, Chambers CD, Gould IC, et al: Simple metric for scaling motor threshold based on scalp-cortex distance: application to studies using transcranial magnetic stimulation. J Neurophysiol 94(6):4520–4527, 2005 16135552

Thut G, Pascual-Leone A: A review of combined TMS-EEG studies to characterize lasting effects of repetitive TMS and assess their usefulness in cognitive and clinical neuroscience. Brain Topogr 22(4):219–232, 2010 19862614

Vickers AJ, Elkin EB: Decision curve analysis: a novel method for evaluating prediction models. Med Decis Making 26(6):565–574, 2006 17099194

Vink JJT, Mandija S, Petrov PI, et al: A novel concurrent TMS-fMRI method to reveal propagation patterns of prefrontal magnetic brain stimulation. Hum Brain Mapp 39(11):4580–4592, 2018 30156743

Wall CA, Croarkin PE, Maroney-Smith MJ, et al: Magnetic resonance imaging-guided, open-label, high-frequency repetitive transcranial magnetic stimulation for adolescents with major depressive disorder. J Child Adolesc Psychopharmacol 26(7):582–589, 2016 26849202

Weigand A, Horn A, Caballero R, et al: Prospective validation that subgenual connectivity predicts antidepressant efficacy of transcranial magnetic stimulation sites. Biol Psychiatry 84(1):28–37, 2018 29274805

Williams NR, Sudheimer KD, Bentzley BS, et al: High-dose spaced theta-burst TMS as a rapid-acting antidepressant in highly refractory depression. Brain 141(3):e18, 2018 29415152

Yang XR, Kirton A, Wilkes TC, et al: Glutamate alterations associated with transcranial magnetic stimulation in youth depression: a case series. J ECT 30(3):242–247, 2014 24820947

Zandvakili A, Philip NS, Jones SR, et al: Use of machine learning in predicting clinical response to transcranial magnetic stimulation in comorbid posttraumatic stress disorder and major depression: a resting state electroencephalography study. J Affect Disord 252:47–54, 2019 30978624

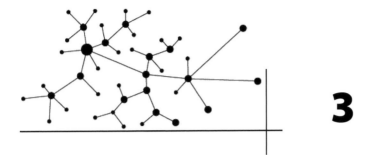

3

Neural Mechanisms of Bipolar Disorder

Toward Personalized Markers of Future Illness Risk

Mary L. Phillips, M.D.

Bipolar disorder is the world's fourth leading cause of psychiatric and neurological disability. It remains a challenge to diagnose, especially in pediatric samples, because of the similarities of its symptoms to those of other disorders. A major problem that has impeded progress in diagnosis—and, as a result, in risk detection—is the absence of objective illness markers that reflect underlying pathophysiological mechanisms of the disorder. Furthermore, there are no established methods of quantifying *individual-level* risk for the development of bipolar disorder using pathophysiologically relevant measures. It is therefore critical to elucidate the underlying pathophysiological mechanisms of bipolar disorder in order to yield measures that reflect these mechanisms that can be used to help characterize individual-level risk for future development of the disorder. In addition, such mechanisms would ultimately serve as targets for novel interventions (e.g., neuromodulation) to delay or even prevent the development of bipolar disorder.

In this chapter, I describe findings from the increasing literature in bipolar disorder that demonstrate that specific abnormalities in the neural circuitries of emotional regulation and reward processing are evident in individuals who have the disorder. I show how these studies provide a foundation for more recent research that examines the extent to which measures of function and structure in these neural circuitries in at-risk youth can predict the future worsening of symptoms that are associated with bipolar disorder, and the future onset of the disorder. I end by highlighting how the combination of machine learning techniques and neuroimaging methodologies has potential to identify neural measures that predict individual-level risk of the disorder in order to provide a way forward to the ultimate goal of a precision psychiatry platform for the assessment and treatment of all individuals with, or at risk for, bipolar disorder.

History

Bipolar disorder is characterized by mood swings, affective lability, episodes of expansive or elevated mood—namely, hypo/mania—and episodes of low mood—namely, depression (First et al. 2016). The disorder is one of the most common and debilitating of all noncommunicable medical illnesses. In the United States, bipolar disorder has a 12-month prevalence of >2.6% (Kessler et al. 2005) and a lifetime prevalence of >4.5% (Angst 1998; Angst et al. 2003; Merikangas et al. 2007, 2011). Bipolar disorder is, in fact, the fourth leading cause of psychiatric and neurological disability in the world (Collins et al. 2011). In the United States, it is associated with 180 million lost workdays and a $25.9 billion salary-equivalent loss in productivity per year (Hirschfeld and Vornik 2005). Worldwide, it is associated with a 9.2-year reduction in expected life span and a suicide risk 20–30 times greater than that found in the general population (Pompili et al. 2013).

A major problem with bipolar disorder is how challenging it is to diagnose, especially in pediatric samples, because of similarities in its symptoms with those of other disorders. While risk for the development of the disorder is best predicted by familial history, with heritability rates ranging from 59% to 87% (Smoller and Finn 2003), the absence of objective illness markers that reflect underlying pathophysiological mechanisms of the disorder has impeded risk detection and the development of new, pathophysiologically based interventions. To date, there are no established methods of quantifying individual-level risk for the development of bipolar disorder using these pathophysiologically relevant measures. Elucidating the underlying pathophysiological mechanisms of bipolar disorder is thus a critical step toward identifying measures that reflect these mechanisms; measures that can help to characterize the individual-level risk for future development of the disorder. The mechanisms could also ultimately serve as targets for novel interventions (e.g., neuromodulation) to delay or even prevent the development of the disorder.

Current Knowledge and Approaches

NEURAL MODELS OF BIPOLAR DISORDER

An increasingly large neuroimaging literature points to a conceptualization of bipolar disorder as dysfunction in the neural circuitries that underlie key information processing abnormalities that characterize the disorder, particularly emotional regulation and reward processing (Figure 3–1). Briefly, emotional regulation circuitry can be considered to be focused on the amygdala, which is important for the perception of emotionally salient cues (Davis and Whalen 2001; Swanson 2003), as well as several prefrontal cortical regions that are implicated in different effortful and automatic (implicit) subprocesses that are important for the regulation of emotional responses to such cues (Phillips et al. 2008). A predominantly lateral prefrontal cortical system (including regions in the dorsolateral and ventrolateral prefrontal cortices) supports effortful subprocesses, including suppression of emotional behaviors, redirection of attention away from emotional cues, and reappraisal of emotional contexts. In parallel, a medial prefrontal cortical system (including the anterior cingulate cortex, mediodorsal prefrontal cortex, and hippocampus) is thought to support automatic subprocesses, including extinction and automatic redirection of attention away from, and automatic reappraisal of, emotional cues (Phillips et al. 2008).

Reward processing circuitry includes several regions, but key among them is the ventral striatum (including the nucleus accumbens), which is critically important for the response to reward cues and reward receipt (Knutson and Wimmer 2007) and, in particular, for coding prediction error and discrepancy between expected and actual outcomes (Kumar et al. 2008; Schultz 2002). Several prefrontal cortical regions are also important for reward processing, including the ventrolateral prefrontal cortex, which links cues to specific reward outcomes (Boorman et al. 2016; Lee et al. 2015) and is implicated in concrete decision making that focuses on immediate rewards (Hill et al. 2017; Smith et al. 2018). The orbitofrontal cortex encodes reward value (Grabenhorst and Rolls 2011), while the mediodorsal prefrontal cortex regulates reward-seeking behaviors in potentially rewarding contexts (Knutson et al. 2003; Schultz 2002), and the rostral-dorsal anterior cingulate cortex guides behavior to incentive stimuli in order to facilitate reward receipt (Grabenhorst and Rolls 2011; Rogers et al. 2004; Rushworth et al. 2011).

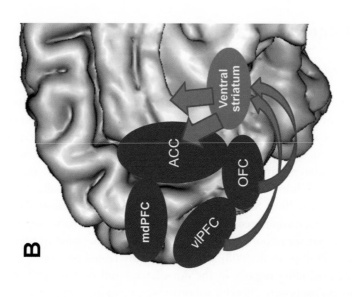

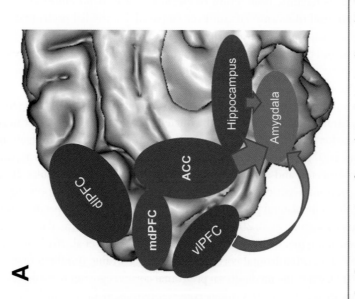

Figure 3–1. Representation of neural circuitries implicated in **(A)** emotional regulation and **(B)** reward processing.

To view this figure in color, see Plate 2 in Color Gallery.

Arrows represent key connectivity among these regions. ACC=anterior cingulate cortex; dlPFC=dorsolateral prefrontal cortex; mdPFC=mediodorsal prefrontal cortex; OFC=orbitofrontal cortex; vlPFC=ventrolateral prefrontal cortex.

Studies have reported functional and structural abnormalities in these core neural circuitries in youth and adults with bipolar disorder. The most commonly reported abnormalities include 1) elevated amygdala and reduced bilateral prefrontal cortical activity, alongside altered functional connectivity among these regions, during emotional regulation (Almeida et al. 2009; Altshuler et al. 2008; Blumberg et al. 2005; Caseras et al. 2015; Delvecchio et al. 2012; Dima et al. 2013; Foland et al. 2008; Foland-Ross et al. 2012; Horacek et al. 2015; Kanske et al. 2015; Keener et al. 2012; Lawrence et al. 2004; Phillips et al. 2003, 2008; Rey et al. 2014; Rosenfeld et al. 2014; Strakowski et al. 2011, 2012; Surguladze et al. 2010; Townsend et al. 2012, 2013; Versace et al. 2010; Wang et al. 2009) and 2) abnormally elevated activity in predominantly left ventral striatal–ventrolateral and orbitofrontal cortical regions during different stages of reward processing (Abler et al. 2008; Bermpohl et al. 2010; Caseras et al. 2013; Chase et al. 2013; Linke et al. 2012; Mason et al. 2014; Nusslock et al. 2012; O'Sullivan et al. 2011; Satterthwaite et al. 2015). However, the elevated ventral striatal response during reward processing is largely absent during depressed episodes (Chase et al. 2013; Satterthwaite et al. 2015). It is thought that these patterns of functional abnormalities may predispose to emotional lability, emotional dysregulation, and heightened reward sensitivity, which are hallmarks of bipolar disorder (Phillips and Swartz 2014). Accompanying these abnormalities are reductions in gray matter in the prefrontal and temporal cortices, amygdala, and hippocampus, and structural abnormalities in white matter tracts that connect prefrontal and subcortical regions in these circuitries (Phillips and Swartz 2014).

CAN NEURAL MEASURES BE USED TO PREDICT FUTURE CLINICAL COURSE IN YOUTH AND YOUNG ADULTS WITH BIPOLAR DISORDER AND THOSE AT RISK OF THE DISORDER?

We need a way to identify neural mechanisms of bipolar disorder and to identify measures that reflect these mechanisms, which are potential predictors of future bipolar disorder development in youth and young adults. One promising way is to identify which specific measures of emotional regulation and reward processing neural circuitry structure and function predict, and which specific changes in these measures over time are associated with worsening mood symptoms in youth at risk for bipolar disorder and individuals who have the disorder.

Few neuroimaging studies have examined whether neural measures can be used to predict future course of illness in individuals with bipolar disorder. Those that have done so suggest that lower gray matter volume in prefrontal cortical and subcortical regions (important for emotional regulation), and white matter lesions in subcortical regions, predict worse outcomes (e.g., greater number of recurrences) in individuals with bipolar disorder (Dusi et al. 2019). The majority of studies have focused on identifying neural measure predictors of response to specific treatments. In one study, lower fractional anisotropy (measuring the longitudinal alignment of fibers in white matter tracts) in the cingulum bundle (hippocampal subsection) predicted poorer clinical response to lithium (Kafantaris et al. 2017). Other studies reported that lower fractional anisotropy in prefrontal cortical regions, together with greater global radial diffusivity, the latter reflecting lower white matter fiber collinearity and/or myelin damage, predicted poorer antidepressant response (Bollettini et al. 2015; Lan et al. 2017). One study reported that lower functional connectivity at rest between the amygdala and anterior insula, and greater functional connectivity at rest between the right ventrolateral prefrontal cortex and anterior insula, were associated with more emotional dysregulation after cognitive-behavioral therapy (Ellard et al. 2018).

Our research team has examined youth across a range of genetic risk for bipolar disorder (Birmaher et al. 2009, 2010; Goldstein et al. 2010), as well as youth who have behavioral and emotional dysregulation and affective lability, who are at symptomatic risk of developing bipolar disorder (Findling et al. 2010; Horwitz et al. 2010). In our neuroimaging studies of these youth, we examined whether neural measures in neural circuitries that underlie emotional regulation and reward processing predicted, or whether changes in these neural measures were associated with, future worsening of bipolar disorder symptoms. We showed the following key relationships across different studies using multimodal neuroimaging techniques. First, in youth at genetic risk of bipolar disorder, hypo/mania severity in the future (29 months postscan) was predicted by greater cortical thickness in the left ventrolateral prefrontal cortex and lower cortical thickness in several regions, including prefrontal cortical regions that are important for emotional regulation (Bertocci et al. 2019). These findings were largely replicated in an independent group of youth who had high levels of emotional dysregulation and were at symptomatic risk of developing bipolar disorder (Bertocci et al. 2019). Second, we reported that in these emotionally dysregulated youth, lower cingulum bundle length, a key white matter tract that connects multiple cortical regions that are important for emotional regulation, was associated with greater positive mood and energy dysregulation at 14.2 months postscan (Bertocci et al. 2016). Third, in youth at risk of bipolar disorder, we showed that increasing amygdala activity, and increasing amygdala–medial prefrontal cortical functional connectivity, during emotional regulation over 2 and 3 years, respectively, were associated with increasing hypo/

mania, depression, and affective lability severity (i.e., increasing severity of mood symptoms in general) (Acuff et al. 2018; Bertocci et al. 2017). Fourth, we showed that in emotionally dysregulated youth, greater functional connectivity among regions in reward circuitry during reward processing was associated with greater positive mood and energy dysregulation at 14.2 months postscan (Figure 3–2) (Bertocci et al. 2016).

INTERIM SUMMARY

Only a small number of studies have examined the extent to which neural measures can predict future clinical course in individuals with bipolar disorder. Their findings show that worse clinical outcomes are predicted by patterns of predominantly lower gray matter volume in prefrontal cortical and subcortical regions, alongside white matter lesions in subcortical regions and altered amygdala and prefrontal cortical resting-state functional connectivity. In parallel, our findings indicate that multimodal neuroimaging measures of cortical thickness, white matter structure and activity, and functional connectivity in emotional regulation and reward processing circuitries predict future clinical course in youth at risk of developing bipolar disorder in the future. Specifically, increases in amygdala activity and amygdala–medial prefrontal cortical functional connectivity over time during emotional regulation predict greater future affective lability and mood severity in general. In contrast, greater thickness in cortical regions that are important for reward processing, lower thickness in cortical regions that are important for emotional regulation, lower length of the cingulum white matter bundle, and greater reward circuitry functional connectivity specifically predict greater future hypo/mania and positive mood and energy dysregulation symptom severity.

These findings thus suggest that specific measures of function and structure in neural circuitries that are relevant to understanding pathophysiological mechanisms of bipolar disorder can help to predict not only future clinical course in individuals who have bipolar disorder but also future worsening, and the polarity, of symptoms in youth at risk of developing bipolar disorder (Table 3–1).

MACHINE LEARNING: MOVING TOWARD PERSONALIZED MARKERS OF RISK FOR BIPOLAR DISORDER

One goal of clinical neuroscience is to identify individual-level measures of neural function and structure, which can provide a measure of personalized risk for the future development of disorders such as bipolar disorder, for the

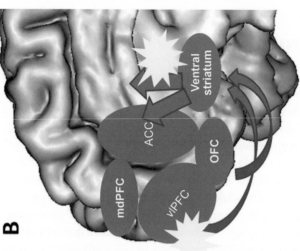

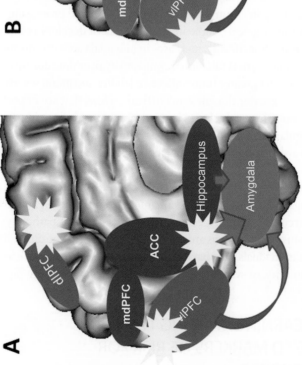

Figure 3–2. Representation of key abnormalities (*yellow bursts*) in **(A)** emotional regulation and **(B)** reward processing circuitries that predict future worsening of bipolar disorder–related psychopathology in youth.

To view this figure in color, see Plate 3 in Color Gallery.

Arrows represent key connectivity among these regions. ACC=anterior cingulate cortex; dlPFC=dorsolateral prefrontal cortex; mdPFC=mediodorsal prefrontal cortex; OFC=orbitofrontal cortex; vlPFC=ventrolateral prefrontal cortex.

TABLE 3–1. Neural measures that have been identified as predictors of future clinical course in individuals with bipolar disorder and in youth and young adults at risk for the disorder

Neural marker	Predicted future mood symptom worsening
Individuals with bipolar disorder	
Lower gray matter volume in subcortical and prefrontal cortical regions	Worse clinical outcomes (e.g., a greater number of recurrences)
White matter lesions in subcortical regions	Worse clinical outcomes (e.g., a greater number of recurrences)
Lower fractional anisotropy in the cingulum bundle and prefrontal cortical regions	Poorer response to lithium and/or antidepressant medications
Lower functional connectivity at rest between the amygdala and anterior insula, greater functional connectivity at rest between right ventrolateral prefrontal cortex and anterior insula	Less improvement in emotional regulation after cognitive-behavioral therapy
Youth at risk of developing bipolar disorder	
Greater cortical thickness in left ventrolateral prefrontal cortex	Greater hypo/mania severity
Lower thickness in cortical regions important for emotional regulation	Greater hypo/mania severity
Lower cingulum bundle length	Greater positive mood and energy dysregulation
Increasing amygdala activity during emotional regulation over time	Increasing severity of mood symptoms in general
Increasing amygdala–medial prefrontal cortical functional connectivity during emotional regulation over time	Increasing severity of mood symptoms in general
Greater functional connectivity among regions in reward circuitry during reward processing	Greater positive mood and energy dysregulation

ultimate goal of guiding precision medicine approaches to interventions and treatments. Identifying patterns of neural activity and functional connectivity that predict the future worsening of symptoms associated with bipolar disorder is a critical step toward this goal but falls short of identifying *individual-level* markers of illness risk.

Pattern recognition approaches can identify multivariate patterns of neural activity that are predictive of diagnosis or future outcomes (Fernandes et al. 2017; Portugal et al. 2016; Stonnington et al. 2010). These approaches consist of two phases: training and testing. During the training phase, the model learns a relationship between a set of patterns (e.g., patterns of neural activity) and labels (e.g., symptom severity score). In the testing phase, given new individual patterns (e.g., patterns of neural activity from new individuals), the model is used to predict the label of each of these new individuals. The model performance is then evaluated by comparing the observed and predicted labels for the new "test" individuals.

Our research team has used machine learning in combination with neuroimaging to identify patterns of neural activity that can identify—at the individual level—the likelihood of a bipolar disorder diagnosis (Almeida et al. 2013; Mourão-Miranda et al. 2012). More recently, we have used such an approach to identify individual-level patterns of neural activity in young adults that can characterize the magnitude of behaviors associated with risk for future bipolar disorder (de Oliveira et al. 2019). We showed that in a first sample of young adults, whole-brain activity during a reward processing task was able to classify each individual regarding risk for future bipolar disorder, as determined by scores on a specific manic symptom relevant to bipolar disorder. The region with the highest contribution to the model was the left ventrolateral prefrontal cortex, a key region that is implicated in reward processing (Boorman et al. 2016; Lee et al. 2015) and was shown to be functionally abnormal in our previous studies of individuals who have bipolar disorder (Bebko et al. 2014; Caseras et al. 2013; Manelis et al. 2019; Nusslock et al. 2012). We replicated these findings in a second independent sample of young adults in which the severity of this symptom was predicted using a bilateral ventrolateral prefrontal cortical mask (de Oliveira et al. 2019). Findings from this study that the severity of a specific bipolar disorder symptom can be predicted from patterns of whole-brain activity in two independent samples. Also, this study provides neural measures that reflect underlying pathophysiological mechanisms of bipolar disorder to aid in the early identification of individual-level risk of this disorder in young adults.

Conclusion and Future Directions

Bipolar disorder is both common and debilitating. Although risk for the development of this disorder can be predicted by genetics, the absence of objective illness markers has impeded progress toward the precision medicine goals of individual-level risk detection and the development of new pathophysiologically based interventions. Neuroimaging studies have identified specific patterns of abnormality in key neural circuitries that are implicated in processes relevant to understanding the pathophysiological basis of the disorder. These studies have provided a foundation for more recent studies examining the extent to which measures of neural circuitry function and structure in at-risk youth can predict the future worsening of symptoms associated with bipolar disorder. Findings from these studies have together provided an array of neural measures that could be used to help predict the future onset of bipolar disorder in at-risk populations. Furthermore, the use of machine learning techniques alongside neuroimaging methodologies holds much promise for identifying neural measures that can predict individual-level risk for the future development of bipolar disorder.

Although we have replicated some of the above findings, further replication in independent samples is clearly needed to establish which specific neural measures are the strongest predictors of future course of illness in at-risk youth and young adults. The inclusion of machine learning methodologies in such studies can help us identify those neural measures that best predict individual-level risk of bipolar disorder. Employing these neural measures in clinical instruments that are currently being developed to help improve bipolar disorder risk detection in individual patients will then be a critical next step toward providing pathophysiologically relevant markers in risk detection algorithms that can be used in clinical contexts. It is our hope that this structured approach to identifying risk markers of bipolar disorder can guide intervention and novel treatment developments for youth and young adults who are at risk of this disorder, and will move the field closer to the ultimate goal of a precision psychiatry platform for the assessment and treatment of individuals with bipolar disorder.

KEY POINTS

- Specific abnormalities in structure and function in emotional regulation and reward circuitry characterize individuals with bipolar disorder.

- Several neural measures that reflect these pathophysiological mechanisms can predict future clinical course in individuals with bipolar disorder.

- These measures can also predict future worsening of symptoms associated with bipolar disorder, and risk of developing the disorder, in youth and young adults.

- Machine learning and neuroimaging have been used in combination to classify individuals into diagnostic groups, and also to predict severity of lifetime risk of bipolar disorder.

- The combination of machine learning and neuroimaging using neural measures can be used to predict both individual-level risk of future worsening of symptoms that are associated with bipolar disorder and individual-level risk of developing the disorder.

References

Abler B, Greenhouse I, Ongur D, et al: Abnormal reward system activation in mania. Neuropsychopharmacology 33(9):2217–2227, 2008 17987058

Acuff HE, Versace A, Bertocci MA, et al: Association of neuroimaging measures of emotion processing and regulation neural circuitries with symptoms of bipolar disorder in offspring at risk for bipolar disorder. JAMA Psychiatry 75(12):1241–1251, 2018 30193355

Almeida JR, Versace A, Mechelli A, et al: Abnormal amygdala-prefrontal effective connectivity to happy faces differentiates bipolar from major depression. Biol Psychiatry 66(5):451–459, 2009 19450794

Almeida JR, Mourao-Miranda J, Aizenstein HJ, et al: Pattern recognition analysis of anterior cingulate cortex blood flow to classify depression polarity. Br J Psychiatry 203(3):310–311, 2013 23969484

Altshuler L, Bookheimer S, Townsend J, et al: Regional brain changes in bipolar I depression: a functional magnetic resonance imaging study. Bipolar Disord 10(6):708–717, 2008 18837865

Angst J: The emerging epidemiology of hypomania and bipolar II disorder. J Affect Disord 50(2–3):143–151, 1998 9858074

Angst J, Gamma A, Benazzi F, et al: Toward a re-definition of subthreshold bipolarity: epidemiology and proposed criteria for bipolar-II, minor bipolar disorders and hypomania. J Affect Disord 73(1–2):133–146, 2003 12507746

Bebko G, Bertocci MA, Fournier JC, et al: Parsing dimensional vs diagnostic category-related patterns of reward circuitry function in behaviorally and emotionally dysregulated youth in the Longitudinal Assessment of Manic Symptoms study. JAMA Psychiatry 71(1):71–80, 2014 24285346

Bermpohl F, Kahnt T, Dalanay U, et al: Altered representation of expected value in the orbitofrontal cortex in mania. Hum Brain Mapp 31(7):958–969, 2010 19950195

Bertocci MA, Bebko G, Versace A, et al: Predicting clinical outcome from reward circuitry function and white matter structure in behaviorally and emotionally dysregulated youth. Mol Psychiatry 21(9):1194–1201, 2016 26903272

Bertocci MA, Bebko G, Dwojak A, et al: Longitudinal relationships among activity in attention redirection neural circuitry and symptom severity in youth. Biol Psychiatry Cogn Neurosci Neuroimaging 2(4):336–345, 2017 28480336

Bertocci MA, Hanford L, Manelis A, et al: Clinical, cortical thickness and neural activity predictors of future affective lability in youth at risk for bipolar disorder: initial discovery and independent sample replication. Mol Psychiatry 24(12):1856–1867, 2019 31628415

Birmaher B, Axelson D, Monk K, et al: Lifetime psychiatric disorders in school-aged offspring of parents with bipolar disorder: the Pittsburgh Bipolar Offspring study. Arch Gen Psychiatry 66(3):287–296, 2009 19255378

Birmaher B, Axelson D, Goldstein B, et al: Psychiatric disorders in preschool offspring of parents with bipolar disorder: the Pittsburgh Bipolar Offspring Study (BIOS). Am J Psychiatry 167(3):321–330, 2010 20080982

Blumberg HP, Donegan NH, Sanislow CA, et al: Preliminary evidence for medication effects on functional abnormalities in the amygdala and anterior cingulate in bipolar disorder. Psychopharmacology (Berl) 183(3):308–313, 2005 16249909

Bollettini I, Poletti S, Locatelli C, et al: Disruption of white matter integrity marks poor antidepressant response in bipolar disorder. J Affect Disord 174:233–240, 2015 25527993

Boorman ED, Rajendran VG, O'Reilly JX, Behrens TE: Two anatomically and computationally distinct learning signals predict changes to stimulus-oOutcome associations in hippocampus. Neuron 89(6):1343–1354, 2016 26948895

Caseras X, Lawrence NS, Murphy K, et al: Ventral striatum activity in response to reward: differences between bipolar I and II disorders. Am J Psychiatry 170(5):533–541, 2013 23558337

Caseras X, Murphy K, Lawrence NS, et al: Emotion regulation deficits in euthymic bipolar I versus bipolar II disorder: a functional and diffusion-tensor imaging study. Bipolar Disord 17(5):461–470, 2015 25771686

Chase HW, Nusslock R, Almeida JR, et al: Dissociable patterns of abnormal frontal cortical activation during anticipation of an uncertain reward or loss in bipolar versus major depression. Bipolar Disord 15(8):839–854, 2013 24148027

Collins PY, Patel V, Joestl SS, et al: Grand challenges in global mental health. Nature 475(7354):27–30, 2011 21734685

Davis M, Whalen PJ: The amygdala: vigilance and emotion. Mol Psychiatry 6(1):13–34, 2001 11244481

de Oliveira L, Portugal LCL, Pereira M, et al: Predicting bipolar disorder risk factors in distressed young adults from patterns of brain activation to reward: a machine learning approach. Biol Psychiatry Cogn Neurosci Neuroimaging 4(8):726–733, 2019 31201147

Delvecchio G, Fossati P, Boyer P, et al: Common and distinct neural correlates of emotional processing in bipolar disorder and major depressive disorder: a voxel-based meta-analysis of functional magnetic resonance imaging studies. Eur Neuropsychopharmacol 22(2):100–113, 2012 21820878

Dima D, Jogia J, Collier D, et al: Independent modulation of engagement and connectivity of the facial network during affect processing by CACNA1C and ANK3 risk genes for bipolar disorder. JAMA Psychiatry 70(12):1303–1311, 2013 24108394

Dusi N, De Carlo V, Delvecchio G, et al: MRI features of clinical outcome in bipolar disorder: a selected review: special section on "Translational and Neuroscience Studies in Affective Disorders." J Affect Disord 243:559–563, 2019 29907266

Ellard KK, Gosai AG, Bernstein EE, et al: Intrinsic functional neurocircuitry associated with treatment response to transdiagnostic CBT in bipolar disorder with anxiety. J Affect Disord 238:383–391, 2018 29909301

Fernandes OJr, Portugal LCL, Alves RCS, et al: Decoding negative affect personality trait from patterns of brain activation to threat stimuli. Neuroimage 145(Pt B):337–345, 2017 26767946

Findling RL, Youngstrom EA, Fristad MA, et al: Characteristics of children with elevated symptoms of mania: the Longitudinal Assessment of Manic Symptoms (LAMS) study. J Clin Psychiatry 71(12):1664–1672, 2010 21034685

First MB, Williams JBW, Karg RS, Spitzer RL: Structured Clinical Interview for DSM-5—Clinician Version (SCID-5-CV). Arlington, VA, American Psychiatric Association Publishing, 2016

Foland LC, Altshuler LL, Bookheimer SY, et al: Evidence for deficient modulation of amygdala response by prefrontal cortex in bipolar mania. Psychiatry Res 162(1):27–37, 2008 18063349

Foland-Ross LC, Bookheimer SY, Lieberman MD, et al: Normal amygdala activation but deficient ventrolateral prefrontal activation in adults with bipolar disorder during euthymia. Neuroimage 59(1):738–744, 2012 21854858

Goldstein BI, Shamseddeen W, Axelson DA, et al: Clinical, demographic, and familial correlates of bipolar spectrum disorders among offspring of parents with bipolar disorder. J Am Acad Child Adolesc Psychiatry 49(4):388–396, 2010 20410731

Grabenhorst F, Rolls ET: Value, pleasure and choice in the ventral prefrontal cortex. Trends Cogn Sci 15(2):56–67, 2011 21216655

Hill PF, Yi R, Spreng RN, et al: Neural congruence between intertemporal and interpersonal self-control: evidence from delay and social discounting. Neuroimage 162:186–198, 2017 28877515

Hirschfeld RM, Vornik LA: Bipolar disorder—costs and comorbidity. Am J Manag Care 11 (3 suppl):S85–S90, 2005 16097719

Horacek J, Mikolas P, Tintera J, et al: Sad mood induction has an opposite effect on amygdala response to emotional stimuli in euthymic patients with bipolar disorder and healthy controls. J Psychiatry Neurosci 40(2):134–142, 2015 25703646

Horwitz SM, Demeter CA, Pagano ME, et al: Longitudinal Assessment of Manic Symptoms (LAMS) study: background, design, and initial screening results. J Clin Psychiatry 71(11):1511–1517, 2010 21034684

Kafantaris V, Spritzer L, Doshi V, et al: Changes in white matter microstructure predict lithium response in adolescents with bipolar disorder. Bipolar Disord 19(7):587–594, 2017 28992395

Kanske P, Schönfelder S, Forneck J, Wessa M: Impaired regulation of emotion: neural correlates of reappraisal and distraction in bipolar disorder and unaffected relatives. Transl Psychiatry 5(1):e497, 2015 25603413

Keener MT, Fournier JC, Mullin BC, et al: Dissociable patterns of medial prefrontal and amygdala activity to face identity versus emotion in bipolar disorder. Psychol Med 42(9):1913–1924, 2012 22273442

Kessler RC, Chiu WT, Demler O, et al: Prevalence, severity, and comorbidity of 12-month DSM-IV disorders in the National Comorbidity Survey Replication. Arch Gen Psychiatry 62(6):617–627, 2005 15939839

Knutson B, Wimmer GE: Splitting the difference: how does the brain code reward episodes? Ann N Y Acad Sci 1104:54–69, 2007 17416922

Knutson B, Fong GW, Bennett SM, et al: A region of mesial prefrontal cortex tracks monetarily rewarding outcomes: characterization with rapid event-related fMRI. Neuroimage 18(2):263–272, 2003 12595181

Kumar P, Waiter G, Ahearn T, et al: Abnormal temporal difference reward-learning signals in major depression. Brain 131(Pt 8):2084–2093, 2008 18579575

Lan MJ, Rubin-Falcone H, Motiwala F, et al: White matter tract integrity is associated with antidepressant response to lurasidone in bipolar depression. Bipolar Disord 19(6):444–449, 2017 28796415

Lawrence NS, Williams AM, Surguladze S, et al: Subcortical and ventral prefrontal cortical neural responses to facial expressions distinguish patients with bipolar disorder and major depression. Biol Psychiatry 55(6):578–587, 2004 15013826

Lee SW, O'Doherty JP, Shimojo S: Neural computations mediating one-shot learning in the human brain. PLoS Biol 13(4):e1002137, 2015 25919291

Linke J, King AV, Rietschel M, et al: Increased medial orbitofrontal and amygdala activation: evidence for a systems-level endophenotype of bipolar I disorder. Am J Psychiatry 169(3):316–325, 2012 22267184

Manelis A, Stiffler R, Lockovich JC, et al: Longitudinal changes in brain activation during anticipation of monetary loss in bipolar disorder. Psychol Med 49(16):2781–2788, 2019 30572969

Mason L, O'Sullivan N, Montaldi D, et al: Decision-making and trait impulsivity in bipolar disorder are associated with reduced prefrontal regulation of striatal reward valuation. Brain 137(Pt 8):2346–2355, 2014 25009169

Merikangas KR, Akiskal HS, Angst J, et al: Lifetime and 12-month prevalence of bipolar spectrum disorder in the National Comorbidity Survey replication. Arch Gen Psychiatry 64(5):543–552, 2007 17485606

Merikangas KR, Jin R, He JP, et al: Prevalence and correlates of bipolar spectrum disorder in the world mental health survey initiative. Arch Gen Psychiatry 68(3):241–251, 2011 21383262

Mourão-Miranda J, Almeida JR, Hassel S, et al: Pattern recognition analyses of brain activation elicited by happy and neutral faces in unipolar and bipolar depression. Bipolar Disord 14(4):451–460, 2012 22631624

Nusslock R, Almeida JR, Forbes EE, et al: Waiting to win: elevated striatal and orbitofrontal cortical activity during reward anticipation in euthymic bipolar disorder adults. Bipolar Disord 14(3):249–260, 2012 22548898

O'Sullivan N, Szczepanowski R, El-Deredy W, et al: fMRI evidence of a relationship between hypomania and both increased goal-sensitivity and positive outcome-expectancy bias. Neuropsychologia 49(10):2825–2835, 2011 21703286

Phillips ML, Swartz HA: A critical appraisal of neuroimaging studies of bipolar disorder: toward a new conceptualization of underlying neural circuitry and a road map for future research. Am J Psychiatry 171(8):829–843, 2014 24626773

Phillips ML, Drevets WC, Rauch SL, et al: Neurobiology of emotion perception II: implications for major psychiatric disorders. Biol Psychiatry 54(5):515–528, 2003 12946880

Phillips ML, Ladouceur CD, Drevets WC: A neural model of voluntary and automatic emotion regulation: implications for understanding the pathophysiology and neurodevelopment of bipolar disorder. Mol Psychiatry 13(9):829, 833–857, 2008 18574483

Pompili M, Gonda X, Serafini G, et al: Epidemiology of suicide in bipolar disorders: a systematic review of the literature. Bipolar Disord 15(5):457–490, 2013 23755739

Portugal LC, Rosa MJ, Rao A, et al: Can emotional and behavioral dysregulation in youth be decoded from functional neuroimaging? PLoS One 11(1):e0117603, 2016 26731403

Rey G, Desseilles M, Favre S, et al: Modulation of brain response to emotional conflict as a function of current mood in bipolar disorder: preliminary findings from a follow-up state-based fMRI study. Psychiatry Res 223(2):84–93, 2014 24862389

Rogers RD, Ramnani N, Mackay C, et al: Distinct portions of anterior cingulate cortex and medial prefrontal cortex are activated by reward processing in separable phases of decision-making cognition. Biol Psychiatry 55(6):594–602, 2004 15013828

Rosenfeld ES, Pearlson GD, Sweeney JA, et al: Prolonged hemodynamic response during incidental facial emotion processing in inter-episode bipolar I disorder. Brain Imaging Behav 8(1):73–86, 2014 23975275

Rushworth MF, Noonan MP, Boorman ED, et al: Frontal cortex and reward-guided learning and decision-making. Neuron 70(6):1054–1069, 2011 21689594

Satterthwaite TD, Kable JW, Vandekar L, et al: Common and dissociable dysfunction of the reward system in bipolar and unipolar depression. Neuropsychopharmacology 40(9):2258–2268, 2015 25767910

Schultz W: Getting formal with dopamine and reward. Neuron 36(2):241–263, 2002 12383780

Smith BJ, Monterosso JR, Wakslak CJ, et al: A meta-analytical review of brain activity associated with intertemporal decisions: evidence for an anterior-posterior tangibility axis. Neurosci Biobehav Rev 86:85–98, 2018 29366699

Smoller JW, Finn CT: Family, twin, and adoption studies of bipolar disorder. Am J Med Genet C Semin Med Genet 123C(1):48–58, 2003 14601036

Stonnington CM, Chu C, Klöppel S, et al: Predicting clinical scores from magnetic resonance scans in Alzheimer's disease. Neuroimage 51(4):1405–1413, 2010 20347044

Strakowski SM, Eliassen JC, Lamy M, et al: Functional magnetic resonance imaging brain activation in bipolar mania: evidence for disruption of the ventrolateral prefrontal-amygdala emotional pathway. Biol Psychiatry 69(4):381–388, 2011 21051038

Strakowski SM, Adler CM, Almeida J, et al: The functional neuroanatomy of bipolar disorder: a consensus model. Bipolar Disord 14(4):313–325, 2012 22631617

Surguladze SA, Marshall N, Schulze K, et al: Exaggerated neural response to emotional faces in patients with bipolar disorder and their first-degree relatives. Neuroimage 53(1):58–64, 2010 20595014

Swanson LW: The amygdala and its place in the cerebral hemisphere. Ann N Y Acad Sci 985:174–184, 2003 12724158

Townsend JD, Bookheimer SY, Foland-Ross LC, et al: Deficits in inferior frontal cortex activation in euthymic bipolar disorder patients during a response inhibition task. Bipolar Disord 14(4):442–450, 2012 22631623

Townsend JD, Torrisi SJ, Lieberman MD, et al: Frontal-amygdala connectivity alterations during emotion downregulation in bipolar I disorder. Biol Psychiatry 73(2):127–135, 2013 22858151

Versace A, Thompson WK, Zhou D, et al: Abnormal left and right amygdala-orbitofrontal cortical functional connectivity to emotional faces: state versus trait vulnerability markers of depression in bipolar disorder. Biol Psychiatry 67(5):422–431, 2010 20159144

Wang F, Kalmar JH, He Y, et al: Functional and structural connectivity between the perigenual anterior cingulate and amygdala in bipolar disorder. Biol Psychiatry 66(5):516–521, 2009 19427632

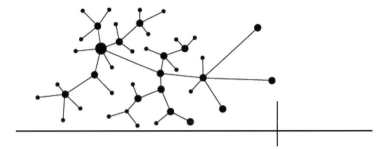

PART 2

NEUROCOGNITION, NEUROPHYSIOLOGY, AND BEHAVIOR

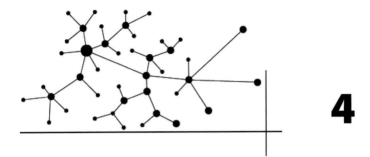

4

Information Processing Impairments as Transdiagnostic Treatment Targets in Psychiatric Disorders

Sophia Vinogradov, M.D.
Jyoti Mishra, Ph.D.
Mor Nahum, Ph.D.
Ian S. Ramsay, Ph.D.

History

Psychiatric disorders have historically been described and defined by subjective symptom reports and abnormalities in observed interpersonal behaviors. Etiological theories in the nineteenth and twentieth centuries focused first on neurological origins and then on psychodynamic and psychological determinants. By the mid–twentieth century, "biological psychiatry" models derived from psychopharmacological treatments emphasized brain neurotransmitter systems as etiopathogenic factors and intervention targets.

Regardless of theoretical orientation, only a handful of twentieth-century scholars explicitly defined the information processing aspects of psychiatric disorders: measurable maladaptive changes in how the brain processes different kinds of information under different circumstances. The exception was schizophrenia, which was labeled "démence" by 1801 and "dementia praecox" by 1893. Despite this early recognition of cognitive failure in schizophrenia, most clinical research into the early 1990s emphasized understanding and treating overt psychotic symptoms rather than identifying the cognitive impairments. Today, schizophrenia is once again understood to be a (heterogeneous) neurocognitive disorder—a disorder of how distributed neural circuits in the brain represent and process information in order to support adaptive behavior.

Schizophrenia serves as a conceptual model that cuts across *all* psychiatric syndromes, which we now know *all* arise from neural circuit dysfunction and maladaptive system-level information processing in the brain (Disner et al. 2011; Gilpin and Weiner 2017; Helm et al. 2018; Kaiser et al. 2015; Kupfer et al. 2012; Malykhin et al. 2012; Pizzagalli 2011; Strakowski et al. 1999). Moreover, like schizophrenia, all psychiatric syndromes have neurodevelopmental origins, with genetic/epigenetic contributors as well as risk factors during gestation, childhood, and adolescence that have a deleterious effect on brain information processing systems and their plastic responses to environmental insults and contingencies (Lima-Ojeda et al. 2018). A range of clinical symptoms may result from information processing impairments but do not have a one-to-one mapping with them.

As described throughout this book, thanks to sophisticated tools from cognitive neuroscience and computational analysis, we can now assess neural circuit changes across different psychiatric disorders and stages of illness. Changes in neural circuits drive alterations in how the brain processes and responds to cognitive and social-emotional information. Yet, as the brain responds to its environment and processes salient information, this in turn drives neural circuit changes.

Current Knowledge and Approaches

WHAT KINDS OF INFORMATION PROCESSING IMPAIRMENTS ARE SEEN IN PSYCHIATRIC DISORDERS?

Multiple impairments in cognitive and social-emotional information processing are observed across psychiatric disorders; they are related to underlying neural circuit dysfunction and correlate with aspects of clinical presentation and illness course. In some disorders, such as schizophrenia and depression, a deep body of knowledge has been established. In others, such as PTSD or eating disorders, the work is still emerging. In many instances, researchers have developed behavioral tasks that capture these impairments. For example, when people with major depression are asked to respond quickly to sad pictures, they show an abnormal allocation of attention to these negative emotional stimuli. This attentional bias is reflected in a slower reaction time to the stimuli, and also in a hyperresponsive late positive potential (LPP), a neural response to attentionally salient stimuli that is observed during electroencephalographic recordings (Auerbach et al. 2015; Benau et al. 2019; Burkhouse et al. 2017; Shestyuk and Deldin 2010; Xie et al. 2018; Zhang et al. 2016) (Figure 4–1). Both the attentional bias and the hyperresponsive LPP normalize during successful treatment, sometimes even before clinical improvement is apparent (Burkhouse et al. 2016).

Although some information processing deficits are more prominent in certain groups of disorders, none are diagnostically specific or pathognomonic (Table 4–1). This is not surprising, as it merely reflects the complex choreography across time, space, and neuro-oscillatory activity among distributed neural circuits that support higher-order functions in the human brain. This lack of diagnostic specificity also reflects the fact that each individual can manifest variants in circuit structure and function across many circuits, as well as develop compensatory activity within and across circuits.

Nonetheless, there do appear to be certain neurocognitive and neuroaffective operations that are critical, if not for fully explaining the development and manifestation of specific psychiatric symptoms and disorders, then at least for indicating an individual's potential for treatment response, recovery, and long-term outcome (Table 4–1). Various combinations of impairments in these core operations are generally present within and across disorders, and the more severe they are, the worse the prognosis and overall treatment responsiveness, regardless of diagnosis.

Although we do not fully understand how these various operations influence one another to determine specific symptom presentations and real-world behaviors at the individual level, it is certain that they interact and influence functioning. For example, in a population-based sample of over 7,000 individuals, Rutter et al. showed that impaired facial emotion recognition was associated with higher self-reported anxiety (Rutter et al. 2019). In healthy individuals, Schad et al. (2014) demonstrated that individual differences in processing speed were related to the use of goal-directed reinforcement learning over habit-based learning. In people with schizophrenia, a rich literature demonstrates an association between early auditory information processing dysfunction, auditory emotional prosody deficits, poorer social functioning, and impaired verbal learning (Javitt and Sweet 2015).

As these examples illustrate, strengths and weaknesses across a range of cognitive and social-emotional operations in the brain interact in complex ways, and their functional significance will be greatly influenced by environ-

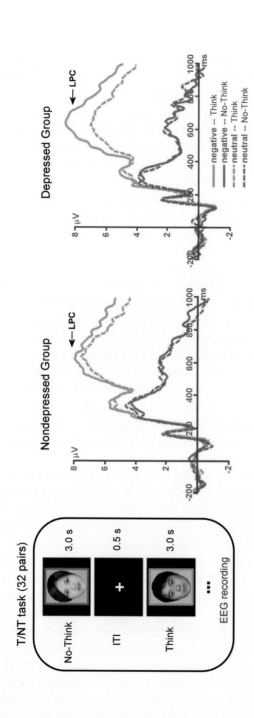

Figure 4–1. An example of a neural correlate of the negative attentional bias in depression.

To view this figure in color, see Plate 4 in Color Gallery.

Participants were instructed to either think about or suppress (not think about) images that were previously associated with positive or negative valence. The group of depressed participants recalled more negative items and had a larger late positive potential (or late positive component [LPC]) for negative "think" items compared with the nondepressed group. These findings reflect abnormal allocation of attentional resources to negative stimuli in the environment, which is believed to arise from increased neural responsivity in prefrontal-parietal attentional circuitry. EEG=electroencephalogram; T/NT=Think/No-Think.

Source. Adapted from Zhang et al. 2016.

TABLE 4–1. Example of the kinds of information processing abnormalities seen in four major groups of psychiatric disorders

Disorder	Processing speed	Attentional control/ Working memory	Inhibitory control	Reinforcement learning	Reward responsivity	Social-emotional cognition	Internal distractions (mind wandering and rumination)
Psychotic disorders	+++ (Blanchard et al. 2010; Lahera et al. 2017; Mesholam-Gately et al. 2009; Rodríguez-Sánchez et al. 2007)	+++ (Erickson et al. 2015; Gold et al. 2018; Karatekin and Asarnow 1998)	+/– Neural but not behavioral deficit (Mayer et al. 2016; Sharma et al. 2017)	+++ (Barch et al. 2016; Maia and Frank 2011; Strauss et al. 2014; Whitton et al. 2015)	+++ (Juckel 2016; Maia and Frank 2017; Rademacher et al. 2017)	+++ (Bora et al. 2017; Fujiwara et al. 2015; Gromann et al. 2013; Lahera et al. 2017; Mier and Kirsch 2017)	+/– (Chen et al. 2015; Phillips et al. 2015; Shin et al. 2015)
ADHD	+++ (Adalio et al. 2018; Cook et al. 2018; Kibby et al. 2019)	+++ (Alderson et al. 2013; Barkley 1997; Karatekin and Asarnow 1998; Lenartowicz et al. 2014)	+++ (Bari and Robbins 2013; Barkley 1997; Dalley and Robbins 2017)	+++ (Kollins and Adcock 2014; Maia and Frank 2011; Tripp and Wickens 2009; Ziegler et al. 2016)	+++ (Luman et al. 2010; Tripp and Wickens 2009; von Rhein et al. 2017)	+/– (Bora and Pantelis 2016; Ibáñez et al. 2014; Miranda et al. 2017)	+++ (Bozhilova et al. 2018; Christoff et al. 2016; Jonkman et al. 2017; Lanier et al. 2019; Mowlem et al. 2019; Seli et al. 2015)

TABLE 4–1. Example of the kinds of information processing abnormalities seen in four major groups of psychiatric disorders *(continued)*

Disorder	Processing speed	Attentional control/ Working memory	Inhibitory control	Reinforcement learning	Reward responsivity	Social-emotional cognition	Internal distractions (mind wandering and rumination)
Anxiety disorders	—	++ (Berggren and Derakshan 2013; Moran 2016)	+++ (Grillon et al. 2017; Nuñez et al. 2017; Ran et al. 2018)	— (Bishop and Gagne 2018)	+++ (Burkhouse et al. 2016)	++ (Plana et al. 2014; van Niekerk et al. 2017)	+ (Makovac et al. 2019)
Depressive disorders	++ (Tsourtos et al. 2002; Vallesi et al. 2015)	+/− (+ adults [McIntyre et al. 2013]; – kids [Vilgis et al. 2015])	++ (Li et al. 2015; Richard-Devantoy et al. 2016; Roca et al. 2015)	+++ (Barch et al. 2016; Chen et al. 2015; Whitton et al. 2015)	+++ (Burkhouse et al. 2016; Peciña et al. 2017)	+++ (Bora and Berk 2016; Ladegaard et al. 2014; Turchi et al. 2017; Zwick and Wolkenstein 2017)	+++ (Christoff et al. 2016; Deng et al. 2014; Hoffmann et al. 2016; Marchetti et al. 2016; Ottaviani et al. 2015)

Note. +++=strong evidence; ++=moderate evidence; +=emerging evidence; +/−=context dependent; —=insufficient evidence.

mental demands. For example, an adolescent who is easily distracted by novel visual stimuli might have functioned very well as a hunter on the alert for game in Paleolithic times, but not as a student in a math classroom in the twenty-first century. An adolescent who develops attentional bias for threatening emotional stimuli after a sexual assault and who experiences disturbing recurrent intrusive imagery along with impaired working memory will likely have maladaptive goal-directed reinforcement learning along with depression, anxiety, and increasingly self-defeating behaviors.

From this emerging evidence, we posit that a forward-thinking precision psychiatry evaluation of patients should routinely include a profile of cognitive and social-emotional processing strengths and weaknesses, with a focus on the major domains listed above (Cuthbert and Insel 2013). Such a profile may well become the basic lab panel for psychiatry (Vinogradov 2017), because it is now possible to carry out such assessments using reliable and scalable digital tools applied remotely, and to develop large normative and comparative data sets (Passell et al. 2019). Like a lab panel, an *information processing profile* can be derived at multiple time points to track changes in cognitive and clinical status and assess response to treatment. Efforts are also under way to map the underlying neural dynamics that represent these diverse cognitive patterns in large samples (Korgaonkar et al. 2013). Ultimately, both neural and behavioral norms in combination have the potential for providing a high degree of predictive precision.

HOW DO WE TREAT INFORMATION PROCESSING IMPAIRMENTS?

A person's *information processing profile* is clinically useful for precision psychiatry only if it provides actionable results. Since 2005, various research groups have developed treatments that target impaired cognitive and social-emotional information processing at the neural systems level with the goal of improving behavior. These treatments make explicit use of intact neuroplasticity mechanisms that enable learning and focus on driving changes in the way brain circuits process the relevant information (Merzenich et al. 2014; Nahum et al. 2013).

Before we delve into these advances, we contrast mechanisms employed in cognitive-behavioral therapy (CBT) and mindfulness-based therapies. These treatments help individuals to *explicitly learn and apply meta-cognitive techniques* to manage their behavior, regardless of any lower-level information processing impairments. In CBT, patients learn to identify and reframe unhelpful interpretations (cognitive distortions) of internal and external events and are taught how such distortions lead to maladaptive feelings and behaviors. For instance, a patient may have difficulties with rapid and accurate social cognition, associated with increased anxiety and a tendency to interpret neutral social interactions as highly critical and humiliating. The patient learns to develop explicit strategies to address such cognitive distortions; that is, they might learn to ask, "Is there another way to interpret the social interaction I just had in which I felt criticized?" Mindfulness-based strategies (Kabat-Zinn 2003) are used to teach active momentary awareness of one's thoughts, feelings, and bodily sensations without judgment ("I am aware of feeling criticized and now I feel butterflies in my stomach"). This nonjudgmental awareness teaches the patient to detach from maladaptive thoughts and feelings, providing subjective relief. Both CBT and mindfulness approaches (and their many derivatives) drive higher-level changes in how the brain handles information (Baioui et al. 2013; Fu et al. 2008; Tang and Posner 2013). Likewise, some baseline aspects of brain information processing capacity are predictive of how well a patient will respond to CBT (Bryant et al. 2008; Siegle et al. 2006).

Complementary to the "top-down" approach of CBT and mindfulness, cognitive training is based on a "bottom-up" view and harnesses *implicit learning mechanisms to focus on direct targeted training of lower-level information processing impairments* (Merzenich et al. 2014; Nahum et al. 2013). Here, we include traditional cognitive training programs as well as attention bias modification training (ABMT) and social cognitive training. In such an approach, the patient with social anxiety who has poor facial emotion recognition abilities and an attentional bias toward threatening faces might undergo computerized training to improve these two abilities. Cognitive training changes neural circuit function in restorative and compensatory directions, though there is still much to be understood and a full review is beyond our scope. Table 4–2 presents a few examples of successful computerized cognitive training approaches for psychiatric disorders.

Successful cognitive interventions can have lasting "sleeper effects" that improve the longer-term trajectory of the illness in a way that medication treatments do not. A 16-session meta-cognitive intervention targeting delusional ideation in schizophrenia showed only modest impact immediately following treatment but drove a significant and sustained improvement in delusional symptoms 6 months and 3 years later (Moritz et al. 2014). In a trial of cognitive training for executive function for schizophrenia, improvements in cognition, functioning, and electrophysiological indices were only observed 3 months *after* the conclusion of treatment (Best et al. 2019). Sleeper effects are likely the result of improved cognitive capacities that lead individuals to better function in their communities, enabling adaptive behavioral and neuroplastic changes.

Cognitive interventions may also have prophylactic effects on psychiatric illness in a way that medications do not (Bar-Haim 2010; Browning et

TABLE 4–2. Examples of successful cognitive training approaches for psychiatric disorders

Disorder	Form of training	Information processing impairments targeted by training	Brief description	Length of intervention	Control group	Outcomes
Psychotic disorders	Combination of computerized targeted cognitive training (TCT) plus social cognitive training (SCT) (Fisher et al. 2017)	Lower-level auditory and visual processing and working memory deficits; lower-level social and emotional processing deficits	*TCT:* Adaptive online exercises focused on auditory and visual speeded discriminations. *SCT:* Adaptive online exercises focused on emotion perception, theory of mind (ToM), social cue perception, and empathy (Nahum et al. 2014)	*TCT:* 50 hours *SCT:* 20 hours (70 hours total)	*TCT* only: 70 hours	Both groups showed significant improvements in multiple cognitive domains and functional capacity. Only the TCT+SCT group showed significant improvements in emotional prosody identification and reward processing.

TABLE 4–2. Examples of successful cognitive training approaches for psychiatric disorders *(continued)*

Disorder	Form of training	Information processing impairments targeted by training	Brief description	Length of intervention	Control group	Outcomes
Anxiety disorders (social anxiety disorder; for review: Linetzky et al. 2015)	Attention bias modification training (ABMT) (Naim et al. 2018)	Abnormal allocation of attentional resources to socially threatening stimuli	Dot probe task: a pair of faces is presented on every trial; a probe replaces the location of the neutral face (rather than the threatening face), to implicitly train attention away from social threat (MacLeod et al. 1986).	8 45-minute sessions over 4 weeks	Cognitive bias modification of interpretation (group cognitive-behavioral therapy) (Murphy et al. 2007)	ABMT yielded greater symptom reduction compared with control intervention.
Depressive disorders (for meta-analysis, see Motter et al. 2016)	Cognitive control training for depression (Iacoviello et al. 2014, 2018)	Abnormal cognitive control during processing of negatively valenced information	Emotional Faces Memory Task (EFMT), designed to enhance cognitive control of emotional information processing. A sequence of emotional faces is presented, and participants must decide whether the emotion of the current face is the same as the emotion *N* faces prior.	18 sessions over 6 weeks	Computerized working memory training (CT)	EFMT group showed a significantly greater reduction in depression symptom severity compared with the CT group.

al. 2012). For example, ABMT trains one's attention either toward or away from threatening stimuli, and has been shown to mitigate anxiety responses by targeting the threat monitoring system (Bar-Haim 2010; MacLeod and Clarke 2015). In a large-scale randomized controlled trial, four sessions of ABMT prior to combat exposure reduced the subsequent incidence of PTSD in deployed soldiers (Wald et al. 2016). ABMT has also been shown to limit the recurrence of depression symptoms in individuals who had previously experienced major depression, suggesting that this intervention may serve as a "cognitive vaccine" against future episodes (Browning et al. 2012).

CLINICAL CASE ILLUSTRATION[1]

Anne W. is a 22-year-old woman who had an acute psychotic episode 4 months ago that required hospitalization. She is now being treated with a second-generation antipsychotic medication plus weekly CBT for psychosis. She feels she is doing much better overall, but at a recent visit, she told her psychiatrist that she has trouble with memory and concentration, and is finding it hard to read, manage her calendar, and remember daily activities and tasks. Though she wants to resume part-time work at a coffee shop and start taking classes at the community college, she worries about keeping up with work and academic demands.

Ms. W. has a high school education and is of average intelligence (Full Scale IQ=99). Her psychiatrist recommends cognitive and neurological evaluation. An MRI scan reveals no overt pathology. Ms. W.'s global neurocognition score, as measured by the MATRICS (Measurement and Treatment Research to Improve Cognition in Schizophrenia) Consensus Cognitive Battery (Nuechterlein et al. 2008), is nearly 1 SD below the average (T=41), driven by large deficits in verbal learning and memory (T=25) and modestly impaired problem-solving (T=43). Her processing speed is only slightly below average (T=47).

Given this cognitive profile, her psychiatrist recommends a course of cognitive training that targets auditory processing with the goal of improving verbal learning and memory. The computerized exercises are designed to improve the speed and accuracy of auditory information processing, maintaining a dense reward schedule (80%–85% accuracy rate on an individually adaptive basis) while remaining challenging enough to drive successful learning. Exercises include speeded frequency modulation sweeps, phoneme distinction, and auditory list learning (Fisher et al. 2009).

Three months later, after completing 20 hours of cognitive training, Ms. W. repeats the tests of cognitive and neurological functioning (Figure 4–2). Her global neurocognitive performance is markedly improved (T=46), driven by strong gains in verbal learning and memory (T=38) as well as strong gains in problem solving (T=53). Volumetric analyses of her follow-

---

[1]This vignette was adapted from data collected on a participant who enrolled in a randomized controlled trial of targeted cognitive training (Fisher et al. 2015).

up MRI scan show small increases in left thalamic volume as well as increases in bilateral middle and superior temporal gyrus volume and thickness, which typically show a reduction in volume when first-episode patients are followed over 2 years (Gutiérrez-Galve et al. 2015; Lee et al. 2016; Ramsay et al. 2018). This is consistent with basic science and clinical literature which suggests that successful cognitive training can be both neuro-restorative and neuro-protective (Eack et al. 2010; Mishra et al. 2014; Ramsay and MacDonald 2015; Ramsay et al. 2017). Ms. W. also shows less depression, anxiety, and irritability, and she feels ready to return to work.

Ms. W. is reassessed 6 months later. She is now working part-time and taking two community college classes and is pleased with her ability to manage her workload. Testing shows sustained gains in global neurocognition, as well as verbal learning and memory, with notable improvement in processing speed. However, her problem-solving score has returned to baseline. Her psychiatrist discusses possible additional cognitive training to focus on problem solving and other executive functioning skills. Ms. W. decides to wait until summer break before trying another course of training.

Conclusion and Future Directions

HOW DO CLINICIANS ASSESS PATIENTS FOR INFORMATION PROCESSING IMPAIRMENTS?

Even as the field of psychiatric neuroscience rapidly moves toward an "information processing" approach for understanding psychopathology, the frontline clinician has almost no tools that enable the reliable and valid assessment of information processing impairments in patients. An ideal information processing panel would be digitized, require low participant burden, be easy for clinicians and patients to interpret, could be applied remotely with high fidelity, and would contain actionable information that is meaningful in the real world. As Germine et al. (2019) note, it is likely that commercialization will be necessary for these platforms to support the continuous updates and norm gathering necessary to validly represent and predict the diversity in individual mental health outcomes.

At present, several digitized cognitive testing platforms are available or are in development for use by clinicians. Examples include TestMyBrain (www.testmybrain.org) (Germine et al. 2019; Passell et al. 2019); Cambridge Neuropsychological Test Automated Battery (CANTAB; www.cambridge-cognition.com); BAC App, a tablet-based version of the Brief Assessment of Cognition in Schizophrenia (Atkins et al. 2017); BrainHQ by Posit Science (Biagianti et al. 2019); the Adaptive Cognitive Evaluation (ACE) battery (www.neuroscape.ucsf.edu/technology/#ace); Mindstrong (Dagum 2018); and the Brain Engagement (BrainE) platform (developed by one of the authors, and also incorporating electroencephalography-based neural

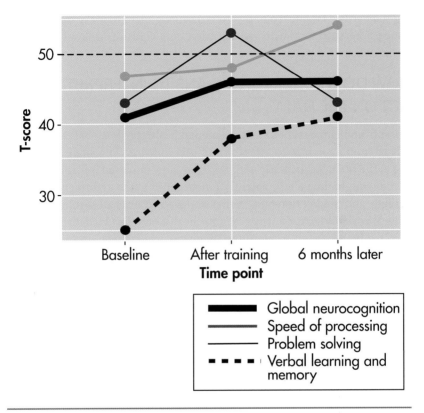

Figure 4–2. Anne W.'s cognitive profile in response to targeted cognitive training.

Anne W. underwent 20 hours of targeted cognitive training of auditory processing to focus on her significant baseline impairments in verbal learning and memory (T=50 reflects the age and gender-normed average). Gains seen after training in verbal learning and memory, and in global neurocognition, were sustained at the 6-month follow-up period. Processing speed showed sleeper effects, with improvement only apparent at the 6-month time point. Gains seen after training in problem solving were not sustained at 6 months, potentially indicating the need for additional targeted training of executive functions.

measures of cognitive function; Balasubramani et al. 2020; Grennan et al. 2021; Misra et al. 2018). The situation is similar to that in the late nineteenth century, when the presence of sugar in the urine was known to indicate diabetes, and multiple chemistry laboratories were being developed to accurately measure it and create standardized measures that would be meaningful to physicians. Recall that in Hippocratic times, doctors made the diagnosis by tasting a patient's urine and perceiving whether it was sweet! This is analogous to our current clinical mental status exam, in which the clinician observes the patient and concludes that "attention is impaired."

Hopefully, the day is not too far off when clinicians become adept at ordering standardized digital cognitive tests, enabling them to make more precise conclusions such as "Sustained attention on a vigilance task was impaired by 1.5 standard deviations."

HOW DO WE TRAIN CLINICIANS TO INTERPRET AND ACT ON THE DATA?

Apart from neuropsychologists, no mental health professional receives any formal training in how to assess or interpret impaired information processing in the brain, particularly with regard to how impaired information processing might impact a patient's functioning, guide treatment decision making, and predict outcome. A first step is to educate all psychiatrists and clinical psychologists on why cognitive health matters (Medalia and Erlich 2017). The next step is to expose clinicians to newly emerging digitized measures of cognitive functioning and how such measures can help to inform clinical decision making at the most straightforward level. For example, if a clinician uses TestMyBrain and uncovers a major working memory impairment in a patient who is not responding to supported employment, this enables the whole team to rethink the treatment strategy. If a patient with major depression shows deficits in executive function, then perhaps he will not be a good candidate for CBT or may require executive function training in addition to standard treatment. Such steps are under way in a few academic centers.

However, the full promise of this field will not occur until clinical scientists and clinicians collaborate with neuroscientists, neural engineers, and software design teams to translate the rapidly evolving scientific knowledge into practical tools for the clinical setting. To use the diabetes analogy again, it is not enough to know how to test urine for the presence of glucose. One must understand how a given test result compares in people with and without diabetes and across various stages of diabetes; one must know all of the factors that can influence a test result for a given patient; one must know when to perform further evaluation; and one must know how to use test results for treatment planning and monitoring. None of this can happen until reliable and highly informative behavioral and neural measures that can easily be acquired in a longitudinal manner in the clinic are normed to comparison groups with and without psychiatric symptoms. In addition, these longitudinal measures must be tethered to treatment options and to longitudinal outcome measures of interest to patients and providers (Gourraud et al. 2014).

With these data sets and tools in place, researchers will be able to identify the interactions among the multiple dimensions of behavioral and neural measures, interventions, and outcomes that occur for patients in real-world treatment settings, and how they relate to measures seen in people without psychiatric illness. The goal is to provide the clinician with interpretable data about which information processing features are the most important to target for any given patient, in terms of choosing interventions that will support an optimal trajectory of clinical improvement and well-being.

Interventional psychiatry may be the best current example of a subdiscipline in which clinicians are continuously acquiring and interpreting complex data in order to guide decision making (Williams et al. 2014). In deep brain stimulation for treatment-refractory obsessive-compulsive disorder, the ideal care team includes neurosurgeons, psychiatrists, and neuropsychologists, who review multiple sources of quantitative assessment data that are relevant to each individual patient before treatment recommendations are made, and who continually monitor patient data for months postsurgery to adjust stimulation parameters as needed (Rappel et al. 2018). At present, outcome measures focus on patient and clinician ratings of obsessive-compulsive symptom severity. However, we are not too far away from being able to add in objective measures of information processing that we know are reflective of adaptive neural system target engagement that leads to better functioning. Ideally, this will be the model for all of psychiatry in the coming years, and for a range of treatment options—all of which, when successful, change the information processing characteristics of the brain.

KEY POINTS

- Psychiatric illnesses have been historically characterized by subjective symptom reports and maladaptive behaviors. However, an abundance of research indicates that these disorders arise from complex patterns of neural circuit dysfunction with changes in cognitive and social-emotional information processing that lead to subjective and behavioral problems.

- We suggest that patients should be evaluated on well-defined information processing measures before, during, and after treatment; such measures could serve as a basic lab panel for psychiatry.

- Several digitized cognitive testing platforms are available or in development for use by clinicians, including TestMyBrain and the Cambridge Neuropsychological Test Automated Battery (CANTAB). However, work still needs to be done to translate these platforms into tools that provide meaningful and actionable data for psychiatric clinicians.

- Interventions that address maladaptive information processing from a "bottom-up" perspective include cognitive training programs, attention bias modification training, and social cognitive training. Psychotherapies and other psychosocial treatments can provide "top-down" influences on brain information processing abilities.

- Translation of rapidly emerging scientific knowledge into clinical tools will require active collaboration among neuroscientists, software design teams, neural engineers, clinicians, and clinical scientists.

References

Adalio CJ, Owens EB, McBurnett K, et al: Processing speed predicts behavioral treatment outcomes in children with attention-deficit/hyperactivity disorder predominantly inattentive type. J Abnorm Child Psychol 46(4):701–711, 2018 28791531

Alderson RM, Kasper LJ, Hudec KL, et al: Attention-deficit/hyperactivity disorder (ADHD) and working memory in adults: a meta-analytic review. Neuropsychology 27(3):287–302, 2013 23688211

Atkins AS, Tseng T, Vaughan A, et al: Validation of the tablet-administered brief assessment of cognition (BAC App). Schizophr Res 181(Mar):100–106, 2017 27771201

Auerbach RP, Stanton CH, Proudfit GH, et al: Self-referential processing in depressed adolescents: a high-density event-related potential study. J Abnorm Psychol 124(2):233–245, 2015 25643205

Baioui A, Pilgramm J, Kagerer S, et al: Neural correlates of symptom reduction after CBT in obsessive-compulsive washers—an fMRI symptom provocation study. J Obsessive Compulsive Relat Disord 2(3):322–330, 2013

Balasubramani PP, Ojeda A, Grennan G, et al: Mapping cognitive brain functions at scale. Neuroimage 231:117641, 2020 33338609

Barch DM, Pagliaccio D, Luking K: Mechanisms underlying motivational deficits in psychopathology: similarities and differences in depression and schizophrenia. Curr Top Behav Neurosci 27:411–449, 2016 26026289

Bar-Haim Y: Research review: attention bias modification (ABM): a novel treatment for anxiety disorders. J Child Psychol Psychiatry 51(8):859–870, 2010 20456540

Bari A, Robbins TW: Inhibition and impulsivity: behavioral and neural basis of response control. Prog Neurobiol 108(Sept):44–79, 2013 23856628

Barkley RA: Behavioral inhibition, sustained attention, and executive functions: constructing a unifying theory of ADHD. Psychol Bull 121(1):65–94, 1997 9000892

Benau EM, Hill KE, Atchley RA, et al: Increased neural sensitivity to self-relevant stimuli in major depressive disorder. Psychophysiology 56(7):e13345, 2019 30793773

Berggren N, Derakshan N: Attentional control deficits in trait anxiety: why you see them and why you don't. Biol Psychol 92(3):440–446, 2013 22465045

Best MW, Milanovic M, Iftene F, et al: A randomized controlled trial of executive functioning training compared with perceptual training for schizophrenia spectrum disorders: effects on neurophysiology, neurocognition, and functioning. Am J Psychiatry 176(4):297–306, 2019 30845819

Biagianti B, Fisher M, Brandrett B, et al: Development and testing of a web-based battery to remotely assess cognitive health in individuals with schizophrenia. Schizophr Res 208(June):250–257, 2019 30733167

Bishop SJ, Gagne C: Anxiety, depression, and decision making: a computational perspective. Annu Rev Neurosci 41(July):371–388, 2018 29709209

Blanchard MM, Jacobson S, Clarke MC, et al: Language, motor and speed of processing deficits in adolescents with subclinical psychotic symptoms. Schizophr Res 123(1):71–76, 2010 20580205

Bora E, Berk M: Theory of mind in major depressive disorder: a meta-analysis. J Affect Disord 191(Feb):49–55, 2016 26655114

Bora E, Pantelis C: Meta-analysis of social cognition in attention-deficit/hyperactivity disorder (ADHD): comparison with healthy controls and autistic spectrum disorder. Psychol Med 46(4):699–716, 2016 26707895

Bora E, Binnur Akdede B, Alptekin K: Neurocognitive impairment in deficit and non-deficit schizophrenia: a meta-analysis. Psychol Med 47(14):2401–2413, 2017 28468693

Bozhilova NS, Michelini G, Kuntsi J, et al: Mind wandering perspective on attention-deficit/hyperactivity disorder. Neurosci Biobehav Rev 92(Sept):464–476, 2018 30036553

Browning M, Holmes EA, Charles M, et al: Using attentional bias modification as a cognitive vaccine against depression. Biol Psychiatry 72(7):572–579, 2012 22579509

Bryant RA, Felmingham K, Kemp A, et al: Amygdala and ventral anterior cingulate activation predicts treatment response to cognitive behaviour therapy for post-traumatic stress disorder. Psychol Med 38(4):555–561, 2008 18005496

Burkhouse KL, Kujawa A, Kennedy AE, et al: Neural reactivity to reward as a predictor of cognitive behavioral therapy response in anxiety and depression. Depress Anxiety 33(4):281–288, 2016 27038409

Burkhouse KL, Owens M, Feurer C, et al: Increased neural and pupillary reactivity to emotional faces in adolescents with current and remitted major depressive disorder. Soc Cogn Affect Neurosci 12(5):783–792, 2017 28008074

Chen C, Takahashi T, Nakagawa S, et al: Reinforcement learning in depression: a review of computational research. Neurosci Biobehav Rev 55(Aug):247–267, 2015 25979140

Christoff K, Irving ZC, Fox KCR, et al: Mind-wandering as spontaneous thought: a dynamic framework. Nat Rev Neurosci 17(11):718–731, 2016 27654862

Cohen N, Ochsner KN: From surviving to thriving in the face of threats: the emerging science of emotion regulation training. Curr Opin Behav Sci 24(Dec):143–155, 2018 31187051

Cook NE, Braaten EB, Surman CBH: Clinical and functional correlates of processing speed in pediatric attention-deficit/hyperactivity disorder: a systematic review and meta-analysis. Child Neuropsychol 24(5):598–616, 2018 28345402

Cuthbert BN, Insel TR: Toward the future of psychiatric diagnosis: the seven pillars of RDoC. BMC Med 11(May):126, 2013 23672542

Dagum P: Digital biomarkers of cognitive function. NPJ Digit Med 1(Mar):10, 2018 31304295

Dalley JW, Robbins TW: Fractionating impulsivity: neuropsychiatric implications. Nat Rev Neurosci 18(3):158–171, 2017 28209979

Deng Y-Q, Li S, Tang Y-Y: The relationship between wandering mind, depression and mindfulness. Mindfulness 5(2):124–128, 2014

Disner SG, Beevers CG, Haigh EAP, et al: Neural mechanisms of the cognitive model of depression. Nat Rev Neurosci 12(8):467–477, 2011 21731066

Eack SM, Hogarty GE, Cho RY, et al: Neuroprotective effects of cognitive enhancement therapy against gray matter loss in early schizophrenia: results from a 2-year randomized controlled trial. Arch Gen Psychiatry 67(7):674–682, 2010 20439824

Erickson MA, Hahn B, Leonard CJ, et al: Impaired working memory capacity is not caused by failures of selective attention in schizophrenia. Schizophr Bull 41(2):366–373, 2015 25031223

Fisher M, Holland C, Merzenich MM, et al: Using neuroplasticity-based auditory training to improve verbal memory in schizophrenia. Am J Psychiatry 166(7):805–811, 2009 19448187

Fisher M, Loewy R, Carter C, et al: Neuroplasticity-based auditory training via laptop computer improves cognition in young individuals with recent onset schizophrenia. Schizophr Bull 41(1):250–258, 2015 24444862

Fisher M, Nahum M, Howard E, et al: Supplementing intensive targeted computerized cognitive training with social cognitive exercises for people with schizophrenia: an interim report. Psychiatr Rehabil J 40(1):21–32, 2017 28368179

Fu CHY, Williams SCR, Cleare AJ, et al: Neural responses to sad facial expressions in major depression following cognitive behavioral therapy. Biol Psychiatry 64(6):505–512, 2008 18550030

Fujiwara H, Yassin W, Murai T: Neuroimaging studies of social cognition in schizophrenia. Psychiatry Clin Neurosci 69(5):259–267, 2015 25418865

Germine L, Reinecke K, Chaytor NS: Digital neuropsychology: challenges and opportunities at the intersection of science and software. Clin Neuropsychol 33(2):271–286, 2019 30614374

Gilpin NW, Weiner JL: Neurobiology of comorbid post-traumatic stress disorder and alcohol-use disorder. Genes Brain Behav 16(1):15–43, 2017 27749004

Gold JM, Robinson B, Leonard CJ, et al: Selective attention, working memory, and executive function as potential independent sources of cognitive dysfunction in schizophrenia. Schizophr Bull 44(6):1227–1234, 2018 29140504

Gourraud P-A, Henry RG, Cree BAC, et al: Precision medicine in chronic disease management: the multiple sclerosis BioScreen. Ann Neurol 76(5):633–642, 2014 25263997

Grennan G, Balasubramani P, Alim F, et al: Cognitive and neural correlates of loneliness and wisdom during emotional bias. Cereb Cortex 2021 33687437 Epub ahead of print

Grillon C, Robinson OJ, Krimsky M, et al: Anxiety-mediated facilitation of behavioral inhibition: threat processing and defensive reactivity during a go/no-go task. Emotion 17(2):259–266, 2017 27642657

Gromann PM, Heslenfeld DJ, Fett A-K, et al: Trust versus paranoia: abnormal response to social reward in psychotic illness. Brain 136 (Pt 6):1968–1975, 2013 23611807

Gutiérrez-Galve L, Chu EM, Leeson VC, et al: A longitudinal study of cortical changes and their cognitive correlates in patients followed up after first-episode psychosis. Psychol Med 45(1):205–216, 2015 24990283

Helm K, Viol K, Weiger TM, et al: Neuronal connectivity in major depressive disorder: a systematic review. Neuropsychiatr Dis Treat 14(Oct):2715–2737, 2018 30425491

Hoffmann F, Banzhaf C, Kanske P, et al: Where the depressed mind wanders: self-generated thought patterns as assessed through experience sampling as a state marker of depression. J Affect Disord 198(July):127–134, 2016 27015160

Iacoviello BM, Wu G, Alvarez E, et al: Cognitive-emotional training as an intervention for major depressive disorder. Depress Anxiety 31(8):699–706, 2014 24753225

Iacoviello BM, Murrough JW, Hoch MM, et al: A randomized, controlled pilot trial of the Emotional Faces Memory Task: a digital therapeutic for depression. NPJ Digit Med 1(June):21, 2018 30854473

Ibáñez A, Aguado J, Baez S, et al: From neural signatures of emotional modulation to social cognition: individual differences in healthy volunteers and psychiatric participants. Soc Cogn Affect Neurosci 9(7):939–950, 2014 23685775

Javitt DC, Sweet RA: Auditory dysfunction in schizophrenia: integrating clinical and basic features. Nat Rev Neurosci 16(9):535–550, 2015 26289573

Jonkman LM, Markus CR, Franklin MS, et al: Mind wandering during attention performance: effects of ADHD-inattention symptomatology, negative mood, ruminative response style and working memory capacity. PLoS One 12(7):e0181213, 2017 28742115

Juckel G: Inhibition of the reward system by antipsychotic treatment. Dialogues Clin Neurosci 18(1):109–114, 2016 27069385

Kabat-Zinn J: Mindfulness-Based Stress Reduction (MBSR). Constr Human Sci 8(2):73, 2003

Kaiser RH, Andrews-Hanna JR, Wager TD, et al: Large-scale network dysfunction in major depressive disorder: a meta-analysis of resting-state functional connectivity. JAMA Psychiatry 72(6):603–611, 2015 25785575

Karatekin C, Asarnow RF: Working memory in childhood-onset schizophrenia and attention-deficit/hyperactivity disorder. Psychiatry Res 80(2):165–176, 1998 9754696

Kibby MY, Vadnais SA, Jagger-Rickels AC: Which components of processing speed are affected in ADHD subtypes? Child Neuropsychol 25(7):964–979, 2019 30558479

Kollins SH, Adcock RA: ADHD, altered dopamine neurotransmission, and disrupted reinforcement processes: implications for smoking and nicotine dependence. Prog Neuropsychopharmacol Biol Psychiatry 52(July):70–78, 2014 24560930

Korgaonkar MS, Grieve SM, Etkin A, et al: Using standardized fMRI protocols to identify patterns of prefrontal circuit dysregulation that are common and specific to cognitive and emotional tasks in major depressive disorder: first wave results from the iSPOT-D study. Neuropsychopharmacology 38(5):863–871, 2013 23303059

Kupfer DJ, Frank E, Phillips ML: Major depressive disorder: new clinical, neurobiological, and treatment perspectives. Lancet 379(9820):1045–1055, 2012 22189047

Ladegaard N, Lysaker PH, Larsen ER, et al: A comparison of capacities for social cognition and metacognition in first episode and prolonged depression. Psychiatry Res 220(3):883–889, 2014 25453639

Lahera G, Ruiz A, Brañas A, et al: Reaction time, processing speed and sustained attention in schizophrenia: impact on social functioning. Rev Psiquiatr Salud Ment 10(4):197–205, 2017 28596126

Lanier J, Noyes E, Biederman J: Mind wandering (internal distractibility) in ADHD: a literature review. J Atten Disord (July):1087054719865781, 2019 31364436

Lee S-H, Niznikiewicz M, Asami T, et al: Initial and progressive gray matter abnormalities in insular gyrus and temporal pole in first-episode schizophrenia contrasted with first-episode affective psychosis. Schizophr Bull 42(3):790–801, 2016 26675295

Lenartowicz A, Delorme A, Walshaw PD, et al: Electroencephalography correlates of spatial working memory deficits in attention-deficit/hyperactivity disorder: vigilance, encoding, and maintenance. J Neurosci 34(4):1171–1182, 2014 24453310

Li Y, Xu Y, Chen Z: Effects of the behavioral inhibition system (BIS), behavioral activation system (BAS), and emotion regulation on depression: a one-year follow-up study in Chinese adolescents. Psychiatry Res 230(2):287–293, 2015 26386601

Lima-Ojeda JM, Rupprecht R, Baghai TC: Neurobiology of depression: a neurodevelopmental approach. World J Biol Psychiatry 19(5):349–359, 2018 28155577

Linetzky M, Pergamin-Hight L, Pine DS, et al: Quantitative evaluation of the clinical efficacy of attention bias modification treatment for anxiety disorders. Depress Anxiety 32(6):383–391, 2015 25708991

Luman M, Tripp G, Scheres A: Identifying the neurobiology of altered reinforcement sensitivity in ADHD: a review and research agenda. Neurosci Biobehav Rev 34(5):744–754, 2010 19944715

MacLeod C, Clarke PJF: The attentional bias modification approach to anxiety intervention. Clin Psychol Sci 3(1):58–78, 2015

MacLeod C, Mathews A, Tata P: Attentional bias in emotional disorders. J Abnorm Psychol 95(1):15–20, 1986 3700842

Maia TV, Frank MJ: From reinforcement learning models to psychiatric and neurological disorders. Nat Neurosci 14(2):154–162, 2011 21270784

Maia TV, Frank MJ: An integrative perspective on the role of dopamine in schizophrenia. Biol Psychiatry 81(1):52–66, 2017 27452791

Makovac E, Fagioli S, Watson DR, et al: Response time as a proxy of ongoing mental state: a combined fMRI and pupillometry study in generalized anxiety disorder. Neuroimage 191(May):380–391, 2019 30798009

Malykhin NV, Carter R, Hegadoren KM, et al: Fronto-limbic volumetric changes in major depressive disorder. J Affect Disord 136(3):1104–1113, 2012 22134041

Marchetti I, Koster EHW, Klinger E, et al: Spontaneous thought and vulnerability to mood disorders: the dark side of the wandering mind. Clin Psychol Sci 4(5):835–857, 2016 28785510

Mayer AR, Hanlon FM, Dodd AB, et al: Proactive response inhibition abnormalities in the sensorimotor cortex of patients with schizophrenia. J Psychiatry Neurosci 41(5):312–321, 2016 26883319

McIntyre RS, Cha DS, Soczynska JK, et al: Cognitive deficits and functional outcomes in major depressive disorder: determinants, substrates, and treatment interventions. Depress Anxiety 30(6):515–527, 2013 23468126

Medalia A, Erlich M: Why cognitive health matters. Am J Public Health 107(1):45–47, 2017 27925815

Merzenich MM, Van Vleet TM, Nahum M: Brain plasticity-based therapeutics. Front Hum Neurosci 8(June):385, 2014 25018719

Mesholam-Gately RI, Giuliano AJ, Goff KP, et al: Neurocognition in first-episode schizophrenia: a meta-analytic review. Neuropsychology 23(3):315–336, 2009 19413446

Mier D, Kirsch P: Social-cognitive deficits in schizophrenia, in Social Behavior From Rodents to Humans: Neural Foundations and Clinical Implications. Edited by Wöhr M, Krach S. Cham, Switzerland, Springer International Publishing, 2017, pp 397–409

Miranda A, Berenguer C, Roselló B, et al: Social cognition in children with high-functioning autism spectrum disorder and attention-deficit/hyperactivity disorder. Front Psychol 8(June):1035, 2017 28690570

Mishra J, de Villers-Sidani E, Merzenich M, et al: Adaptive training diminishes distractibility in aging across species. Neuron 84(5):1091–1103, 2014 25467987

Misra A, Ojeda A, Mishra J: BrainE: A Digital Platform for Evaluating, Engaging and Enhancing Brain Function. Regents of the University of California Copyright SD2018-816, 2018

Moran TP: Anxiety and working memory capacity: a meta-analysis and narrative review. Psychol Bull 142(8):831–864, 2016 26963369

Moritz S, Veckenstedt R, Andreou C, et al: Sustained and "sleeper" effects of group metacognitive training for schizophrenia: a randomized clinical trial. JAMA Psychiatry 71(10):1103–1111, 2014 25103718

Motter JN, Pimontel MA, Rindskopf D, et al: Computerized cognitive training and functional recovery in major depressive disorder: a meta-analysis. J Affect Disord 189(Jan):184–191, 2016 26437233

Mowlem FD, Skirrow C, Reid P, et al: Validation of the mind excessively wandering scale and the relationship of mind wandering to impairment in adult ADHD. J Atten Disord 23(6):624–634, 2019 27255536

Murphy R, Hirsch CR, Mathews A, et al: Facilitating a benign interpretation bias in a high socially anxious population. Behav Res Ther 45(7):1517–1529, 2007 17349970

Nahum M, Lee H, Merzenich MM: Principles of neuroplasticity-based rehabilitation. Prog Brain Res 207:141–171, 2013 24309254

Nahum M, Fisher M, Loewy R, et al: A novel, online social cognitive training program for young adults with schizophrenia: a pilot study. Schizophr Res Cogn 1(1):e11–e19, 2014 25267937

Naim R, Kivity Y, Bar-Haim Y, et al: Attention and interpretation bias modification treatment for social anxiety disorder: a randomized clinical trial of efficacy and synergy. J Behav Ther Exp Psychiatry 59(June):19–30, 2018 29127945

Nuechterlein KH, Green MF, Kern RS, et al: The MATRICS Consensus Cognitive Battery, part 1: test selection, reliability, and validity. Am J Psychiatry 165(2):203–213, 2008 18172019

Nuñez M, Gregory J, Zinbarg RE: Anxiety and retrieval inhibition: support for an enhanced inhibition account. Cogn Emotion 31(2):349–359, 2017 26437374

Ottaviani C, Shahabi L, Tarvainen M, et al: Cognitive, behavioral, and autonomic correlates of mind wandering and perseverative cognition in major depression. Front Neurosci 8:433, 2015 25601824

Passell E, Dillon DG, Baker JT, et al: Digital cognitive assessment: results from the TestMyBrain NIMH Research Domain Criteria (RDoC) Field Test Battery Report. 2019. Available at: psyarxiv.com/dcszr/. Accessed February 15, 2021.

Peciña M, Sikora M, Avery ET, et al: Striatal dopamine D2/3 receptor-mediated neurotransmission in major depression: Implications for anhedonia, anxiety and treatment response. Eur Neuropsychopharmacol 27(10):977–986, 2017 28870407

Phillips RC, Salo T, Carter CS: Distinct neural correlates for attention lapses in patients with schizophrenia and healthy participants. Front Hum Neurosci 9(Oct):502, 2015 26500517

Pizzagalli DA: Frontocingulate dysfunction in depression: toward biomarkers of treatment response. Neuropsychopharmacology 36(1):183–206, 2011 20861828

Plana I, Lavoie M-A, Battaglia M, et al: A meta-analysis and scoping review of social cognition performance in social phobia, posttraumatic stress disorder and other anxiety disorders. J Anxiety Disord 28(2):169–177, 2014 24239443

Rademacher L, Schulte-Rüther M, Hanewald B, et al: Reward: from basic reinforcers to anticipation of social cues. Curr Top Behav Neurosci 30:207–221, 2017 26728170

Ramsay IS, MacDonald AW III: Brain correlates of cognitive remediation in schizophrenia: activation likelihood analysis shows preliminary evidence of neural target engagement. Schizophr Bull 41(6):1276–1284, 2015 25800249

Ramsay IS, Nienow TM, MacDonald AW III: Increases in intrinsic thalamocortical connectivity and overall cognition following cognitive remediation in chronic schizophrenia. Biol Psychiatry Cogn Neurosci Neuroimaging 2(4):355–362, 2017 28584882

Ramsay IS, Fryer S, Boos A, et al: Response to targeted cognitive training correlates with change in thalamic volume in a randomized trial for early schizophrenia. Neuropsychopharmacology 43(3):590–597, 2018 28895568

Ran G, Zhang Q, Huang H: Behavioral inhibition system and self-esteem as mediators between shyness and social anxiety. Psychiatry Res 270(Dec):568–573, 2018 30347379

Rappel P, Marmor O, Bick AS, et al: Subthalamic theta activity: a novel human subcortical biomarker for obsessive compulsive disorder. Transl Psychiatry 8(1):118, 2018 29915200

Richard-Devantoy S, Ding Y, Lepage M, et al: Cognitive inhibition in depression and suicidal behavior: a neuroimaging study. Psychol Med 46(5):933–944, 2016 26670261

Roca M, Vives M, López-Navarro E, et al: Cognitive impairments and depression: a critical review. Actas Esp Psiquiatr 43(5):187–193, 2015 26320897

Rodríguez-Sánchez JM, Crespo-Facorro B, González-Blanch C, et al: Cognitive dysfunction in first-episode psychosis: the processing speed hypothesis. Br J Psychiatry Suppl 51(Dec):s107–s110, 2007 18055925

Rutter LA, Scheuer L, Vahia IV, et al: Emotion sensitivity and self-reported symptoms of generalized anxiety disorder across the lifespan: a population-based sample approach. Brain Behav 9(6):e01282, 2019 30993908

Schad DJ, Jünger E, Sebold M, et al: Processing speed enhances model-based over model-free reinforcement learning in the presence of high working memory functioning. Front Psychol 5(Dec):1450, 2014 25566131

Seli P, Smallwood J, Cheyne JA, et al: On the relation of mind wandering and ADHD symptomatology. Psychon Bull Rev 22(3):629–636, 2015 25561417

Sharma A, Vogel M, Weisbrod M, et al: Pronounced inhibition-related hypofrontal dysfunction in early onset schizophrenia as indexed by NoGo-P300 amplitude. Schizophr Res 189(Nov):213–214, 2017 28174035

Shestyuk AY, Deldin PJ: Automatic and strategic representation of the self in major depression: trait and state abnormalities. Am J Psychiatry 167(5):536–544, 2010 20360316

Shin D-J, Lee TY, Jung WH, et al: Away from home: the brain of the wandering mind as a model for schizophrenia. Schizophr Res 165(1):83–89, 2015 25864955

Siegle GJ, Carter CS, Thase ME: Use of FMRI to predict recovery from unipolar depression with cognitive behavior therapy. Am J Psychiatry 163(4):735–738, 2006 16585452

Strakowski SM, DelBello MP, Sax KW, et al: Brain magnetic resonance imaging of structural abnormalities in bipolar disorder. Arch Gen Psychiatry 56(3):254–260, 1999 10078503

Strauss ME, McLouth CJ, Barch DM, et al: Temporal stability and moderating effects of age and sex on CNTRaCS task performance. Schizophr Bull 40(4):835–844, 2014 23817024

Tang Y-Y, Posner MI: Special issue on mindfulness neuroscience. Soc Cogn Affect Neurosci 8(1):1–3, 2013 22956677

Tripp G, Wickens JR: Neurobiology of ADHD. Neuropharmacology 57(7–8):579–589, 2009 19627998

Tsourtos G, Thompson JC, Stough C: Evidence of an early information processing speed deficit in unipolar major depression. Psychol Med 32(2):259–265, 2002 11866321

Turchi F, Cuomo A, Amodeo G, et al: [The neural bases of social cognition in major depressive disorder: a review] [in Italian]. Riv Psichiatr 52(4):137–149, 2017 28845862

Vallesi A, Canalaz F, Balestrieri M, et al: Modulating speed-accuracy strategies in major depression. J Psychiatr Res 60(Jan):103–108, 2015 25294698

van Niekerk RE, Klein AM, Allart-van Dam E, et al: The role of cognitive factors in childhood social anxiety: social threat thoughts and social skills perception. Cognit Ther Res 41(3):489–497, 2017 28515542

Vilgis V, Silk TJ, Vance A: Executive function and attention in children and adolescents with depressive disorders: a systematic review. Eur Child Adolesc Psychiatry 24(4):365–384, 2015 25633323

Vinogradov S: The golden age of computational psychiatry is within sight. Nature Human Behaviour 1:0047, 2017

von Rhein D, Beckmann CF, Franke B, et al: Network-level assessment of reward-related activation in patients with ADHD and healthy individuals. Hum Brain Mapp 38(5):2359–2369, 2017 28176434

Wald I, Fruchter E, Ginat K, et al: Selective prevention of combat-related post-traumatic stress disorder using attention bias modification training: a randomized controlled trial. Psychol Med 46(12):2627–2636, 2016 27377418

Whitton AE, Treadway MT, Pizzagalli DA: Reward processing dysfunction in major depression, bipolar disorder and schizophrenia. Curr Opin Psychiatry 28(1):7–12, 2015 25415499

Williams NR, Taylor JJ, Kerns S, et al: Interventional psychiatry: why now? J Clin Psychiatry 75(8):895–897, 2014 25191910

Xie H, Jiang D, Zhang D: Individuals with depressive tendencies experience difficulty in forgetting negative material: two mechanisms revealed by ERP data in the directed forgetting paradigm. Sci Rep 8(1):1113, 2018 29348422

Zhang D, Xie H, Liu Y, Luo Y: Neural correlates underlying impaired memory facilitation and suppression of negative material in depression. Sci Rep 6(Nov):37556, 2016 27857199

Ziegler S, Pedersen ML, Mowinckel AM, et al: Modelling ADHD: a review of ADHD theories through their predictions for computational models of decision-making and reinforcement learning. Neurosci Biobehav Rev 71(Dec):633–656, 2016 27608958

Zwick JC, Wolkenstein L: Facial emotion recognition, theory of mind and the role of facial mimicry in depression. J Affect Disord 210(Mar):90–99, 2017 28024224

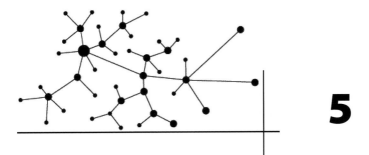

5

State-Sensitive Biomarkers of Specific Computational Processes for Monitoring Symptoms and Predicting Outcomes in People With Schizophrenia

Steven M. Silverstein, Ph.D.
Docia L. Demmin, M.S.
Samantha I. Fradkin, M.S.

History

Although *precision psychiatry* is a relatively new term, the concept was perhaps best articulated over 50 years ago by Gordon Paul with the following question: "Which treatment, prescribed by whom, and in which circumstances, is the most effective for this particular individual with this specific problem?" (Paul 1967, p. 111). Despite many years of research on psychological and biological aspects of mental illnesses and their treatment, however, it has been argued that psychiatry lags behind many other fields of medicine when it comes to our understanding of the causes of these conditions, their prevention, and the development of effective treatments (Insel 2010). For example, although there have been modest gains made on some issues, we currently have no clinical tests for diagnoses, there has been no change in prevalence and premature mortality rates (Cuthbert and Insel 2013), and levels of self-reported psychiatric disability, suicide, and drug overdose have increased dramatically in recent years (Centers for Disease Control and Prevention 2011; Hedegaard et al. 2018; Mojtabai 2011).

It is often noted that the lack of progress in understanding, preventing, and treating psychiatric disorders is rooted in psychiatry's overreliance on traditional and questionably valid diagnostic categories at the expense of focusing on the assessment and targeted treatment of relevant psychological and pathophysiological mechanisms (Cuthbert and Insel 2013). Of course, this is not entirely true, because much work has been based—to varying degrees—on theoretical mechanistic constructs and on biological data as applied to individual symptoms and behaviors. Examples would be work done in psychoanalysis, behavior therapy, the development of families of dopamine receptor–blocking medications, the prefrontal lobotomy, and other areas. Nevertheless, as Wang and Krystal (2014) noted: "There is not a single symptom of a single psychiatric disorder for which we fully understand its physiologic basis at a molecular, cellular, and microcircuit level" (p. 639). The same can be stated for the psychological basis of symptoms and disorders. As a result, "we have only a somewhat vague idea of how the brain generates the cognitive, emotional, and behavioral problems that lead people to seek treatment by psychiatrists and other mental health clinicians" (Wang and Krystal 2014, p. 639).

It has recently been argued that one solution to this problem would be to focus on computational mechanisms, since this could bridge the gap between psychological and biological levels of understanding and provide formal, rigorous, and precise quantitative metrics for mechanistic constructs (Adams et al. 2016; Silverstein et al. 2017; Teufel and Fletcher 2016). While attempts to mathematically model behavior in terms of relationships between relevant core parameters are not new (e.g., Hull 1943; Payne 1958; Wiener 1948), the current hope is that our understanding of how the brain works, along with the processing capacity of computers, has advanced to the point where real progress can now be made using this approach. We believe this approach can succeed in clarifying important aspects of mental illness, but with a few important caveats.

Formally defining variables in terms of parameters that represent aspects of neural function—and for which the relationships can be expressed mathematically—is superior to simply mapping biological findings onto test scores without an understanding of intermediate-level mechanisms. However, there is already a well-developed but underutilized tradition within experimental psychopathology research that approaches experimentation in a theory-driven fashion. In this tradition, precisely specified patterns of scores across conditions are used to test strong hypotheses about core mechanisms in mental functioning (see, e.g., Knight 1984, 1992; Knight and Silverstein 1998, 2001; Silverstein 2008). Stated differently, the critical aspects are that 1) clear hypotheses regarding different mechanisms are tested against each other, and against the performance pattern that would be expected to result from a generalized performance deficit; and 2) tests are designed to allow for the emergence of different patterns of performance that can be understood in terms of these different mechanisms (Bennett et al. 2019). There is nothing magical about mathematical equations. In the absence of strong experimental designs and adequate controls for confounding factors (e.g., poor attention and motivation, anxiety, sedation), computational model parameters can be just as useless as behavioral findings and functional MRI (fMRI) data that are obtained from poorly designed studies.

Current Knowledge and Approaches

In this chapter, we provide examples of experimental data and computational methods that have been, or can be, used to develop biomarkers of CNS processes that we believe represent the basis of each of the three primary symptom clusters in schizophrenia (disorganized, positive, negative). The examples we discuss are from vision science—the most studied and understood area of neuroscience—because many visual tasks are particularly good at isolating specific processes independent of generalized deficit confounds (Knight 1984; Silverstein 2016; Silverstein and Keane 2011a, 2011b; Silverstein and Thompson 2015). One point we wish to emphasize throughout the discussion is that, at least in the study of schizophrenia, the development of biomarkers for outcomes such as conversion to psychosis, early treatment response, impending relapse, and so forth requires measures that tap into the processes whose changes are the basis of symptom emergence and remission. That is, these biomarkers must be state sensitive.

While much work, especially in the 1980s and 1990s, focused on identifying vulnerability markers for schizophrenia (i.e., those that could be observed in patients regardless of illness phase or clinical state, and in unaffected family members) (Nuechterlein and Dawson 1984b; Nuechterlein et al. 1986, 1994), these markers are unlikely to be sensitive to outcomes that involve changes in clinical presentation. This is not to say that vulnerability markers cannot be useful for precision psychiatry efforts. They are likely to be useful for characterizing heterogeneity and specifying genetic contributions. But there has been far less work done in identifying state-sensitive measures or *episode markers* (Nuechterlein and Dawson 1984a). Therefore, we believe that the time is right to increase efforts to develop them.

One reason for the relative lack of focus on state-sensitive measures is misconceptions about using measures that, because of state sensitivity, have lower test-retest reliability. However, a state-sensitive measure that can isolate specific mechanisms can have excellent validity (construct, concurrent, and predictive) even when reliability is low, when the reason for low reliability is valid measurement of the current state of a process that is naturally characterized by instability (Knight and Silverstein 2001; Silverstein 2008). While this issue has traditionally been discussed within the context of generalized deficit confounds, it is clearly critical for precision psychiatry, which emphasizes defining relevant mechanisms and developing measures of these mechanisms (with minimal confounds from other mechanisms) that can be used in real-world clinical settings.

Clinical Illustrations

DISORGANIZED SYMPTOMS

For over 20 years, studies in our lab and in other labs around the world, using psychophysics, event-related potentials, and fMRI, have indicated that people diagnosed with schizophrenia have a reduced ability to organize visual features into perceptual wholes (Butler et al. 2008, 2013; Uhlhaas and Silverstein 2005b) (Figure 5–1). Moreover, this impairment in perceptual organization is related to reduced conceptual organization (reviewed in Phillips and Silverstein 2003, 2013; Silverstein 2016; Silverstein and Uhlhaas 2004; Uhlhaas and Mishara 2007; Uhlhaas and Silverstein 2005a; Uhlhaas et al. 2006). The latter findings have been interpreted as having two implications. The first is the presence of a canonical cortical processing algorithm in which context disambiguates and highlights the behavioral relevance or meaning of a target stimulus. For example, the presence of closely spaced edge features with similar orientations leads to lateral excitation among neurons that signal those features, which increases the likelihood of the perception of an edge, surface, or object that is distinguished from other features; words preceding the current spoken word generate expectations about the likely meaning of the current and following words, thereby facilitating the generation and maintenance of coherent linguistic representations (Phillips 2017; Phillips and Silverstein 2013; Phillips and Singer 1997; Phillips et al. 2015, 2016). The second implication is the presence of a widespread failure of this contextual modulation process in schizophrenia that accounts for multiple manifestations of "processing stimuli out of context,"

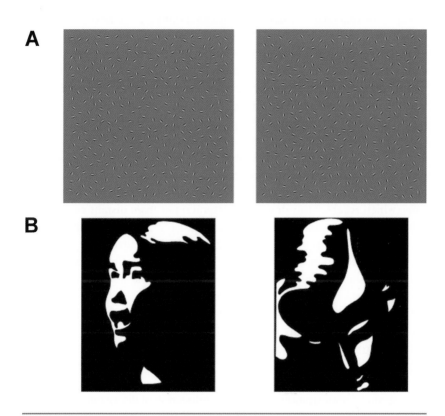

Figure 5–1. Examples of stimuli used in multiple studies of perceptual organization in schizophrenia.

A) Stimuli from the Jittered Orientation Visual Integration (JOVI) task. The left panel is an example of a leftward-pointing oval with a smooth contour (i.e., no orientational jitter applied to the Gabor elements that make up the oval contour) embedded within a field of randomly oriented noise Gabors. The right panel is an example of a rightward-pointing oval with orientational jitter of ±13° applied to each contour element. This disrupts collinearity and the smoothness of the contour and makes perception of the shape more difficult. The participant's task on each trial is to determine whether the oval is pointing to the left or to the right. Multiple conditions of orientational jitter are typically used within a single task. Accuracy levels and their slope across conditions indicate sensitivity to the grouping manipulation. **B)** Stimuli from the Mooney Faces task, in which all features are rendered as pure black or white. The left panel is an example of a face that is easy to perceive. The right panel is a face that is difficult to perceive due to the light-dark rendering seriously disrupting the ability to achieve perceptual closure. In this task, participants are typically asked to report whether or not they see a face, or sometimes to make a determination about the face they see (e.g., child/adult, male/female).

including reduced perceptual organization and sometimes a better-than-controls ability to identify single features that are strongly grouped with others (see, e.g., Place and Gilmore 1980; Silverstein et al. 1996), and thought disorder characterized by fragmented thinking and associative loose-ness (for review, see Phillips and Silverstein 2003, 2013; Phillips et al. 2015).

Recent work has emphasized the ability to account for these findings within an information theoretic framework in which failures of contextual modulation can be understood in terms of concepts such as mutual (shared) information (i.e., coherent infomax), entropy (uncertainty), coding with syn-ergy (i.e., output activity that is dependent on receiving a specific pattern of input across multiple axons), and noise (Kay and Phillips 2011; Kay et al. 2019; Phillips et al. 2015; Silverstein et al. 2017; Wibral et al. 2017). Recent work has also emphasized the implementation of these functions via the in-teraction of the independent contributions of input from apical dendritic tufts (which receive "top-down" and lateral input from distant cortical and subcortical regions that can be conceptualized as representing context), and input to the cell soma's dendrites that can be conceptualized as feedforward processing that corresponds to that cell's receptive field (Phillips et al. 2015, 2016). The ability of information theoretic metrics to accurately model both biological data on contextual modulation in vision (Phillips and Singer 1997; Phillips et al. 1998) and the modifying influence of apical dendritic activity on neuronal firing rates (Kay et al. 2019) demonstrates the utility of this approach for bridging psychological and biological levels of under-standing, and for using computational metrics to account for specific im-pairments in schizophrenia.

A second demonstration of a visual manifestation of disorganization comes from the Ebbinghaus illusion task. In this task, the perceived size of a circle is smaller if it is surrounded by larger circles, and larger if it is surrounded by smaller circles (Figure 5–2). Although the factors that contribute to this effect are not agreed on, it clearly involves a contribution of perceptual or-ganization, since moving context circles further from the center circle (thereby reducing grouping strength within the overall stimulus) reduces the effects of the illusion (Roberts et al. 2005). Using a computerized ver-sion of this task, we have shown that reduced illusion effects (i.e., *more accu-rate perception* of the size of the center circles) are found to a striking degree among schizophrenia patients upon short-term hospital admission, whereas illusion effects return to normal levels by hospital discharge, and the degree of veridical perception on admission is positively related to the level of dis-organized symptoms (Silverstein et al. 2013). The primary metric on this task, which involves the difference in accuracy between the condition in which context is helpful (i.e., enhances size discrimination) and the condi-tion in which context is misleading, can be generated in under 4 minutes. Therefore, this task would be convenient to use with a laptop computer in nearly any clinical or residential setting.

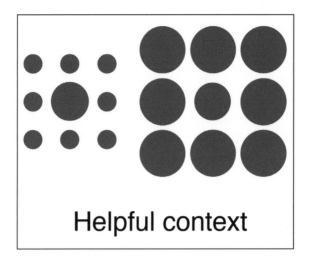

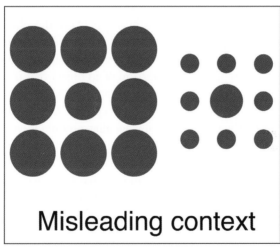

Figure 5–2. Sample stimuli from two conditions of the Ebbinghaus illusion task.

The participant's task is to indicate, on each trial (in which stimuli from only one of the three conditions is presented), which target circle is larger. In this illusion, the perceived size of a target circle is magnified when surrounded by smaller circles and reduced when surrounded by larger circles. In the examples in this figure, the target/inner circle on the left is 2% larger than the one on the right. Therefore, surrounding it with smaller circles amplifies the real difference (i.e., Helpful context), whereas surrounding it with larger circles reduces the chance of an accurate size judgment (Misleading context).

POSITIVE SYMPTOMS

A currently influential model of positive symptoms is that they reflect abnormalities in predictive coding, or are the consequences of mismatches between incoming sensory information and prior beliefs (Clark 2013; Corlett et al. 2007, 2009, 2016; Sterzer et al. 2018). For example, hallucinations can be conceptualized as being due to the excessive influence of prior sensory experiences and beliefs about what kinds of sensations are likely to be experienced. Delusions may involve a similar mechanism for conceptual information. This view is not without controversies, as data indicate both stronger and weaker influences of prior beliefs in people with psychotic disorders (Sterzer et al. 2018). Therefore, current work is focusing on issues such as potential differences in the manifestations of predictive coding alterations as a function of different sensory/cognitive domains, the level of processing at which mismatches may occur, and the distinction between symptom genesis and symptom maintenance (Sterzer et al. 2018).

In our work, we have shown what we believe to be clear examples of the reduced effects of priors, and the relationship between this phenomenon and psychotic symptoms. For example, depth inversion illusions (DIIs) provide conceptually clear and visually compelling examples of the effects of priors. In this class of illusion, a concave version of an object that is found only in convex form in nature (e.g., a face) is presented to the participants, and the typical response is to perceive the object as convex. That is, in determining what is perceived, the expectation of what a face should look like overrides the actual sensory information that is presented to the participant.

Studies from several laboratories since the 1980s have demonstrated that schizophrenia patients are less likely to perceive a concave face stimulus as convex (i.e., they are less susceptible to the illusion, and are perceiving the stimulus *more accurately* than control subjects) (Dima et al. 2009, 2010, 2011; Keane et al. 2013; Koethe et al. 2006; Schneider et al. 2002). It has also been demonstrated, using dynamic causal modeling of both fMRI and electroencephalography (EEG) data, that 1) the normal illusion effect with concave face stimuli is due to a suppressive effect on the output of visual regions (e.g., the lateral occipital complex, which is involved in generating full object representations) by a frontoparietal network which is presumably carrying high-level information related to expectations about what faces, in this case, should look like; and 2) in people with schizophrenia, there is a reduced suppressive effect from frontal and parietal activity and a relatively greater level of output from the lateral occipital complex (Dima et al. 2009, 2010). The reduced DII effect was not observed in people with bipolar disorder (Keane et al. 2016). Among people with schizophrenia, reduced illusion effects (i.e., more veridical perception of concave face stimuli) are related to a higher level of positive symptoms, less time since the last hospitalization ($r=0.41$; $P=0.02$), and a greater likelihood of being in a more structured (e.g., partial hospital) versus less structured (e.g., outpatient) treatment program ($r=0.51$; $P=0.004$) (Keane et al. 2013).

These cross-sectional data support the hypothesis that our DII task is tapping into a general (i.e., not just perceptual) predictive coding process in which dysregulation is related to both perception and the genesis of psychotic symptoms. This is consistent with the view that perception, like belief formation, is a dynamic process that involves the generation of predictions that are most likely to fit incoming sensory data (Clark 2013; Gregory 1997).

We are currently carrying out a longitudinal study—across the time frame of short-term inpatient unit admission to discharge—to determine the extent to which changes in DII task performance covary with and precede, co-occur, or follow changes in hallucinations and delusions. Importantly, while prior studies have used three-dimensional stimuli or computer-generated pseudoscopic images, we are currently piloting a completely portable setup in which participants view the stimuli via a virtual reality headset and the experiment is run on a smartphone, with data being saved via WiFi either on a second smartphone or a computer server (Figure 5–3). If our hypothesized results are obtained, this would establish the feasibility of DII assessment in many real-world settings.

NEGATIVE SYMPTOMS

A defining characteristic of negative symptoms of schizophrenia is a reduced level of reactivity. This is observed in facial affect, expressive gestures, anticipation of pleasure, volition, and rates of speech and movement (Marder and Galderisi 2017). Reduced reactivity can also be observed in electrophysiological recordings, in which attenuated amplitudes and longer latencies in waveforms are commonly reported (Erickson et al. 2016; Onitsuka et al. 2013). This has also been demonstrated in the form of smaller and delayed waveform activity in retinal responses, using electroretinography (ERG) (Balogh et al. 2008; Demmin et al. 2018; Hébert et al. 2015, 2020).

We recently demonstrated that in schizophrenia patients, reduced photoreceptor, bipolar cell, and ganglion cell activation to weak light stimuli was related to higher levels of negative symptoms (Demmin et al. 2018). This raises the possibility that these ERG findings reflect a reduced ability to represent change in the environment or to signal that a new relevant event has occurred, which is consistent with prior data on a relationship between reduced salience attribution and negative symptoms (Katthagen et al. 2016).

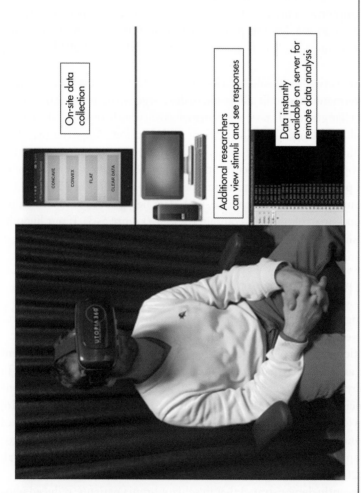

Figure 5–3. Aspects of the portable depth inversion illusion task.

Stimuli are perceived via a virtual reality headset into which the smartphone that generates the images is inserted. Stimulus presentation is controlled by the experimenter via a second smartphone. Data can be stored on that phone or sent via WiFi to a remote server in the experimenter's lab.

We then extended these findings by demonstrating that 1) while ERG amplitudes varied as a function of the salience of a food reward in healthy control subjects, this pattern of activation was significantly attenuated in people with schizophrenia; and 2) degree of changes in amplitudes as a function of reward salience was related to negative symptoms in patients, and to self-reports of hedonic capacity, in both groups (Demmin et al. 2020). These data suggest that ERG responses could serve as a proxy for reward sensitivity, which has consistently been found to be reduced in the disorder (Gold et al. 2012, 2013; Waltz et al. 2018) and the reduction of which is considered to be a prototypical negative symptom.

In both of our studies that demonstrated links between attenuated ERG response and negative symptoms, ERG was recorded using a portable hand-held device, stimuli presentation was brief (typically under 1 minute), and signals were detected using skin electrodes (i.e., with no direct eye contact) (Figure 5–4). This suggests that ERG testing could be used in clinic settings to detect levels of neural responsivity, which would be less time consuming and expensive compared with assessment using measures such as fMRI or EEG.

Consideration of Individual Differences and Trajectories

Nearly all studies of schizophrenia (and other conditions) explore patient-control differences by comparing group means, with little regard to how participants differ in their intra-individual variability during task performance. As a result, a great deal of information about trial-to-trial behavior is discarded. However, parameters related to such variation can provide unique information about brain and computational function (Li and Sikström 2002; Li et al. 2006; MacDonald et al. 2009; Nguyen et al. 2016; Northoff et al. 2018; Russell et al. 2006; Torres et al. 2016; Weinger et al. 2014), and excessive (trial-to-trial) intra-individual variability has been demonstrated in behavior and electrophysiological recordings in both schizophrenia patients and individuals considered to be at risk (Rentrop et al. 2010; Shin et al. 2015). We recently demonstrated that trial-to-trial variability/randomness (e.g., increased Fano factor) in target-directed movements relative to non-target-directed movements can reliably differentiate schizophrenia patients from control subjects (Nguyen et al. 2016). This same approach has characterized other conditions such as autism and Parkinson's disease (Torres et al. 2016). These data suggest that schizophrenia involves increased noise and randomness across processing domains, and that it is best conceptualized as more than a primarily cognitive (Kahn and Keefe 2013) disorder.

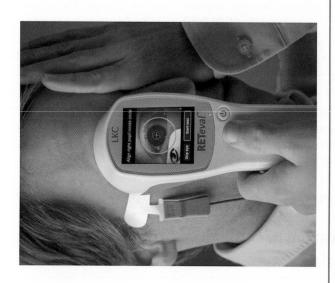

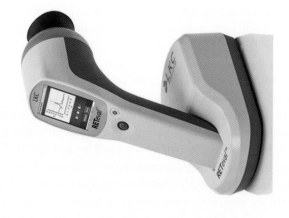

Figure 5–4. A portable electroretinography device, RET*eval* (LKC Technologies, Gaithersburg, Maryland), in use.

Right panel shows a portion of the skin electrode, which is placed 2 mm under the lower eyelid (and is visible in the device window).

Source.   Images courtesy of LKC Technologies.

A final important issue is that just as the identification of state markers will help to advance precision psychiatry, so will tasks that are sensitive to long-term illness trajectory. An excellent example of this is visual contrast sensitivity, in which unmedicated first-episode schizophrenia patients have been shown to have greater-than-normal sensitivity, whereas chronically ill patients—whether medicated or unmedicated—have consistently demonstrated reduced sensitivity (for review, see Silverstein 2016). Perceptual organization may also be enhanced in the high-risk state (Parnas et al. 2001), but is for the most part normal after a first episode of psychosis (Silverstein et al. 2006b) and then is often severely impaired after multiple episodes (Butler et al. 2008, 2012, 2013; Silverstein 2016; Silverstein and Keane 2011a; Silverstein et al. 2000, 2005, 2006a, 2009, 2012, 2015; Uhlhaas and Silverstein 2005a, 2005b). The latter finding may reflect both retinal and visual cortical atrophy or other forms of progressive structural pathology—features of poor outcome and chronic schizophrenia (Dorph-Petersen et al. 2007; Lee et al. 2013; Mitelman and Buchsbaum 2007; Onitsuka et al. 2006, 2007; Schultz et al. 2013; Selemon et al. 1995; Silverstein and Rosen 2015; Silverstein et al. 2018)—which could contribute to excessive noise, reduced contextual modulation, and broadened orientation tuning.

Conclusion and Future Directions

Methods from vision science have advanced our understanding of basic processing mechanisms that occur throughout the CNS, are altered in schizophrenia, and can be sensitively, rapidly and non-invasively quantified using psychophysical and psychophysiological tasks. Ongoing studies are extending past data on illness state sensitivity and stage sensitivity, and this will refine the predictive validity of these visual biomarkers. The modeling of both latent task parameters and indices of intra-individual variability can complement traditional mean-based data analysis techniques for characterizing and comparing patients, and for predicting important clinical outcomes. Ultimately, we expect that multivariate prediction, using brief measures that can be implemented in clinical and residential settings, will be necessary to fully achieve the vision of precision psychiatry.

KEY POINTS

- Despite many years of research investigating the psychological and biological underpinnings of mental illness, we still heavily rely on questionably valid diagnostic categories, and we have made little progress in improving the understanding, prevention, and treatment of psychiatric disorders.

- A proposed solution includes focusing on computational mechanisms that provide formal, rigorous, and precise quantitative metrics for mechanistic constructs.

- Experimental data and computational methods, such as those derived from vision science research as outlined in this chapter, can be utilized to create state-sensitive biomarkers for each of the three symptom clusters in schizophrenia (positive, negative, and disorganized).

- Methods from vision science have enhanced our understanding of basic cortical processing mechanisms that are maladaptive in schizophrenia. The modeling of latent task parameters and indices of intra-individual variability, in combination with traditional mean-based data analysis approaches, has the potential to improve prediction of clinical outcomes.

References

Adams RA, Huys QJ, Roiser JP: Computational psychiatry: towards a mathematically informed understanding of mental illness. J Neurol Neurosurg Psychiatry 87(1):53–63, 2016 26157034

Balogh Z, Benedek G, Kéri S: Retinal dysfunctions in schizophrenia. Prog Neuropsychopharmacol Biol Psychiatry 32(1):297–300, 2008 17889979

Bennett D, Silverstein SM, Niv Y: The two cultures of computational psychiatry. JAMA Psychiatry 76(6):563–564, 2019 31017638

Butler PD, Silverstein SM, Dakin SC: Visual perception and its impairment in schizophrenia. Biol Psychiatry 64(1):40–47, 2008 18549875

Butler PD, Chen Y, Ford JM, et al: Perceptual measurement in schizophrenia: promising electrophysiology and neuroimaging paradigms from CNTRICS. Schizophr Bull 38(1):81–91, 2012 21890745

Butler PD, Abeles IY, Silverstein SM, et al: An event-related potential examination of contour integration deficits in schizophrenia. Front Psychol 4:132, 2013 23519476

Centers for Disease Control and Prevention: Vital signs: overdoses of prescription opioid pain relievers—United States, 1999–2008. MMWR Morb Mortal Wkly Rep 60(43):1487–1492, 2011 22048730

Clark A: Whatever next? Predictive brains, situated agents, and the future of cognitive science. Behav Brain Sci 36(3):181–204, 2013 23663408

Corlett PR, Honey GD, Fletcher PC: From prediction error to psychosis: ketamine as a pharmacological model of delusions. J Psychopharmacol 21(3):238–252, 2007 17591652

Corlett PR, Frith CD, Fletcher PC: From drugs to deprivation: a Bayesian framework for understanding models of psychosis. Psychopharmacology (Berl) 206(4):515–530, 2009 19475401

Corlett PR, Honey GD, Fletcher PC: Prediction error, ketamine and psychosis: an updated model. J Psychopharmacol 30(11):1145–1155, 2016 27226342

Cuthbert BN, Insel TR: Toward the future of psychiatric diagnosis: the seven pillars of RDoC. BMC Med 11:126, 2013 23672542

Demmin DL, Davis Q, Roché M, Silverstein SM: Electroretinographic anomalies in schizophrenia. J Abnorm Psychol 127(4):417–428, 2018 29745706

Demmin DL, Mote J, Beaudette DM, et al: Retinal functioning and reward processing in schizophrenia. Schizophr Res 219:25–33, 2020 31280976

Dima D, Roiser JP, Dietrich DE, et al: Understanding why patients with schizophrenia do not perceive the hollow-mask illusion using dynamic causal modelling. Neuroimage 46(4):1180–1186, 2009 19327402

Dima D, Dietrich DE, Dillo W, et al: Impaired top-down processes in schizophrenia: a DCM study of ERPs. Neuroimage 52(3):824–832, 2010 20056155

Dima D, Dillo W, Bonnemann C, et al: Reduced P300 and P600 amplitude in the hollow-mask illusion in patients with schizophrenia. Psychiatry Res 191(2):145–151, 2011 21236647

Dorph-Petersen KA, Pierri JN, Wu Q, et al: Primary visual cortex volume and total neuron number are reduced in schizophrenia. J Comp Neurol 501(2):290–301, 2007 17226750

Erickson MA, Ruffle A, Gold JM: A meta-analysis of mismatch negativity in schizophrenia: from clinical risk to disease specificity and progression. Biol Psychiatry 79(12):980–987, 2016 26444073

Gold JM, Waltz JA, Matveeva TM, et al: Negative symptoms and the failure to represent the expected reward value of actions: behavioral and computational modeling evidence. Arch Gen Psychiatry 69(2):129–138, 2012 22310503

Gold JM, Strauss GP, Waltz JA, et al: Negative symptoms of schizophrenia are associated with abnormal effort-cost computations. Biol Psychiatry 74(2):130–136, 2013 23394903

Gregory RL: Eye and Brain: The Psychology of Seeing, 5th Edition. Princeton, NJ, Princeton University Press, 1997

Hébert M, Mérette C, Paccalet T, et al: Light evoked potentials measured by electroretinogram may tap into the neurodevelopmental roots of schizophrenia. Schizophr Res 162(1–3):294–295, 2015 25579051

Hébert M, Mérette C, Gagné AM, et al: The electroretinogram may differentiate schizophrenia from bipolar disorder. Biol Psychiatry 87(3):263–270, 2020 31443935

Hedegaard H, Curtin SC, Warner M: Suicide rates in the United States continue to increase. NHCS Data Brief (309):1–8, 2018 30312151

Hull CL: Principles of Behavior. New York, Appleton-Century, 1943

Insel TR: Rethinking schizophrenia. Nature 468(7321):187–193, 2010 21068826

Kahn RS, Keefe RS: Schizophrenia is a cognitive illness: time for a change in focus. JAMA Psychiatry 70(10):1107–1112, 2013 23925787

Katthagen T, Dammering F, Kathmann N, et al: Validating the construct of aberrant salience in schizophrenia—behavioral evidence for an automatic process. Schizophr Res Cogn 6:22–27, 2016 28740821

Kay JW, Phillips WA: Coherent Infomax as a computational goal for neural systems. Bull Math Biol 73(2):344–372, 2011 20821064

Kay J, Phillips W, Aru J, et al: A Bayesian decomposition of BAC firing as a mechanisms for apical amplification in neocortical pyramidal neurons. bioRxiv April 15, 2019. Available at: www.biorxiv.org/content/10.1101/604066v1. Accessed February 15, 2021.

Keane BP, Silverstein SM, Wang Y, et al: Reduced depth inversion illusions in schizophrenia are state-specific and occur for multiple object types and viewing conditions. J Abnorm Psychol 122(2):506–512, 2013 23713504

Keane BP, Silverstein SM, Wang Y, et al: Seeing more clearly through psychosis: depth inversion illusions are normal in bipolar disorder but reduced in schizophrenia. Schizophr Res 176(2–3):485–492, 2016 27344363

Knight R: Converging models of cognitive deficits in schizophrenia, in Nebraska Symposium on Motivation: Theories of Schizophrenia and Psychosis, Vol 31. Edited by Spaulding W, Coles J. Lincoln, University of Nebraska Press, 1984, pp 93–156

Knight RA: Specifying cognitive deficiencies in poor premorbid schizophrenics, in Progress in Experimental Psychology and Psychopathology Research, Vol 15. Edited by Walker EF, Dworkin R, Cornblatt B. New York, Springer, 1992, pp 252–289

Knight RA, Silverstein SM: The role of cognitive psychology in guiding research on cognitive deficits in schizophrenia, in Origins and Development of Schizophrenia: Advances in Experimental Psychopathology. Edited by Lenzenweger M, Dworkin RH. Washington, DC, American Psychological Association, 1998, pp 247–295

Knight RA, Silverstein SM: A process-oriented approach for averting confounds resulting from general performance deficiencies in schizophrenia. J Abnorm Psychol 110(1):15–30, 2001 11261389

Koethe D, Gerth CW, Neatby MA, et al: Disturbances of visual information processing in early states of psychosis and experimental delta-9-tetrahydrocannabinol altered states of consciousness. Schizophr Res 88(1–3):142–150, 2006 17005373

Lee WW, Tajunisah I, Sharmilla K, et al: Retinal nerve fiber layer structure abnormalities in schizophrenia and its relationship to disease state: evidence from optical coherence tomography. Invest Ophthalmol Vis Sci 54(12):7785–7792, 2013 24135757

Li SC, Sikström S: Integrative neurocomputational perspectives on cognitive aging, neuromodulation, and representation. Neurosci Biobehav Rev 26(7):795–808, 2002 12470691

Li SC, von Oertzen T, Lindenberger U: A neurocomputational model of stochastic resonance and aging. Neurocomputing 69(13–15):1553–1560, 2006

MacDonald SW, Li SC, Bäckman L: Neural underpinnings of within-person variability in cognitive functioning. Psychol Aging 24(4):792–808, 2009 20025396

Marder SR, Galderisi S: The current conceptualization of negative symptoms in schizophrenia. World Psychiatry 16(1):14–24, 2017 28127915

Mitelman SA, Buchsbaum MS: Very poor outcome schizophrenia: clinical and neuroimaging aspects. Int Rev Psychiatry 19(4):345–357, 2007 17671868

Mojtabai R: National trends in mental health disability, 1997–2009. Am J Public Health 101(11):2156–2163, 2011 21940913

Nguyen J, Majmudar U, Papathomas TV, et al: Schizophrenia: the micro-movements perspective. Neuropsychologia 85:310–326, 2016 26951932

Northoff G, Magioncalda P, Martino M, et al: Too fast or too slow? Time and neuronal variability in bipolar disorder—a combined theoretical and empirical investigation. Schizophr Bull 44(1):54–64, 2018 28525601

Nuechterlein KH, Dawson ME: A heuristic vulnerability/stress model of schizophrenic episodes. Schizophr Bull 10(2):300–312, 1984a 6729414

Nuechterlein KH, Dawson ME: Information processing and attentional functioning in the developmental course of schizophrenic disorders. Schizophr Bull 10(2):160–203, 1984b 6729409

Nuechterlein KH, Edell WS, Norris M, et al: Attentional vulnerability indicators, thought disorder, and negative symptoms. Schizophr Bull 12(3):408–426, 1986 3764359

Nuechterlein KH, Dawson ME, Green MF: Information-processing abnormalities as neuropsychological vulnerability indicators for schizophrenia. Acta Psychiatr Scand Suppl 384:71–79, 1994 7879647

Onitsuka T, Niznikiewicz MA, Spencer KM, et al: Functional and structural deficits in brain regions subserving face perception in schizophrenia. Am J Psychiatry 163(3):455–462, 2006 16513867

Onitsuka T, McCarley RW, Kuroki N, et al: Occipital lobe gray matter volume in male patients with chronic schizophrenia: a quantitative MRI study. Schizophr Res 92(1–3):197–206, 2007 17350226

Onitsuka T, Oribe N, Nakamura I, et al: Review of neurophysiological findings in patients with schizophrenia. Psychiatry Clin Neurosci 67(7):461–470, 2013 24102977

Parnas J, Vianin P, Saebye D, et al: Visual binding abilities in the initial and advanced stages of schizophrenia. Acta Psychiatr Scand 103(3):171–180, 2001 11240573

Paul GL: Strategy of outcome research in psychotherapy. J Consult Psychol 31(2):109–118, 1967 5342732

Payne RB: An extension of Hullian theory to response decrements resulting from drugs. J Exp Psychol 55(4):342–346, 1958 13539315

Phillips WA: Cognitive functions of intracellular mechanisms for contextual amplification. Brain Cogn 112:39–53, 2017 26428863

Phillips WA, Silverstein SM: Convergence of biological and psychological perspectives on cognitive coordination in schizophrenia. Behav Brain Sci 26(1):65–82, discussion 82–137, 2003 14598440

Phillips WA, Silverstein SM: The coherent organization of mental life depends on mechanisms for context-sensitive gain-control that are impaired in schizophrenia. Front Psychol 4:307, 2013 23755035

Phillips WA, Singer W: In search of common foundations for cortical computation. Behav Brain Sci 20(4):657–683, discussion 683–722, 1997 10097008

Phillips WA, Floreano D, Kay J: Contextually guided unsupervised learning using local multivariate binary processors. Neural Netw 11(1):117–140, 1998 12662852

Phillips WA, Clark A, Silverstein SM: On the functions, mechanisms, and malfunctions of intracortical contextual modulation. Neurosci Biobehav Rev 52:1–20, 2015 25721105

Phillips WA, Larkum ME, Harley CW: The effects of arousal on apical amplification and conscious state. Neurosci Conscious 2016(1):niw015, 2016 29877512

Place EJ, Gilmore GC: Perceptual organization in schizophrenia. J Abnorm Psychol 89(3):409–418, 1980 7410708

Rentrop M, Rodewald K, Roth A, et al: Intra-individual variability in high-functioning patients with schizophrenia. Psychiatry Res 178(1):27–32, 2010 20447695

Roberts B, Harris MG, Yates TA: The roles of inducer size and distance in the Ebbinghaus illusion (Titchener circles). Perception 34(7):847–856, 2005 16124270

Russell VA, Oades RD, Tannock R, et al: Response variability in attention-deficit/hyperactivity disorder: a neuronal and glial energetics hypothesis. Behav Brain Funct 2:30, 2006 16925830

Schneider U, Borsutzky M, Seifert J, et al: Reduced binocular depth inversion in schizophrenic patients. Schizophr Res 53(1–2):101–108, 2002 11728843

Schultz CC, Wagner G, Koch K, et al: The visual cortex in schizophrenia: alterations of gyrification rather than cortical thickness—a combined cortical shape analysis. Brain Struct Funct 218(1):51–58, 2013 22200883

Selemon LD, Rajkowska G, Goldman-Rakic PS: Abnormally high neuronal density in the schizophrenic cortex. A morphometric analysis of prefrontal area 9 and occipital area 17. Arch Gen Psychiatry 52(10):805–818, discussion 819–820, 1995 7575100

Shin KS, Kim JS, Kim SN, et al: Intraindividual neurophysiological variability in ultra-high-risk for psychosis and schizophrenia patients: single-trial analysis. NPJ Schizophr 1:15031, 2015 27336039

Silverstein SM: Measuring specific, rather than generalized, cognitive deficits and maximizing between-group effect size in studies of cognition and cognitive change. Schizophr Bull 34(4):645–655, 2008 18468987

Silverstein SM: Visual perception disturbances in schizophrenia: a unified model. Nebr Symp Motiv 63:77–132, 2016 27627825

Silverstein SM, Keane BP: Perceptual organization impairment in schizophrenia and associated brain mechanisms: review of research from 2005 to 2010. Schizophr Bull 37(4):690–699, 2011a 21700589

Silverstein SM, Keane BP: Vision science and schizophrenia research: toward a review of the disorder. Editors' introduction to special section. Schizophr Bull 37(4):681–689, 2011b 21700588

Silverstein SM, Rosen R: Schizophrenia and the eye. Schizophr Res Cogn 2(2):46–55, 2015 26345525

Silverstein SM, Thompson JL: A vision science perspective on schizophrenia. Schizophr Res Cogn 2(2):39–41, 2015 26345386

Silverstein SM, Uhlhaas PJ: Gestalt psychology: the forgotten paradigm in abnormal psychology. Am J Psychol 117(2):259–277, 2004 15209373

Silverstein SM, Knight RA, Schwarzkopf SB, et al: Stimulus configuration and context effects in perceptual organization in schizophrenia. J Abnorm Psychol 105(3):410–420, 1996 8772011

Silverstein SM, Kovács I, Corry R, et al: Perceptual organization, the disorganization syndrome, and context processing in chronic schizophrenia. Schizophr Res 43(1):11–20, 2000 10828411

Silverstein SM, Bakshi S, Nuernberger S, et al: Effects of stimulus structure and target-distracter similarity on the development of visual memory representations in schizophrenia. Cogn Neuropsychiatry 10(3):215–229, 2005 16571460

Silverstein SM, Hatashita-Wong M, Schenkel LS, et al: Reduced top-down influences in contour detection in schizophrenia. Cogn Neuropsychiatry 11(2):112–132, 2006a 16537237

Silverstein SM, Uhlhaas PJ, Essex B, et al: Perceptual organization in first episode schizophrenia and ultra-high-risk states. Schizophr Res 83(1):41–52, 2006b 16497484

Silverstein SM, Berten S, Essex B, et al: An fMRI examination of visual integration in schizophrenia. J Integr Neurosci 8(2):175–202, 2009 19618486

Silverstein SM, Keane BP, Barch DM, et al: Optimization and validation of a visual integration test for schizophrenia research. Schizophr Bull 38(1):125–134, 2012 22021658

Silverstein SM, Harms MP, Carter CS, et al: Cortical contributions to impaired contour integration in schizophrenia. Neuropsychologia 75:469–480, 2015 26160288

Silverstein SM, Keane BP, Wang Y, et al: Effects of short-term inpatient treatment on sensitivity to a size contrast illusion in first-episode psychosis and multiple-episode schizophrenia. Front Psychol 4:466, 2013 23898311

Silverstein SM, Wibral M, Phillips WA: Implications of information theory for computational modeling of schizophrenia. Comput Psychiatr 1:82–101, 2017 29601053

Silverstein SM, Paterno D, Cherneski L, et al: Optical coherence tomography indices of structural retinal pathology in schizophrenia. Psychol Med 48(12):2023–2033, 2018 29233210

Sterzer P, Adams RA, Fletcher P, et al: The predictive coding account of psychosis. Biol Psychiatry 84(9):634–643, 2018 30007575

Teufel C, Fletcher PC: The promises and pitfalls of applying computational models to neurological and psychiatric disorders. Brain 139(Pt 10):2600–2608, 2016 27543973

Torres EB, Isenhower RW, Nguyen J, et al: Toward precision psychiatry: statistical platform for the personalized characterization of natural behaviors. Front Neurol 7:8, 2016 26869988

Uhlhaas PJ, Mishara AL: Perceptual anomalies in schizophrenia: integrating phenomenology and cognitive neuroscience. Schizophr Bull 33(1):142–156, 2007 17118973

Uhlhaas PJ, Silverstein SM: Perceptual organization in schizophrenia spectrum disorders: empirical research and theoretical implications. Psychol Bull 131(4):618–632, 2005a 16060805

Uhlhaas PJ, Silverstein SM: Phenomenology, biology, and specificity of dysfunctions in gestalt perception in schizophrenia. Gestalt Theory 27:57–69, 2005b

Uhlhaas PJ, Phillips WA, Mitchell G, Silverstein SM: Perceptual grouping in disorganized schizophrenia. Psychiatry Res 145(2–3):105–117, 2006 17081620

Waltz JA, Xu Z, Brown EC, et al: Motivational deficits in schizophrenia are associated with reduced differentiation between gain and loss-avoidance feedback in the striatum. Biol Psychiatry Cogn Neurosci Neuroimaging 3(3):239–247, 2018 29486865

Wang XJ, Krystal JH: Computational psychiatry. Neuron 84(3):638–654, 2014 25442941

Weinger PM, Zemon V, Soorya L, et al: Low-contrast response deficits and increased neural noise in children with autism spectrum disorder. Neuropsychologia 63:10–18, 2014 25107679

Wibral M, Priesemann V, Kay JW, et al: Partial information decomposition as a unified approach to the specification of neural goal functions. Brain Cogn 112:25–38, 2017 26475739

Wiener N: Cybernetics. New York, Wiley, 1948

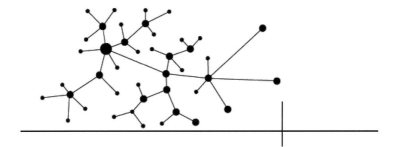

PART 3

BLOOD **M**ARKERS

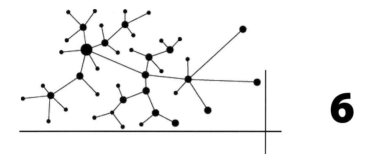

6

Using Inflammatory Biomarkers to Identify and Treat Transdiagnostic Subtypes in Psychiatric Disorders

Carolina Medeiros Da Frota Ribeiro, M.D.
Jennifer C. Felger, Ph.D.
Michael T. Treadway, Ph.D.
David R. Goldsmith, M.D.
Ebrahim Haroon, M.D.
Andrew H. Miller, M.D.

History

A large and developing literature has identified a link between chronic activation of the inflammatory response and a variety of psychiatric disorders (Miller and Raison 2016). The best-studied disorder in this regard is depression, in which reliable increases in markers of inflammation, including inflammatory cytokines, acute-phase reactants, chemokines, and cellular adhesion molecules, have been described (Miller and Raison 2016). In meta-analyses of these studies, the inflammatory cytokines tumor necrosis factor (TNF), interleukin (IL)-1β and IL-6, and the acute-phase reactant C-reactive protein (CRP) in the peripheral blood appear to be the most reproducibly elevated (Dowlati et al. 2010; Goldsmith et al. 2016; Howren et al. 2009; Osimo et al. 2019). Postmortem samples from depressed individuals who died from suicide also demonstrate evidence of increased inflammation in the brain, including activation of inflammatory signaling molecules in brain parenchyma (Pandey 2017), increased microglial density and priming (Steiner et al. 2008; Torres-Platas et al. 2014), trafficking of immune cells to the brain as reflected by perivascular macrophages (Torres-Platas et al. 2014), and decreased molecules associated with blood-brain barrier integrity in key brain regions related to reward processing (Menard et al. 2017). Interestingly, immune activation has also been described in multiple other psychiatric disorders, including bipolar disorder, anxiety disorders, PTSD, and psychotic disorders such as schizophrenia (Goldsmith et al. 2016; Michopoulos et al. 2017). It should be noted, however, that none of these disorders are considered inflammatory disorders, because in each case only a subgroup of individuals exhibit markers of increased inflammation. For example, in depression approximately 25%–30% of individuals exhibit increased inflammation, depending on the sample and relevant risk factors (Osimo et al. 2019).

Many factors have been associated with the risk for increased inflammation in psychiatric disease. These include obesity (and the metabolic syndrome) (Shelton et al. 2015), childhood maltreatment (Danese et al. 2007), treatment resistance (Haroon et al. 2018b; Strawbridge et al. 2015), dysbiosis (e.g., "leaky gut" and alterations in the gut microbiome) (Dinan and Cryan 2017), and medical disorders, including cardiovascular disease, diabetes, cancer, and autoimmune and inflammatory disorders, and their treatments (Xiao et al. 2017).

Taken together, these data suggest that increased inflammation represents a transdiagnostic pathology that may contribute to specific symptom clusters in subgroups of patients with psychiatric and other disorders. With this in mind, the possibility exists that these subgroups of individuals can be identified by relevant inflammatory markers and may ultimately warrant targeted treatments that address inflammation itself or its downstream effects on the brain.

Current Knowledge and Approaches

A great deal of information has been amassed on how inflammation can target the brain to influence behavior. In vitro and in vivo studies have elucidated the effects of inflammation on neurotransmitter systems as well as neural plasticity, including effects on growth factors and neurogenesis (Miller and Raison 2016). In addition, data on the neurocircuits affected by inflammation have been derived from studies that involve examination of the brain using neuroimaging strategies after the administration of inflammatory stimuli (Miller and Raison 2016). Neuroimaging studies have relied on individuals chronically exposed to an inflammatory stimulus (almost exclusively patients administered interferon [IFN]–α for infectious diseases or cancer) or healthy volunteers exposed acutely to either typhoid vaccination or endotoxin. Few studies have examined the relationship between endogenous inflammation and functional neuroimaging parameters in patients with psychiatric disorders.

INFLAMMATION TARGETS NEUROTRANSMITTER SYSTEMS

Cell culture and laboratory animal and human studies demonstrate that inflammation has effects on the synthesis, release, and reuptake of neurotransmitters, including monoamines and glutamate (Miller and Raison 2016). For example, inflammatory cytokines have been shown to decrease tetrahydrobiopterin (BH4), an enzyme cofactor that supports the activity of all the major enzymes that are responsible for the synthesis of serotonin (5-HT), norepinephrine (NE), and dopamine (DA) (Haroon et al. 2012). In addition to effects on synthesis, chronic administration of the inflammatory cytokine IFN-α reduces DA release in the basal ganglia (especially striatum) as measured by in vivo microdialysis in nonhuman primates and as reflected by reduced DA turnover in humans using PET neuroimaging (Capuron et al. 2012; Felger et al. 2013). Interestingly, administration of levodopa, the immediate precursor of DA, via reverse microdialysis restores DA release in the striatum of IFN-α-treated nonhuman primates, supporting the notion that effects of inflammation on DA synthesis may be involved (Felger et al. 2015). Data also indicate that the inflammatory cytokines TNF and IL-1β increase the expression and activity of 5-HT and NE reuptake pumps through activation of p38 mitogen activated protein kinase (MAPK) (Zhu et al. 2005). Indeed, lipopolysaccharide-induced depressive-like behavior is associated with increased expression of 5-HT transporters as well as 5-HT clearance, which is reversible by a p38 MAPK antagonist (Zhu et al. 2010). Similar effects on DA reuptake by activation of MAPK pathways have been described (Morón et al. 2003).

Inflammation and inflammatory mediators, including reactive nitrogen and oxygen species, also affect astrocytes, leading to increased release and decreased reuptake of glutamate through effects on glutamate transporters as well as exchange pumps involved in the synthesis of the antioxidant glutathione (Haroon et al. 2017). Excessive glutamate in turn can spill over into the extrasynaptic space, binding to extrasynaptic glutamate (*N*-methyl-D-aspartate [NMDA]) receptors that, unlike intrasynaptic NMDA receptors, lead to decreased production of growth factors such as brain-derived neurotrophic factor (BDNF) and ultimately neurotoxicity (Haroon et al. 2017). In addition, inflammatory cytokines can lead to the activation of the enzyme indoleamine 2,3-dioxygenase (IDO), which converts tryptophan to kynurenine, which is then transported to the brain and converted to quinolinic acid and kynurenic acid (Savitz 2020). Quinolinic acid stimulates glutamate release and blocks reuptake while activating extrasynaptic NMDA receptors. Kynurenic acid leads to reduced extracellular DA through allosteric effects on the NMDA receptor and ultimately decreased glutamate-stimulated DA release (Savitz 2020; Wu et al. 2007). Finally, inflammatory cytokines such as IL-1β can have direct effects on growth factor production and neurogenesis, which in turn has been associated with depressive-like behavior in laboratory animals (Barrientos et al. 2003; Koo and Duman 2008).

INFLAMMATION TARGETS SPECIFIC NEUROCIRCUITS

Evolutionary theories regarding the relationship between inflammation and behavior posit that the increased immunometabolic demands of infection and wounding lead to a reallocation of energy resources away from exploratory behavior to the immune system, while promoting a posture of hypervigilance and arousal to protect against future attack (Miller et al. 2013; Treadway et al. 2019). Consistent with these notions, effects of inflammation on neurocircuits in the brain have focused on circuits involved in motivation and motor activity as well as anxiety, arousal, and alarm.

Reward Networks

One of the most reproducible findings of the impact of inflammation on neurocircuits in the brain is the inhibitory effects of inflammatory stimuli on the activation of the DA-rich ventral striatum (Felger and Treadway 2017; Treadway et al. 2019). These results are consistent with the reliable effects of inflammation on DA in the striatum as described above. At least three different immune stimuli, including chronic administration of IFN-α and acute administration of endotoxin and typhoid vaccination, reduce ventral striatal activation in response to reward in association with behavioral changes including anhedonia, a core symptom of depression (Capuron et al. 2012; Eisenberger et al. 2010; Harrison et al. 2016). These effects are consistent with studies in depressed patients demonstrating that increased CRP as an index of inflammation (see "Clinical Illustrations") is related to decreased connectivity within reward circuitry, including decreased connectivity between ventral striatum and ventromedial prefrontal cortex in association with symptoms of anhedonia (Felger et al. 2016). In addition, decreased connectivity between dorsal striatum and cortical regions is associated with decreased psychomotor speed (Felger et al. 2016). Increased CRP in depressed patients has also been associated with increased basal ganglia glutamate in association with decreased local and regional homogeneity (a measure of coherence of neuronal activity) in brain networks associated with motivation and motor activity (Haroon et al. 2018a).

These effects of inflammation on reward circuitry following administration of inflammatory stimuli in association with decreases in motivated behavior have also been observed in laboratory animal models, in which it is clear that while the capacity for pleasure remains intact, the amount of effort expenditure for reward is reduced (Felger et al. 2013; Treadway et al. 2019; Vichaya et al. 2014; Yohn et al. 2016a). These findings, in conjunction with findings from human studies, indicate that inflammation has relatively specific effects on positive valence systems related to reward processing as outlined in the Research Domain Criteria (RDoC) developed by the National Institute of Mental Health. Inflammation effects on the dorsal striatum and substantia nigra affecting motor speed relate to negative valence systems involving psychomotor slowing/retardation. Finally, recent work suggests there may be sex differences in the ventral striatal response to inflammatory stimuli, with females being more sensitive to these effects than males (Moieni et al. 2019).

Networks Involved in Anxiety, Arousal, and Alarm

Several studies have identified inflammation-induced activation of neural networks involving the dorsal anterior cingulate cortex, insula, hippocampus, and amygdala in association with increased sensitivity to environmental stimuli, including social rejection; task-related errors; and emotional facial expressions (Capuron et al. 2005; Inagaki et al. 2012; Slavich et al. 2010). These findings have been complemented by one depression study in which increased inflammation as indexed by CRP was related to decreased functional connectivity between the ventromedial prefrontal cortex and amygdala in association with symptoms of anxiety, especially in depressed patients with comorbid anxiety disorders and PTSD (Mehta et al. 2018).

Clinical Illustrations

INFLAMMATORY MARKERS AS PREDICTORS OF TREATMENT RESPONSE TO ANTIDEPRESSANT AND ANTI-INFLAMMATORY MEDICATIONS

A rich literature has examined the relationship between inflammatory biomarkers and the response to antidepressant treatment in patients with depression (Table 6–1). However, few studies have examined this relationship in other psychiatric disorders. In a meta-analysis of the literature in depression, data were extracted from 35 studies that examined inflammatory biomarkers before and after treatment in depressed patients (Strawbridge et al. 2015). Sufficient data were available to evaluate CRP, TNF and IL-6, and the treatments were almost exclusively pharmacological in nature, primarily conventional antidepressant medications. Although none of the inflammatory biomarkers alone predicted treatment outcome, when a composite measure of inflammation was used (including CRP, TNF, IL-6 plus IL-1α/β and IFN-α/β), increased inflammation was found to be a significant predictor of treatment nonresponse in ambulatory depressed patients and in studies with a higher quality rating. In addition, persistent elevations in TNF were associated with prospectively determined treatment nonresponse. This latter finding is consistent with recent reports that patients with treatment-resistant depression exhibit increased markers of inflammation, including CRP, TNF, soluble TNF receptor 2, and IL-6 (Chamberlain et al. 2019; Haroon et al. 2018b).

In contrast to inflammation predicting a poor response to conventional antidepressants, there is some evidence that inflammatory biomarkers may predict a positive response to ketamine and electroconvulsive therapy (ECT). Indeed, higher baseline concentrations of IL-6 were found to be associated with lower end-of-treatment depressive symptom severity scores for patients treated with ECT (Kruse et al. 2018). In patients receiving ketamine, higher IL-6 was significantly associated with treatment response (50% reduction in depressive symptoms) (Yang et al. 2015). These latter data are consistent with findings indicating that increased body mass index and lower plasma adiponectin (both associated with an inflammatory metabolic state) predict response to ketamine (Machado-Vieira et al. 2017). In addition, these findings are supported by laboratory animal studies demonstrating that CRP and TNF predict an antidepressant response to ketamine in an animal model of treatment-resistant depression (Walker et al. 2015).

Based on the data described above, the evidence suggests that depressed patients with increased inflammatory biomarkers may be less likely to respond to conventional antidepressant medications, and preliminary evidence suggests that these patients may respond better to ECT or ketamine. Nevertheless, emerging data suggest that inflammatory biomarkers, especially CRP, may be able to identify subpopulations of depressed patients that differentially respond to specific classes of conventional antidepressant medications. At least three clinical trials have addressed this possibility (Jha et al. 2017; Uher et al. 2014; Zhang et al. 2019) (see Table 6–1). In all three, post hoc analyses indicated that depressed patients with a CRP ≥1 mg/L demonstrated a significantly worse response to selective serotonin reuptake inhibitors (SSRIs) or

TABLE 6–1. Representative examples of inflammatory biomarkers predicting treatment response[a]

Biomarker	Treatment	Finding	Reference
CRP	SSRI, SSRI+nortriptyline	Baseline CRP ≥1 mg/L predicted poor response to SSRI.	Uher et al. 2014
CRP	SSRI, SNRI+bupropion	Baseline CRP ≥1 mg/L predicted poor response to SSRI.	Jha et al. 2017
CRP	SSRI, SNRI	CRP ≥1 mg/L predicted poor response to SSRI and SNRI.	Zhang et al. 2019
CRP	Infliximab	CRP >5 mg/L predicted lower depression severity at study endpoint.	Raison et al. 2013
CRP	Sirukumab	Higher baseline CRP was associated with lower anhedonia scores at study endpoint.	Salvadore et al. 2018
IL-6	Minocycline	Higher baseline IL-6 was associated with greater response at study endpoint.	Savitz et al. 2018
IL-6	ECT	Higher baseline IL-6 was associated with lower depression severity at study endpoint.	Kruse et al. 2018
IL-6	Ketamine	Baseline IL-6 was higher in treatment responders.	Yang et al. 2015
MIF and IL-1β mRNA	SSRI, nortriptyline	Increased baseline MIF and IL-1β predicted treatment nonresponse.	Cattaneo et al. 2016

Note. CRP=C-reactive protein; ECT=electroconvulsive therapy; IL=interleukin; MIF=macrophage inhibitory factor; SSRI=selective serotonin reuptake inhibitor; SNRI=serotonin-norepinephrine reuptake inhibitor.
[a]See also Strawbridge et al. 2015 and Liu et al. 2020 for meta-analyses of this literature.

serotonin-norepinephrine reuptake inhibitors (SNRIs) compared with individuals with a CRP <1 mg/L. Interestingly, in one of these trials, bupropion (plus escitalopram) (Jha et al. 2017), and in another trial, nortriptyline (Uher et al. 2014), showed a superior response compared with the SSRI escitalopram alone in patients with a CRP ≥1 mg/L. For example, in the trial with bupropion, depressed patients with a CRP≥1 mg/L who received escitalopram alone had a 29.7% remission rate, compared with a remission rate of 57.1% in escitalopram-treated patients with a CRP <1 mg/L (Jha et al. 2017). In contrast, in patients with a CRP ≥1 mg/L who received escitalopram plus bupropion, the remission rate was 51.4%, similar to the remission rate in those with low inflammation who received escitalopram alone. A follow-up analysis of these data further indicated that the effect of inflammation on treatment response to escitalopram and escitalopram plus bupropion may be most apparent in females versus males (Jha et al. 2019). Taken together, these data suggest that inflammatory biomarkers such as CRP may help guide treatment selection, indicating that patients with higher inflammation may respond less well to SSRIs and SNRIs, and may preferentially respond to drugs such as bupropion or nortriptyline.

Bupropion (and potentially nortriptyline) might have increased efficacy in depressed patients who have increased inflammation, in part related to its impact on DA as described earlier. In human studies using displacement of radiolabeled DA transporter (DAT) ligands, bupropion (300 mg/day) was shown to occupy the DAT by as much as 25% (Argyelán et al. 2005; Learned-Coughlin et al. 2003). Of note, a study of nonhuman primates administered an acute intravenous bolus of 5 mg/kg of bupropion found ~85% DAT occupancy in the striatum (Eriksson et al. 2011). In addition, several studies in rodents have demonstrated that bupropion increases extracellular DA in the striatum and nucleus accumbens in a dose- and time-dependent manner (Nomikos et al. 1992). Moreover, intraperitoneal administration of bupropion has been shown to increase effort-based motivation for food rewards in association with pre- and postsynaptic markers of increased DA transmission (Randall et al. 2014). Finally, bupropion (but not fluoxetine or desipramine) was shown to reverse the inhibitory effects on effort-based motivation by tetrabenazine, a drug that depletes accumbens DA (Yohn et al. 2016b). It should be noted that although nortriptyline has also exhibited efficacy in depressed patients with high inflammation, this may be related to reported effects of nortriptyline-mediated NE transporter inhibition on increasing DA release in frontal cortex (Valentini et al. 2004). Moreover, in a systematic review of conventional antidepressants for smoking cessation, only bupropion and nortriptyline exhibited significant efficacy (Hughes et al. 2014), suggesting some overlap of their effects on reward-related pathways (likely involving DA).

CRP AS A VIABLE BIOMARKER OF INFLAMMATION AND SUBGROUPING PSYCHIATRIC PATIENTS

A number of biomarkers for inflammation have been proposed for evaluating the role of chronic inflammation in a myriad of disorders, including cardiovascular disease, metabolic disorders, and cancer. Consensus recommendations from a 2017 National Institutes of Health workshop on chronic inflammation biomarkers in disease development and prevention suggested that several inflammatory factors, including CRP, TNF, and IL-6, may be part of a screening panel for chronic inflammation (Liu et al. 2017). As noted previously, all of these inflammatory markers have been found to be reliably elevated in depression and other psychiatric disorders.

These recommendations occurred in the context of another set of guidelines proposed in a foundational report by the Institute of Medicine (IOM) in 2010 that set forth parameters for the determination of a viable biomarker (Wagner and Ball 2015). In the IOM report, it was suggested that the evaluation process of a biomarker includes three critical considerations: analytic validity, clinical validity, and clinical utility (Table 6–2). These considerations can be found, in one way or another, in the rich and varied literature on what is a useful biomarker (Biomarkers Definitions Working Group 2001). Indeed, before a biomarker can become a standard of care, it is essential to establish that the biomarker can be accurately and reliably measured (analytic validity), that it has a well-established connection to the disease of interest and/or its outcome (clinical validity), and that it demonstrates that it can result in improved patient care (clinical utility). As suggested above, a number of inflammatory biomarkers have been associated with antidepressant treatment response (see Table 6–1). However, of the inflammatory markers recommended for the panel of markers of chronic inflammation, CRP appears to be in the best position for further scrutiny at this time.

CRP is already measured under standardized, high-quality conditions in clinical laboratories throughout the United States as regulated by the Centers for Medicare & Medicaid Services through the Clinical Laboratory Improvement Amendments of 1988 regulations, which include federal standards applicable to all U.S. facilities or sites that test human specimens for the diagnosis, prevention, or treatment of disease. Thus, CRP fits the criterion of a biomarker that has analytic validity. It should be noted that CRP (through finger-stick blood sampling) is also beginning to be used in point-of-care testing (Bukve et al. 2016), indicating its promise for use in the primary care settings for rapid CRP assessment and clinical decision-making. TNF is not routinely measured in clinical laboratories, and IL-6, which highly correlates with CRP, has important measurement stipulations that include the

TABLE 6–2.   Suggested criteria for a biomarker of disease

Criteria	Definition
Analytic validity	The biomarker should be assayed under standardized conditions that give accurate, reliable, and reproducible results with good sensitivity and specificity across multiple laboratories and clinical settings.
Clinical validity	The biomarker should be reliably associated with the disease state, including data on interventions on both the biomarker and clinical outcome.
Clinical utility	Use of the biomarker should impact disease outcome as either a surrogate endpoint or a positive or negative predictor.

Source.   Wagner and Ball 2015.

timing of blood draw based on the marked circadian variation of this cytokine as well as its sensitivity to stress, factors that are not relevant to the more stable CRP, which has a half-life of ~19 hours (Pepys and Hirschfield 2003) compared with the ~1-hour half-life of IL-6 (Castell et al. 1988).

Relative to clinical validity, there is evidence to support that CRP is linked to the development of depression, its pathophysiology, and its response to treatment. Longitudinal studies in large cohorts of patients have demonstrated an increased odds ratio for the development of depression in patients with increased CRP. For example, in the English Longitudinal Study of Ageing, patients with a CRP >3 mg/L had an odds ratio of 1.49 for developing depression during a follow-up period of ~3–4 years (Au et al. 2015). Similar results have been found in participants with cardiovascular disease (Sforzini et al. 2019). Moreover, as noted above, increased CRP has been linked to decreased functional connectivity within reward-related neurocircuits as well as increased glutamate neurotransmission in association with anhedonia and psychomotor slowing in patients with major depression (Felger et al. 2016; Haroon et al. 2015, 2018a). In addition, increased CRP has been shown to predict treatment response to SSRIs as well as response to the anti-TNF antibody infliximab, in which patients with increased CRP (CRP >5 mg/L) exhibited the most prominent decreases in symptoms of anhedonia, psychomotor retardation, and psychic anxiety (consistent with the impact of inflammation on the neural networks described above) (Jha et al. 2017; Raison et al. 2013). Similar results on anhedonia were found regarding the effects of the anti-IL-6 antibody sirukumab in depressed patients with a CRP >3 mg/L (Salvadore et al. 2018), although a recent trial using infliximab in patients with bipolar depression found effects only in participants with childhood maltreatment, not directly related to CRP

(McIntyre et al. 2019). Finally, recent data indicate that increased plasma CRP is associated with higher concentrations of multiple inflammatory markers and their composite scores in both the peripheral blood and cerebrospinal fluid (Felger et al. 2020).

Other inflammatory biomarkers have also been examined relative to antidepressant treatment response (see Table 6–1). However, the clinical utility of these biomarkers as well as CRP has yet to be established. Indeed, most studies to date have been post hoc in nature. Thus, the relevance of inflammatory markers to improving patient outcome by a priori (prospectively) identifying a subgroup of patients who might benefit from drugs targeting inflammation or its downstream effects on the brain remains to be determined. This is a critical area for future studies.

Conclusion and Future Directions

GUIDELINES FOR FUTURE CLINICAL TRIALS

Targeting Inflammation

Despite the availability of inflammatory markers, including CRP, no clinical trial to date has a priori stratified patients on the basis of any inflammatory biomarker. There have been studies that have focused solely on patients with high inflammation (McIntyre et al. 2019; Salvadore et al. 2018). Nevertheless, without a low inflammation comparator group, it is impossible to know whether the treatment would have been equally as effective in individuals without inflammation. Optimal clinical trial designs that warrant consideration in this regard include the match/mismatch design, in which individuals with low and high inflammation are assigned to a treatment that targets inflammation with the hypothesis that those with high inflammation will respond and those with low inflammation will not (Miller et al. 2017).

Although the obvious target for addressing the impact of inflammation on the brain is inflammation itself, what is least known at this point are the immunological and other mechanisms that drive inflammatory responses in psychiatric disorders. Indeed, current data support both myeloid (e.g., monocyte) and lymphoid (T cell) processes in inflammation in depression, including a host of associated mediators, such as TNF and IL-6 as well as IL-17, respectively (Beurel and Lowell 2018; Miller 2010; Miller and Raison 2016). In addition, the roles of immune cell trafficking, microglial activation, and alterations in blood-brain barrier integrity in key brain regions, including the striatum, have yet to be resolved (Menard et al. 2017; Miller and Raison 2016). Moreover, given the role of stress in psychiatric illnesses, autonomic and neuroendocrine processes involving the sympathetic and parasympathetic nervous systems and hypothalamic-pituitary axis, both potent regulators of the inflammatory response, are also likely involved (Miller et al. 2009). In addition, metabolic dysregulation, including alterations in immunometabolism as well as the gut microbiome, is an important source of inflammation (Dinan and Cryan 2017; Miller and Raison 2016; Treadway et al. 2019). Taken together, the myriad possibilities for intervening at the level of the inflammatory response suggest that inhibiting inflammation itself, whatever the cause(s), may be somewhat premature until more research has revealed the most high-value immune and immunoregulatory targets (Figure 6–1).

Targeting Downstream Effects of Inflammation on the Brain

Few studies have taken advantage of what is known about how inflammation affects the brain in terms of the neurotransmitter systems involved as well as the neurocircuits that are affected. Given the above-noted effects of inflammation on DA and glutamate as well as reward circuitry, studies examining drugs that target these neurotransmitter systems may represent "low-hanging fruit" in clinical trials using inflammatory biomarkers for stratification coupled with match/mismatch trial designs (Figure 6–1). In addition, given neuroimaging correlates of the impact of inflammation on these neurotransmitter systems (e.g., functional connectivity within reward circuitry and regional homogeneity in striatal brain regions), there exist "targets in the brain" that can serve to reflect target engagement as well as proximal measures potentially predictive of long-term outcome. Moreover, there is an opportunity to combine inflammatory biomarkers and the neuroimaging of other downstream consequences of inflammation (e.g., kynurenine metabolites) as well as behavior (e.g., anhedonia) to identify subgroups within subgroups of psychiatric patients with increased inflammation, further enhancing precision medicine strategies (Haroon et al. 2018a).

IMPLICATIONS FOR CLINICAL PRACTICE

Given the state of the science, it is clear that increased inflammation is reliably associated with several psychiatric disorders, and in some disorders—notably depression—it is associated with a poor response to treatment. Thus, in depressed patients who are responding poorly to conventional antidepressants, there may be value in measuring inflammation as reflected by CRP. In individuals with high inflammation (CRP >1 mg/L or higher), there is a rationale for ensuring that sources of inflammation are mitigated

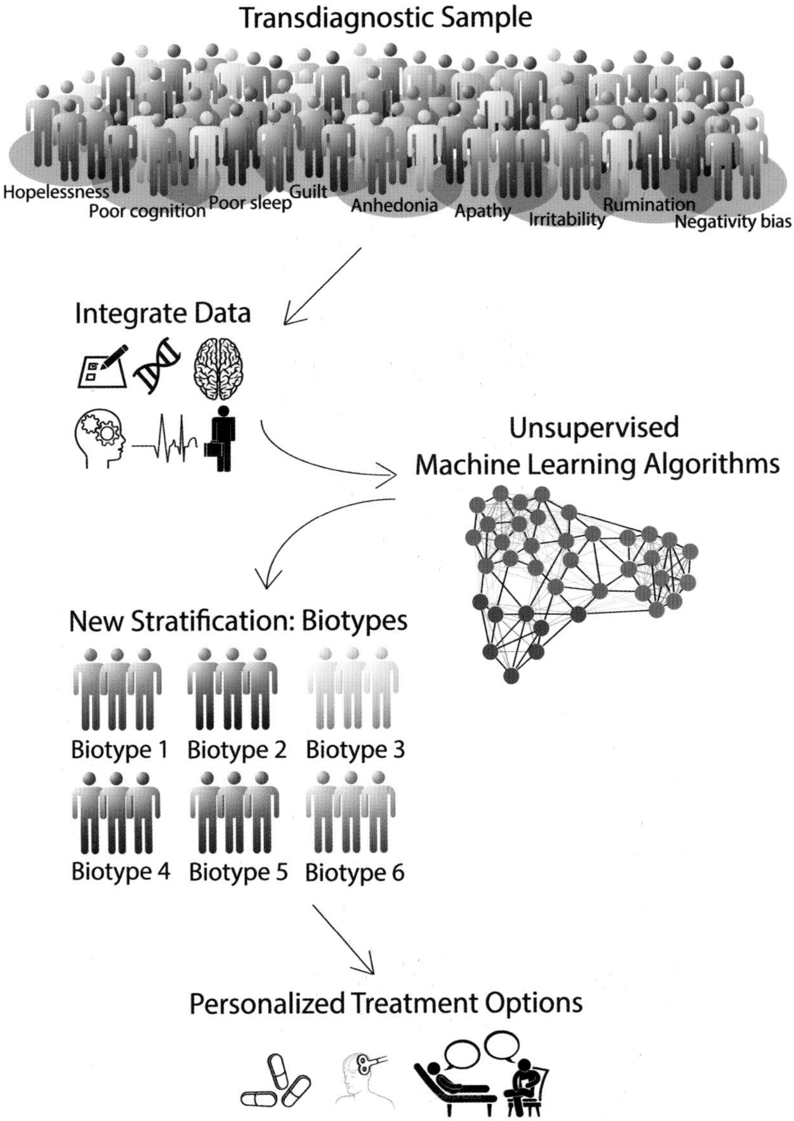

PLATE 1. *(Figure 1–1)* Example of how multimodal data and data-driven techniques may be used to help define the optimal number of biotypes accounting for the heterogeneity of mood and anxiety disorders.

The biotypes thus identified could then be utilized to guide patients to targeted treatments.

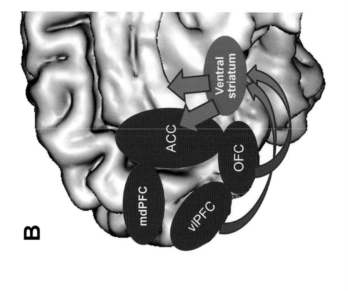

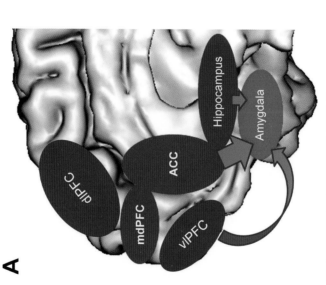

PLATE 2. *(Figure 3–1)* Representation of neural circuitries implicated in **(A)** emotional regulation and **(B)** reward processing.

Arrows represent key connectivity among these regions. ACC = anterior cingulate cortex; dlPFC = dorsolateral prefrontal cortex; mdPFC = mediodorsal prefrontal cortex; OFC = orbitofrontal cortex; vlPFC = ventrolateral prefrontal cortex.

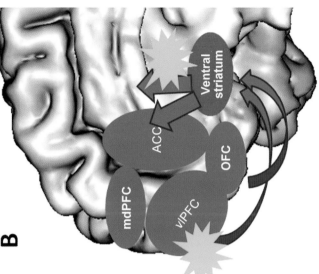

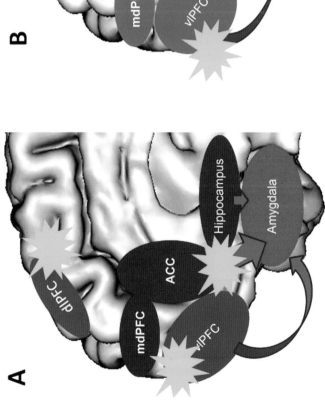

PLATE 3. *(Figure 3–2)* Representation of key abnormalities *(yellow bursts)* in **(A)** emotional regulation and **(B)** reward processing circuitries that predict future worsening of bipolar disorder–related psychopathology in youth.

Arrows represent key connectivity among these regions. ACC = anterior cingulate cortex; dlPFC = dorsolateral prefrontal cortex; mdPFC = mediodorsal prefrontal cortex; OFC = orbitofrontal cortex; vlPFC = ventrolateral prefrontal cortex.

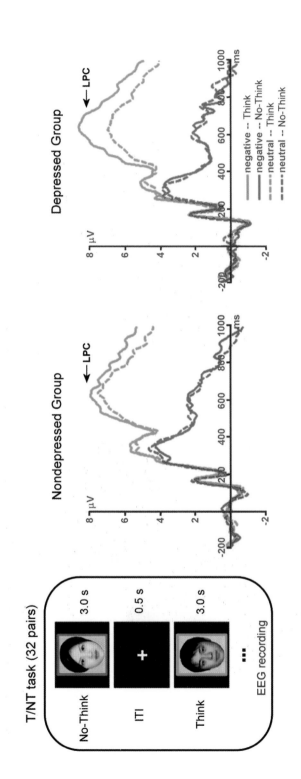

PLATE 4. *(Figure 4–1)* An example of a neural correlate of the negative attention bias in depression.

Participants were instructed to either think about or suppress (not think about) images that were previously associated with positive or negative valence. The group of depressed participants recalled more negative items and had a larger late positive potential (or late positive component [LPC]) for negative "think" items compared with the nondepressed group. These findings reflect abnormal allocation of attentional resources to negative stimuli in the environment, which is believed to arise from increased neural responsivity in prefrontal-parietal attentional circuitry. EEG = electroencephalogram; T/NT = Think/No-Think.

Source. Adapted from Zhang et al. 2016.

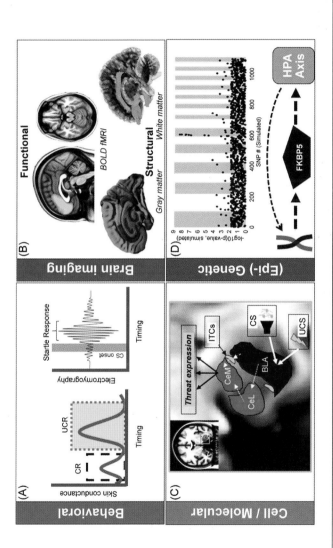

PLATE 5. *(Figure 9–1)* Schematic overview of translational levels for understanding fear and threat.

(A) Behavioral correlates of the conditioned response (CR) and unconditioned response (UCR) can be probed through physiological recording. **(B)** Neural substrates that support fear and threat conditioning may be probed through both functional (to index neural activity) and structural (to index gray and white matter morphology) brain imaging. **(C)** Cell and molecular approaches allow for investigation of specific microcircuits, such as those within the amygdala, that support threat conditioning processes. **(D)** Insights from both genomic and epigenomic approaches can identify individual risk factors and potential physiological pathways that can modulate fear and threat processing. BLA=basolateral nucleus of the amygdala; CeL=lateral central amygdala; CeM=centromedial amygdala; CS=conditioned stimulus; fMRI=functional MRI; HPA=hypothalamic-pituitary-adrenal; ITCs=intercalated cells; SNP=single nucleotide polymorphism; UCS=unconditioned stimulus.

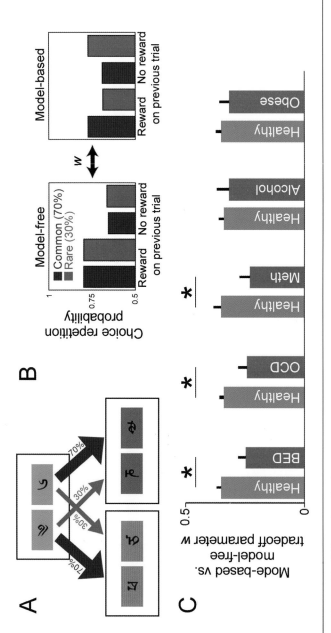

PLATE 6. *(Figure 11–1)* Two-step task.

(A) Participants must first choose among two of the green stimuli. Each of the stimuli probabilistically leads to one of the second-stage stimulus sets with high probability, and to the other set with low probability. Participants then choose one of the two resulting second-stage stimuli and obtain a reward or not. **(B)** A model-free strategy here corresponds to repeating the first-stage (green) choice if the second-stage choice was rewarded, irrespective of the frequency of the transition observed. A model-based strategy takes the transition probability into account: after a rare transition, a reward leads to a switch at the first stage. Consider choosing the left green choice, but transitioning to the blue second stage and then obtaining a reward. In order to gain another reward from the same blue stimulus, the best strategy takes the transition probability into account and leads to a switch of the unchosen first-stage stimulus. Individuals typically use a mixture of these two strategies, which can be measured by the parameter w. **(C)** Patients who have binge-eating disorder (BED), obsessive-compulsive disorder (OCD), or methamphetamine dependence (Meth), but not obesity or alcohol dependence, show a reduction in the parameter w that trades off between these strategies (i.e., they show a shift toward mode-free decision making).

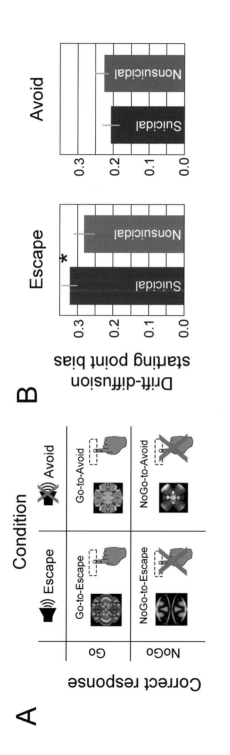

PLATE 7. *(Figure 11–2)* Affective Go-NoGo task.

(A) Individuals were taught to choose whether to Go or NoGo (respond on a button) for different stimuli. With some stimuli (fractals), an unpleasant tone could be escaped or entirely avoided by a Go response (top row). With other stimuli, the unpleasant tone could be escaped or avoided by a NoGo response (bottom row). **(B)** A computational model fitted to the data extracts a key parameter on which groups differed. Participants with a lifetime history of suicidal ideation showed a selective bias toward actively escaping, but did not show a bias in the avoid condition. The bias here was the starting point of a drift-diffusion model (Ratcliff and Smith 2004).

Source. Adapted from Millner et al. 2019.

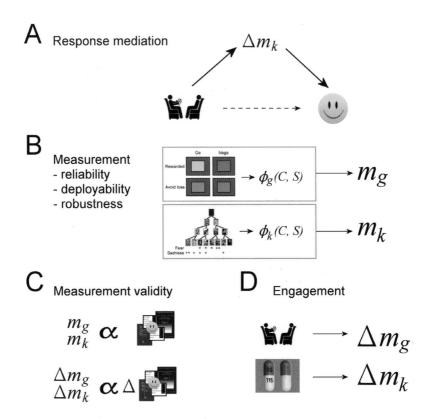

PLATE 8. *(Figure 11–3)* Measuring mechanisms for the clinic.

(A) For precision targeting, the measures derived from computational probes should mediate the effect of interventions. The measure m_k can be used to decide whether to apply intervention k if intervention k reduces measure m_k, and this measure m_k relates in a mechanistic or causal way to the illness. For instance, if antibiotics reduce certain bacterial cell counts, and these bacterial cell counts cause symptoms such as fever, then applying this antibiotic is likely to lead to an improvement in symptoms via its impact on the bacteria. **(B)** To be useful for precision targeting, computational probes, which might involve the results of a task being analyzed with some computational model and producing a measure m_k or m_g, must be reliable at the individual level. The probes must also be deployable in clinical settings and be robust to typical clinical situations. **(C)** Measurements derived from computational probes must be valid (i.e., changes in these measurements should covary with changes in other measures of illness within individuals over time and between individuals). **(D)** Treatments, be they novel or established, should impact the measurement.

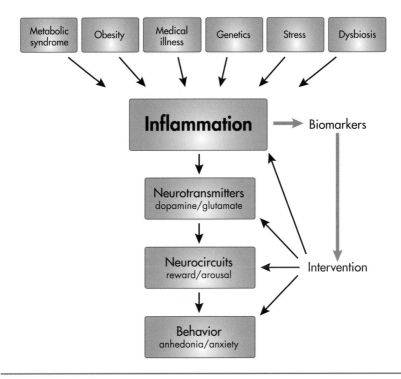

Figure 6–1. Use of inflammatory biomarkers to inform intervention strategies to mitigate the impact of inflammation on the brain.

Multiple factors contribute to the development of chronic inflammation that in turn can influence neurotransmitter systems and neurocircuits that mediate the effects of inflammation on behavior. Biomarkers of inflammation can help identify patients for relevant interventions that target inflammation itself or its downstream effects on the brain.

by lifestyle measures including diet and exercise, which have both been shown to reduce the inflammatory response (Dai et al. 2008; Paolucci et al. 2018). Another important consideration is the evaluation and aggressive treatment of comorbid medical conditions. Although anti-inflammatory treatments have shown some efficacy in meta-analyses of the literature (Kappelmann et al. 2018; Köhler-Forsberg et al. 2019), the data are most clear in patients with autoimmune and inflammatory disorders. However, as noted above, because of limitations in study designs, the utility of anti-inflammatory drugs in depression or other psychiatric disorders has yet to be established. Using drugs that target DA in patients with increased CRP may represent a reasonable first step in the application of principles of precision medicine to the treatment of patients. Inflammation has reliable effects on DA (Felger and Treadway 2017; Treadway et al. 2019), and post hoc evidence indicates that drugs targeting DA may be more efficacious in depressed patients with increased inflammation as reflected by CRP (Jha et al. 2017). Moreover, there is some suggestion that increased inflammation may predict a better response to ECT or ketamine (Kruse et al. 2018; Yang et al. 2015). Nevertheless, much more data are needed to fully translate the emerging literature on the immune system and inflammation in psychiatric disease. However, from the knowledge that has been gained, there is considerable hope that biomarkers of inflammation can identify patients with specific pathologies, which will help guide treatment development and selection, and ultimately support precision medicine.

KEY POINTS

- A large body of research has demonstrated that subgroups of patients with depression, bipolar disorder, anxiety disorders, PTSD, and schizophrenia show chronic activation of the immune system.

- The most compelling evidence exists for a relationship between depression and reproducible elevations in markers of inflammation, particularly the inflammatory cytokines tumor necrosis factor, interleukin (IL)-1β and IL-6, and the acute-phase reactant C-reactive protein (CRP).

- Preclinical and human studies suggest that inflammation alters the synthesis, release, and reuptake of monoamines and glutamate as well as modulates activity in neurocircuits, including those that underlie reward and anxiety.

- Post hoc analysis of three clinical trials showed that depressed patients with higher inflammation (CRP ≥ 1 mg/L) responded significantly worse to selective serotonin reuptake inhibitors or serotonin-norepinephrine reuptake inhibitors compared with individuals with a CRP < 1 mg/L.

- Inflammation has reliable effects on dopamine signaling, and medications that target dopamine, including bupropion, have shown efficacy in depressed patients with high inflammation.

References

Argyelán M, Szabó Z, Kanyó B, et al: Dopamine transporter availability in medication free and in bupropion treated depression: a 99mTc-TRODAT-1 SPECT study. J Affect Disord 89(1–3):115–123, 2005 16213028

Au B, Smith KJ, Gariépy G, et al: The longitudinal associations between C-reactive protein and depressive symptoms: evidence from the English Longitudinal Study of Ageing (ELSA). Int J Geriatr Psychiatry 30(9):976–984, 2015 25537199

Barrientos RM, Sprunger DB, Campeau S, et al: Brain-derived neurotrophic factor mRNA downregulation produced by social isolation is blocked by intrahippocampal interleukin-1 receptor antagonist. Neuroscience 121(4):847–853, 2003 14580934

Beurel E, Lowell JA: Th17 cells in depression. Brain Behav Immun 69:28–34, 2018 28779999

Biomarkers Definitions Working Group: Biomarkers and surrogate endpoints: preferred definitions and conceptual framework. Clin Pharmacol Ther 69(3):89–95, 2001 11240971

Bukve T, Stavelin A, Sandberg S: Effect of participating in a quality improvement system over time for point-of-care C-reactive protein, glucose, and hemoglobin testing. Clin Chem 62(11):1474–1481, 2016 27591289

Capuron L, Pagnoni G, Demetrashvili M, et al: Anterior cingulate activation and error processing during interferon-alpha treatment. Biol Psychiatry 58(3):190–196, 2005 16084839

Capuron L, Pagnoni G, Drake DF, et al: Dopaminergic mechanisms of reduced basal ganglia responses to hedonic reward during interferon alfa administration. Arch Gen Psychiatry 69(10):1044–1053, 2012 23026954

Castell JV, Geiger T, Gross V, et al: Plasma clearance, organ distribution and target cells of interleukin-6/hepatocyte-stimulating factor in the rat. Eur J Biochem 177(2):357–361, 1988 3263918

Cattaneo A, Ferrari C, Uher R, et al: Absolute measurements of macrophage migration inhibitory factor and interleukin-1-β mRNA levels accurately predict treatment response in depressed patients. Int J Neuropsychopharmacol 19(10):pyw045, 2016 27207917

Chamberlain SR, Cavanagh J, de Boer P, et al: Treatment-resistant depression and peripheral C-reactive protein. Br J Psychiatry 214(1):11–19, 2019 29764522

Dai J, Miller AH, Bremner JD, et al: Adherence to the mediterranean diet is inversely associated with circulating interleukin-6 among middle-aged men: a twin study. Circulation 117(2):169–175, 2008 18086924

Danese A, Pariante CM, Caspi A, et al: Childhood maltreatment predicts adult inflammation in a life-course study. Proc Natl Acad Sci USA 104(4):1319–1324, 2007 17229839

Dinan TG, Cryan JF: Microbes, immunity, and behavior: psychoneuroimmunology meets the microbiome. Neuropsychopharmacology 42(1):178–192, 2017 27319972

Dowlati Y, Herrmann N, Swardfager W, et al: A meta-analysis of cytokines in major depression. Biol Psychiatry 67(5):446–457, 2010 20015486

Eisenberger NI, Berkman ET, Inagaki TK, et al: Inflammation-induced anhedonia: endotoxin reduces ventral striatum responses to reward. Biol Psychiatry 68(8):748–754, 2010 20719303

Eriksson O, Långström B, Josephsson R: Assessment of receptor occupancy-over-time of two dopamine transporter inhibitors by [(11)C]CIT and target controlled infusion. Ups J Med Sci 116(2):100–106, 2011 21443419

Felger JC, Treadway MT: Inflammation effects on motivation and motor activity: role of dopamine. Neuropsychopharmacology 42(1):216–241, 2017 27480574

Felger JC, Mun J, Kimmel HL, et al: Chronic interferon-α decreases dopamine 2 receptor binding and striatal dopamine release in association with anhedonia-like behavior in nonhuman primates. Neuropsychopharmacology 38(11):2179–2187, 2013 23657438

Felger JC, Hernandez CR, Miller AH: Levodopa reverses cytokine-induced reductions in striatal dopamine release. Int J Neuropsychopharmacol 18(4):pyu084, 2015 25638816

Felger JC, Li Z, Haroon E, et al: Inflammation is associated with decreased functional connectivity within corticostriatal reward circuitry in depression. Mol Psychiatry 21(10):1358–1365, 2016 26552591

Felger JC, Haroon E, Patel TA, et al: What does plasma CRP tell us about peripheral and central inflammation in depression? Mol Psychiatry 25(6):1301–1311, 2020 29895893

Goldsmith DR, Rapaport MH, Miller BJ: A meta-analysis of blood cytokine network alterations in psychiatric patients: comparisons between schizophrenia, bipolar disorder and depression. Mol Psychiatry 21(12):1696–1709, 2016 26903267

Haroon E, Raison CL, Miller AH: Psychoneuroimmunology meets neuropsychopharmacology: translational implications of the impact of inflammation on behavior. Neuropsychopharmacology 37(1):137–162, 2012 21918508

Haroon E, Felger JC, Jung MY, et al: Increased inflammation is associated with increased glutamate in the basal ganglia of depressed patients. Brain Behav Immun 49:e24, 2015

Haroon E, Miller AH, Sanacora G: Inflammation, glutamate, and glia: a trio of trouble in mood disorders. Neuropsychopharmacology 42(1):193–215, 2017 27629368

Haroon E, Chen X, Li Z, et al: Increased inflammation and brain glutamate define a subtype of depression with decreased regional homogeneity, impaired network integrity, and anhedonia. Transl Psychiatry 8(1):189, 2018a 30202011

Haroon E, Daguanno AW, Woolwine BJ, et al: Antidepressant treatment resistance is associated with increased inflammatory markers in patients with major depressive disorder. Psychoneuroendocrinology 95:43–49, 2018b 29800779

Harrison NA, Voon V, Cercignani M, et al: A neurocomputational account of how inflammation enhances sensitivity to punishments versus rewards. Biol Psychiatry 80(1):73–81, 2016 26359113

Howren MB, Lamkin DM, Suls J: Associations of depression with C-reactive protein, IL-1, and IL-6: a meta-analysis. Psychosom Med 71(2):171–186, 2009 19188531

Hughes JR, Stead LF, Hartmann-Boyce J, et al: Antidepressants for smoking cessation. Cochrane Database Syst Rev (1):CD000031, 2014 24402784

Inagaki TK, Muscatell KA, Irwin MR, et al: Inflammation selectively enhances amygdala activity to socially threatening images. Neuroimage 59(4):3222–3226, 2012 22079507

Jha MK, Minhajuddin A, Gadad BS, et al: Can C-reactive protein inform antidepressant medication selection in depressed outpatients? Findings from the CO-MED trial. Psychoneuroendocrinology 78:105–113, 2017 28187400

Jha MK, Minhajuddin A, Chin-Fatt C, et al: Sex differences in the association of baseline C-reactive protein (CRP) and acute-phase treatment outcomes in major depressive disorder: findings from the EMBARC study. J Psychiatr Res 113:165–171, 2019 30959227

Kappelmann N, Lewis G, Dantzer R, et al: Antidepressant activity of anti-cytokine treatment: a systematic review and meta-analysis of clinical trials of chronic inflammatory conditions. Mol Psychiatry 23(2):335–343, 2018 27752078

Köhler-Forsberg O, Lydholm CN, Hjorthøj C, et al: Efficacy of anti-inflammatory treatment on major depressive disorder or depressive symptoms: meta-analysis of clinical trials. Acta Psychiatr Scand 139(5):404–419, 2019 30834514

Koo JW, Duman RS: IL-1beta is an essential mediator of the antineurogenic and anhedonic effects of stress. Proc Natl Acad Sci USA 105(2):751–756, 2008 18178625

Kruse JL, Congdon E, Olmstead R, et al: Inflammation and improvement of depression following electroconvulsive therapy in treatment-resistant depression. J Clin Psychiatry 79(2):17m11597, 2018 29489077

Learned-Coughlin SM, Bergström M, Savitcheva I, et al: In vivo activity of bupropion at the human dopamine transporter as measured by positron emission tomography. Biol Psychiatry 54(8):800–805, 2003 14550679

Liu CH, Abrams ND, Carrick DM, et al: Biomarkers of chronic inflammation in disease development and prevention: challenges and opportunities. Nat Immunol 18(11):1175–1180, 2017 29044245

Liu JJ, Wei YB, Strawbridge R, et al: Peripheral cytokine levels and response to antidepressant treatment in depression: a systematic review and meta-analysis. Mol Psychiatry 25(2):339–350, 2020 31427752

Machado-Vieira R, Gold PW, Luckenbaugh DA, et al: The role of adipokines in the rapid antidepressant effects of ketamine. Mol Psychiatry 22(1):127–133, 2017 27046644

McIntyre RS, Subramaniapillai M, Lee Y, et al: Efficacy of adjunctive infliximab vs placebo in the treatment of adults with bipolar I/II depression: a randomized clinical trial. JAMA Psychiatry 76(8):783–790, 2019 31066887

Mehta ND, Haroon E, Xu X, et al: Inflammation negatively correlates with amygdala-ventromedial prefrontal functional connectivity in association with anxiety in patients with depression: preliminary results. Brain Behav Immun 73:725–730, 2018 30076980

Menard C, Pfau ML, Hodes GE, et al: Social stress induces neurovascular pathology promoting depression. Nat Neurosci 20(12):1752–1760, 2017 29184215

Michopoulos V, Powers A, Gillespie CF, et al: Inflammation in fear- and anxiety-based disorders: PTSD, GAD, and beyond. Neuropsychopharmacology 42(1):254–270, 2017 27510423

Miller AH: Depression and immunity: a role for T cells? Brain Behav Immun 24(1):1–8, 2010 19818725

Miller AH, Raison CL: The role of inflammation in depression: from evolutionary imperative to modern treatment target. Nat Rev Immunol 16(1):22–34, 2016 26711676

Miller AH, Maletic V, Raison CL: Inflammation and its discontents: the role of cytokines in the pathophysiology of major depression. Biol Psychiatry 65(9):732–741, 2009 19150053

Miller AH, Haroon E, Raison CL, et al: Cytokine targets in the brain: impact on neurotransmitters and neurocircuits. Depress Anxiety 30(4):297–306, 2013 23468190

Miller AH, Haroon E, Felger JC: Therapeutic implications of brain-immune interactions: treatment in translation. Neuropsychopharmacology 42(1):334–359, 2017 27555382

Moieni M, Tan KM, Inagaki TK, et al: Sex differences in the relationship between inflammation and reward sensitivity: a randomized controlled trial of endotoxin. Biol Psychiatry Cogn Neurosci Neuroimaging 4(7):619–626, 2019 31103547

Morón JA, Zakharova I, Ferrer JV, et al: Mitogen-activated protein kinase regulates dopamine transporter surface expression and dopamine transport capacity. J Neurosci 23(24):8480–8488, 2003 13679416

Nomikos GG, Damsma G, Wenkstern D, et al: Effects of chronic bupropion on interstitial concentrations of dopamine in rat nucleus accumbens and striatum. Neuropsychopharmacology 7(1):7–14, 1992 1381923

Osimo EF, Baxter LJ, Lewis G, et al: Prevalence of low-grade inflammation in depression: a systematic review and meta-analysis of CRP levels. Psychol Med 49(12):1958–1970, 2019 31258105

Pandey GN: Inflammatory and Innate Immune markers of neuroprogression in depressed and teenage suicide brain. Mod Trends Pharmacopsychiatry 31:79–95, 2017 28738369

Paolucci EM, Loukov D, Bowdish DME, et al: Exercise reduces depression and inflammation but intensity matters. Biol Psychol 133:79–84, 2018 29408464

Pepys MB, Hirschfield GM: C-reactive protein: a critical update. J Clin Invest 111(12):1805–1812, 2003 12813013

Raison CL, Rutherford RE, Woolwine BJ, et al: A randomized controlled trial of the tumor necrosis factor antagonist infliximab for treatment-resistant depression: the role of baseline inflammatory biomarkers. JAMA Psychiatry 70(1):31–41, 2013 22945416

Randall PA, Lee CA, Podurgiel SJ, et al: Bupropion increases selection of high effort activity in rats tested on a progressive ratio/chow feeding choice procedure: implications for treatment of effort-related motivational symptoms. Int J Neuropsychopharmacol 18(2):pyu017, 2014 25575584

Salvadore G, Nash A, Bleys C, et al: A double-blind, placebo-controlled, multicenter study of sirukumab as adjunctive treatment to a monoaminergic antidepressant in adults with major depressive disorder. Paper presented at the annual meeting of the American College of Neuropsychopharmacology, Hollywood, FL, December 9–13, 2018

Savitz J: The kynurenine pathway: a finger in every pie. Mol Psychiatry 25(1):131–147, 2020 30980044

Savitz JB, Teague TK, Misaki M, et al: Treatment of bipolar depression with minocycline and/or aspirin: an adaptive, 2×2 double-blind, randomized, placebo-controlled, phase IIA clinical trial. Transl Psychiatry 8(1):27, 2018 29362444

Sforzini L, Pariante CM, Palacios JE, et al: Inflammation associated with coronary heart disease predicts onset of depression in a three-year prospective follow-up: a preliminary study. Brain Behav Immun 81:659–664, 2019 31344494

Shelton RC, Pencina MJ, Barrentine LW, et al: Association of obesity and inflammatory marker levels on treatment outcome: results from a double-blind, randomized study of adjunctive L-methylfolate calcium in patients with MDD who are inadequate responders to SSRIs. J Clin Psychiatry 76(12):1635–1641, 2015 26613389

Slavich GM, Way BM, Eisenberger NI, et al: Neural sensitivity to social rejection is associated with inflammatory responses to social stress. Proc Natl Acad Sci USA 107(33):14817–14822, 2010 20679216

Steiner J, Bielau H, Brisch R, et al: Immunological aspects in the neurobiology of suicide: elevated microglial density in schizophrenia and depression is associated with suicide. J Psychiatr Res 42(2):151–157, 2008 17174336

Strawbridge R, Arnone D, Danese A, et al: Inflammation and clinical response to treatment in depression: a meta-analysis. Eur Neuropsychopharmacol 25(10):1532–1543, 2015 26169573

Torres-Platas SG, Cruceanu C, Chen GG, et al: Evidence for increased microglial priming and macrophage recruitment in the dorsal anterior cingulate white matter of depressed suicides. Brain Behav Immun 42:50–59, 2014 24858659

Treadway MT, Cooper JA, Miller AH: Can't or won't? Immunometabolic constraints on dopaminergic drive. Trends Cogn Sci 23(5):435–448, 2019 30948204

Uher R, Tansey KE, Dew T, et al: An inflammatory biomarker as a differential predictor of outcome of depression treatment with escitalopram and nortriptyline. Am J Psychiatry 171(12):1278–1286, 2014 25017001

Valentini V, Frau R, Di Chiara G: Noradrenaline transporter blockers raise extracellular dopamine in medial prefrontal but not parietal and occipital cortex: differences with mianserin and clozapine. J Neurochem 88(4):917–927, 2004 14756813

Vichaya EG, Hunt SC, Dantzer R: Lipopolysaccharide reduces incentive motivation while boosting preference for high reward in mice. Neuropsychopharmacology 39(12):2884–2890, 2014 24917202

Wagner JA, Ball JR: Implications of the Institute of Medicine report: evaluation of biomarkers and surrogate endpoints in chronic disease. Clin Pharmacol Ther 98(1):12–15, 2015 25833004

Walker AJ, Foley BM, Sutor SL, et al: Peripheral proinflammatory markers associated with ketamine response in a preclinical model of antidepressant-resistance. Behav Brain Res 293:198–202, 2015 26209292

Wu HQ, Rassoulpour A, Schwarcz R: Kynurenic acid leads, dopamine follows: a new case of volume transmission in the brain? J Neural Transm (Vienna) 114(1):33–41, 2007 16932989

Xiao C, Miller AH, Felger J, et al: Depressive symptoms and inflammation are independent risk factors of fatigue in breast cancer survivors. Psychol Med 47(10):1733–1743, 2017 28193310

Yang JJ, Wang N, Yang C, et al: Serum interleukin-6 is a predictive biomarker for ketamine's antidepressant effect in treatment-resistant patients with major depression. Biol Psychiatry 77(3):e19–e20, 2015 25104172

Yohn SE, Arif Y, Haley A, et al: Effort-related motivational effects of the proinflammatory cytokine interleukin-6: pharmacological and neurochemical characterization. Psychopharmacology (Berl) 233(19–20):3575–3586, 2016a 27497935

Yohn SE, Collins SL, Contreras-Mora HM, et al: Not all antidepressants are created equal: differential effects of monoamine uptake inhibitors on effort-related choice behavior. Neuropsychopharmacology 41(3):686–694, 2016b 26105139

Zhang J, Yue Y, Thapa A, et al: Baseline serum C-reactive protein levels may predict antidepressant treatment responses in patients with major depressive disorder. J Affect Disord 250:432–438, 2019 30878656

Zhu CB, Carneiro AM, Dostmann WR, et al: p38 MAPK activation elevates serotonin transport activity via a trafficking-independent, protein phosphatase 2A-dependent process. J Biol Chem 280(16):15649–15658, 2005 15728187

Zhu CB, Lindler KM, Owens AW, et al: Interleukin-1 receptor activation by systemic lipopolysaccharide induces behavioral despair linked to MAPK regulation of CNS serotonin transporters. Neuropsychopharmacology 35(13):2510–2520, 2010 20827273

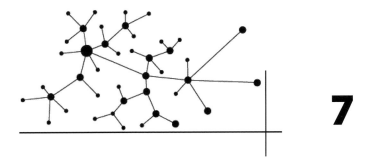

7

Pharmacogenetic Testing

A Tool for Precision Prescribing in Psychiatry

Chad A. Bousman, Ph.D.
Malcolm P. Forbes, M.B.B.S.
Boadie W. Dunlop, M.D.

Aligned with the aims of precision psychiatry, pharmacogenetic testing provides an approach for addressing the variability in drug response (e.g., efficacy, optimal dose and adverse drug reactions) via identification and tailoring of treatment for an individual based on their genetic information. This approach is based on the premise that medications do not always work and in some instances could be harmful to individuals, despite the high evidentiary standards and rigorous regulations placed on drugs used in clinical practice. Indeed, although marketed drugs are generally both tolerable and efficacious when assessed at the population level, for any given individual in a population the tolerability and efficacy of these same drugs can substantially vary. Thus, it is not surprising that since 2000 pharmacogenetic testing options have grown exponentially (Bousman and Hopwood 2016; Haga and Kantor 2018) and that attitudes toward testing are favorable among the general public (Haga et al. 2012), patients (McKillip et al. 2017), and health care providers (Stanek et al. 2012; Walden et al. 2015). Notably, much of the early implementation of pharmacogenetic testing in the clinic has occurred in psychiatry (Müller et al. 2013; Ramsey et al. 2019; Volpi et al. 2018) and continues to evolve alongside the pharmacogenetic evidence base. In this chapter, we begin with a brief summary of the current knowledge underpinning the provision of pharmacogenetic testing in psychiatry and then address common questions related to the implementation of testing before concluding with clinical cases that illustrate the utility of pharmacogenetic testing in practice.

Current Knowledge

Pharmacogenetics evidence can be divided into pharmacokinetic (i.e., absorption, distribution, metabolism, and elimination of drugs), pharmacodynamic (i.e., biochemical, cellular, and physiological effects of drugs and their mechanism of action), and immune-related (i.e., human leukocyte antigen [HLA]) processes. These processes require an array of enzymes, transporters, receptors, and immune modulators that are encoded by hundreds of genes expressed in a range of tissues (e.g., liver, brain). For some individuals these genes contain genetic variants that can alter the function of these processes, ultimately leading to variation in drug response.

From a pharmacokinetic perspective, genetic variation in the cytochrome P450 (CYP) metabolizing enzymes have received the most attention in psychiatry, with the evidence pointing to the CYP2C19, CYP2C9, and CYP2D6 as the most clinically relevant to commonly used psychiatric medications. In fact, 21 psychiatric drugs have prescribing guidelines associated with one or more of these three genes (Table 7–1) (Caudle et al. 2014; Hicks et al. 2015, 2017).

For each of the guidelines associated with CYP2C19, CYP2C9, and CYP2D6, recommendations are made according to an individual's genotype-predicted metabolizer phenotype. Metabolizer phenotypes are determined by genotyping sets (haplotypes) of genetic variants, known as star ("*") alleles. Each individual has two star alleles that are collectively referred to as a *diplotype* or *genotype* (e.g., *1/*17). Each star allele is then assigned a function (i.e., no, decreased, normal, or increased) or activity score (in the case of CYP2D6) based on the current evidence, such as that curated by the Pharmacogene Variation Consortium (PharmVar) (Gaedigk et al. 2018) or established activity score procedures (Gaedigk et al. 2008) (Figure 7–1A). An individual's allele functions or activity scores are then combined to derive a metabolizer phenotype (i.e., poor, intermediate, normal, rapid, ultra-

TABLE 7–1. Gene-drug pairs with clinical prescribing guidelines[a] relevant to psychiatry

Gene	Drugs
CYP2C19	Amitriptyline, citalopram, clomipramine, doxepin, escitalopram, imipramine, sertraline, trimipramine
CYP2C9	Phenytoin
CYP2D6	Amitriptyline, aripiprazole, atomoxetine, clomipramine, desipramine, doxepin, fluvoxamine, haloperidol, imipramine, nortriptyline, paroxetine, pimozide, trimipramine, venlafaxine, zuclopenthixol
HLA-A	Carbamazepine
HLA-B	Carbamazepine, oxcarbazepine, phenytoin

[a]Guidelines published as of September 10, 2019, from the Clinical Pharmacogenetics Implementation Consortium, Dutch Pharmacogenetics Working Group, or Canadian Pharmacogenomics Network for Drug Safety.

rapid) (Figures 7–1B and 7–1C). For example, an individual with a *CYP2C19* *1/*17 genotype carries one normal (*1) and one increased (*17) allele, translating to a rapid metabolizer phenotype. An individual with a *CYP2D6* *4/*5 genotype would be classified as a poor metabolizer because both the *4 and *5 alleles have an activity score of zero (i.e., no function).

Relative to pharmacokinetics, the evidence base for pharmacodynamic genes is less robust. Historically, research in this area has focused on variation in genes that encode receptors and transporters implicated in the actions of psychiatric medications, such as those involved in dopaminergic (e.g., dopamine D_2 receptor; *DRD2*), serotonergic (e.g., serotonin transporter; *SLC6A4*), or glutamatergic (e.g., glutamate ionotropic receptor kainate type subunit 4 [*GRIK4*]) signaling. However, genes involved in hypothalamic-pituitary-adrenal axis function (e.g., FK506 binding protein 5; *FKBP5*) and the leptin-melanocortin pathway (e.g., melanocortin 4 receptor; *MC4R*), to name only two, have emerged as potential harbors of informative genetic markers for psychiatric drug response (Fabbri et al. 2018; Zhang et al. 2016). That said, no pharmacodynamic gene has been implicated in a prescribing guideline relevant to psychiatry because evidence supporting their use in clinical settings is limited.

The final class of pharmacogenetic evidence involves genes involved in immune system function, particularly the HLA system. HLA genes have been implicated in hypersensitivity reactions to a number of drugs relevant to psychiatry (Crettol et al. 2014). The most well-known and robust associations involve the *HLA-A**31:01 and *HLA-B**15:02 alleles, which substan-

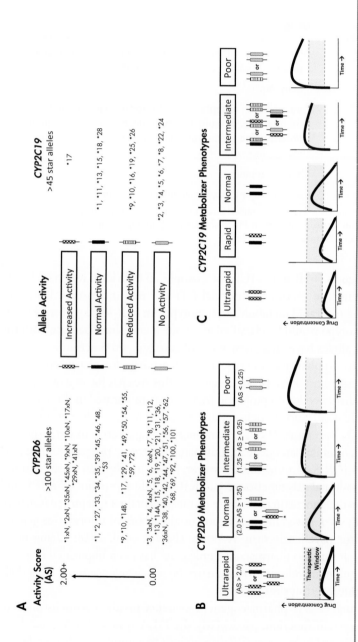

Figure 7–1. Overview of *CYP2D6* and *CYP2C19* star ("*") allele function **(A)** and their translation into metabolizer phenotypes **(B, C)**.

Only a select number of star alleles are shown for *CYP2D6* and *CYP2C19*. A comprehensive list of alleles and their function can be found on the Pharmacogene Variation Consortium website (pharmvar.org). xN=number of copies of an increased allele.

*Individuals carrying more than two copies of an increased activity allele will be defined as ultrarapid metabolizers regardless of other alleles present.

tially increase the risk of severe cutaneous adverse reactions (SCARs) following exposure to carbamazepine (Tangamornsuksan et al. 2013; Yip and Pirmohamed 2017). In addition, carriers of the *HLA-B**15:02 allele are at higher risk of SCARs following exposure to oxcarbazepine or phenytoin (Dean 2012). Based on this evidence, prescribing guidelines have been developed for these gene-drug pairs (Amstutz et al. 2014; Caudle et al. 2014; Phillips et al. 2018; Swen et al. 2011) and routine screening has been implemented in Taiwan (Chen et al. 2011) and Thailand (Sukasem and Chantratita 2016), where the frequency of these alleles are most prevalent.

Collectively, current pharmacogenetics knowledge supports the use of *CYP2C19*, *CYP2C9*, *CYP2D6*, *HLA-A*, and *HLA-B* genetic information to guide drug selection and dosing in psychiatry. Guidelines to assist with the translation of this information into clinical recommendations are freely available (Caudle et al. 2014; Hicks et al. 2015, 2017; Phillips et al. 2018), and their implementation into practice is encouraged by the International Society of Psychiatric Genetics (Bousman et al. 2021), Association for Molecular Pathology (2019), Royal College of Pathologists of Australasia (2018), and American Society of Health-System Pharmacists (2015). Notably, the evidence base is quite dynamic and will continue to evolve rapidly. As such, to remain updated on the current pharmacogenetic evidence we encourage readers to regularly consult the pharmacogenomics knowledge base PharmGKB (www.pharmgkb.org), a comprehensive resource encompassing guidelines, drug labels, and genotype-phenotype relationships (Whirl-Carrillo et al. 2012).

Current Approach

As highlighted in the previous section, the current evidence suggests that several gene-drug associations are sufficiently robust to warrant clinical implementation. However, for many psychiatrist and other health care providers, the implementation of pharmacogenetic testing can be overwhelming and often raises practical questions related to the where, what, when, and whom to test. In this section, we briefly address these questions and provide an overview of the clinical implementation of pharmacogenetic testing in psychiatry.

WHERE IS TESTING PERFORMED?

The provision of pharmacogenetic testing varies by geography but, for most regions of the world, commercial laboratories are the predominant testing provider. This is particularly the case in the United States, where recent estimates suggest 76 commercial laboratories offer pharmacogenetic testing

(Haga and Kantor 2018). In addition, there are at least 45 health care organizations around the world providing pharmacogenetic testing, according to the Clinical Pharmacogenetics Implementation Consortium (CPIC) website (cpicpgx.org) (Clinical Pharmacogenetics Implementation Consortium 2019). The main differences between these two types of test providers relate to testing access and interpretation of test results. Commercial laboratories provide testing via a gatekeeper or via a direct-to-consumer process, whereas testing provided by health care organizations employs only a gatekeeper model. The gatekeeper model requires the involvement of a health care provider to order and interpret test results. In contrast, the direct-to-consumer model does not require involvement of a health care provider, though in some cases commercial labs will offer consultations delivered by in-house health professionals. Although the optimal model for offering pharmacogenetic testing has not been established, there is general consensus that the involvement of a health care provider—preferably a provider known to the individual being tested—is essential for proper interpretation and implementation of pharmacogenetic testing results; the risks are not negligible if results are provided in the absence of a health care provider.

WHAT SHOULD BE TESTED?

There is no gold standard by which to evaluate the quality of content included on a particular pharmacogenetic test. However, the current evidence base would suggest that a pharmacogenetic test for psychiatry would ideally include *CYP2C19*, *CYP2C9*, *CYP2D6*, *HLA-A*, and *HLA-B* (Bousman et al. 2019a). That said, *CYP2C19* and *CYP2D6* enable implementation of 82% (23 gene-drug pairs) of the prescribing guidelines relevant to psychiatry (Fan and Bousman 2020), including all guidelines related to antidepressants, antipsychotics, and the ADHD medication atomoxetine (see Table 7–1). Inclusion of *CYP2C9*, *HLA-A*, and *HLA-B* facilitates implementation of prescribing guidelines for drugs less commonly prescribed (carbamazepine, oxcarbazepine, and phenytoin).

Beyond the individual genes included on a pharmacogenetic testing panel, the specific alleles being tested within these genes are also important. Comparative studies have shown that multiple tests may include the same gene, but the alleles tested vary substantially (Bousman et al. 2017), which can lead to differences in phenotype predictions and prescribing recommendations (Bousman and Dunlop 2018). Recommended allele sets have been developed to assist with the complex task of evaluating the allele content of a test panel (Bousman et al. 2019a; Pratt et al. 2018, 2019). To allow utilization of these recommendations, test manufacturers are encouraged to be transparent about the alleles they include on their panels or provide such information upon request. Additional information on what to consider when selecting a pharmacogenetic test, including a decision tree, has been published elsewhere (Bousman et al. 2019b).

TO WHOM AND WHEN SHOULD TESTING BE OFFERED?

Pharmacogenetic testing presumably would have the greatest impact if offered to everyone in early life, before drug therapy is required. This approach is referred to as *preemptive testing* and is one of three main approaches for determining to whom and when testing should be offered (Figure 7–2). Although there are not yet longitudinal data to unequivocally support widespread adoption of preemptive testing, epidemiological findings estimate that 80% of the population carries at least one actionable (functional) genetic variant relevant to at least one of the 100 most prescribed medications (Schärfe et al. 2017), and that about two-thirds (67%) of physician office visits and 80% of emergency department visits involve a prescription medication (Centers for Disease Control and Prevention 2016). Consequently, most people will be exposed to multiple drug therapies during their lifetime, and there is a high probability that one or more of these drugs will have pharmacogenetic implications. However, preemptive testing is a long-game approach that can be difficult for third-party payers to adopt without solid supporting evidence (Keeling et al. 2019). As a result, point-of-care and reactive approaches to pharmacogenetic testing are currently favored.

The point-of-care approach targets individuals commencing drug therapy for which pharmacogenetic testing could be informative (e.g., initiation of antidepressant therapy). The strength of this approach is that it allows for adjustments to selected drug therapies and can guide future treatment planning. Unfortunately, it can take up to 21 days to receive pharmacogenetic testing results (Bousman and Hopwood 2016). Thus, the point-of-care approach is limited in its ability to guide initial drug selection and dosing, particularly in acute psychiatric settings, and has restricted utility to identify risk for adverse drug reactions that occur within the first weeks of treatment. In contrast, the reactive approach is reserved for individuals with a history of inadequate response or adverse drug reactions to drug therapy—the premise for this approach being that these individuals are more likely to carry actionable pharmacogenetic variants and as such, testing is more likely to be informative for future treatment planning. However, the cost savings of this approach are questionable because it requires potentially costly and avoidable outcomes to occur before the benefits of pharmacogenetics can be realized. Nevertheless, reactive testing, as illustrated in the next section, is currently the most utilized approach in psychiatry.

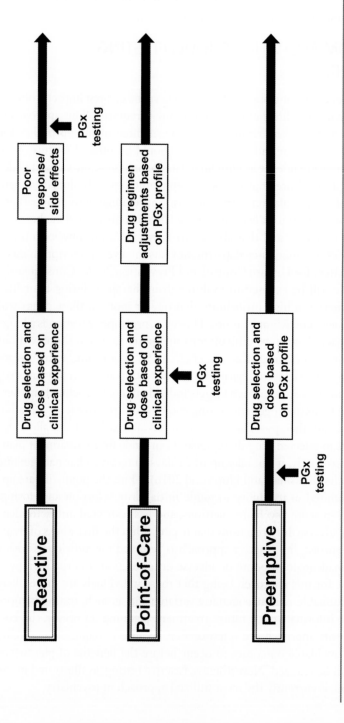

Figure 7–2. The three most common pharmacogenetic (PGx) testing approaches.

Clinical Case Illustrations

CASE 1: GENERALIZED ANXIETY DISORDER

A 72-year-old woman presented for a second opinion regarding her pharmacological regimen for anxiety and insomnia. She had suffered from generalized anxiety disorder for about 20 years and had initially been treated unsuccessfully with nefazodone, mirtazapine, and amitriptyline. The amitriptyline had caused intolerable dissociative side effects of derealization and depersonalization. She reported that a 2004 consultation concluded that she was a "slow metabolizer" (enzyme unspecified) based on clinical history, without the aid of genetic testing. She was subsequently prescribed paroxetine 10 mg daily, which was helpful for her anxiety, along with quetiapine 150 mg nightly for insomnia, a combination she continued for 14 years. Approximately 8 months prior to the consultation, she initiated a slow taper off the paroxetine due to side effects of emotional blunting and low libido. Around this time, she was also diagnosed with sciatica and prescribed gabapentin 900 mg/day. Two months after the paroxetine was discontinued (and 2 months prior to the consultation), she experienced the return of intense anxiety and insomnia. The paroxetine was restarted, but, fearful of her "slow metabolizer" status, her psychiatrist began titrating her dose in 1-mg increments every 2 weeks using liquid paroxetine; she had reached 6 mg/day at the time of the consultation. To simplify her regimen, she had simultaneously been lowering her gabapentin dose down to 300 mg daily. She described her anxiety as daily worry, insomnia, and "feeling gripped in the chest, feeling quivery inside, and my scalp being tightened." The consultant ordered pharmacogenetic testing to inform the treatment approach. While they awaited the results, the consultant advised the patient to immediately increase her gabapentin dose to 900 mg daily, based on the clinical timeline and because the genetic results would not inform gabapentin dosing because of it being excreted unchanged by the renal system.

Pharmacogenetic testing determined the patient to be a *CYP2D6* and *CYP2C19* intermediate metabolizer, and a normal metabolizer for other tested genes (Table 7–2). The increase in gabapentin resolved the patient's somatic anxiety symptoms within 3 days, though worry and insomnia continued. Because she was not a poor metabolizer at *CYP2D6*, the primary enzyme responsible for paroxetine's metabolism, and was a normal metabolizer at *CYP3A4* and *CYP1A2*, paroxetine's minor metabolic pathways, she was advised to increase the dose to 10 mg daily. The consultant advised her that the increased somatic anxiety symptoms she had been experiencing most likely stemmed from the lowering of gabapentin, not the slow up-titration of paroxetine. However, she remained fearful that a higher dose of paroxetine would cause worsening anxiety and chose instead to increase it by 2-mg increments. In 4 weeks, the patient had reached a dose of 10 mg daily and remitted soon thereafter. The patient's history of dissociative symptoms with amitriptyline may be explained by the patient's reduced function at both *CYP2C19* (the primary pathway for amitriptyline metabolism) and *CYP2D6* (the secondary pathway). In fact, CPIC guidelines for amitriptyline suggest a 25% reduction of the starting dose among individuals who are both *CYP2C19* and *CYP2D6* intermediate metabolizers (Hicks et al. 2017).

CASE 2: MAJOR DEPRESSIVE DISORDER

A 67-year-old man on a disability pension for osteoarthritis who lived with his son was admitted with major depressive disorder with anxious distress. He had been diagnosed with major depression 6 months prior to his admission by his primary care physician. His liver function and renal function were normal for his age. Trials of citalopram and escitalopram at maximum doses had been tried for approximately 3 weeks, with inadequate resolution of his symptoms, before a referral was made to a psychiatrist. He was admitted to the hospital with suicidal ideation and catatonic symptoms and received a course of electroconvulsive therapy. His mental state improved, and he was changed from escitalopram to sertraline prior to discharge from hospital. Shortly after discharge his depressive symptoms recurred and he was readmitted to the hospital. At this point a pharmacogenetic test was performed.

Pharmacogenetic testing showed he was a *CYP2C19* rapid metabolizer and *CYP2D6* normal metabolizer (Table 7–3). CYP2C19 is the primary enzyme involved in the metabolism of citalopram, escitalopram, and sertraline, all of which are implicated in *CYP2C19* prescribing guidelines developed by CPIC (Hicks et al. 2015). For *CYP2C19* rapid metabolizers, CPIC guidelines recommend using an alternative drug that is not predominantly metabolized by *CYP2C19* (e.g., paroxetine, fluvoxamine, venlafaxine). As a result, the patient was changed to paroxetine, which is predominantly metabolized by *CYP2D6*, and the dose increased quickly to 50 mg daily. He was discharged from hospital 3 weeks later and remains well in the community with no further relapses.

CLINICAL CONSIDERATIONS

These cases illustrate the impact pharmacogenetic information can have on treatment planning and patient outcomes. Case 1 highlights how pharmacogenetic testing can help explain drug tolerability issues and facilitate shared decision-making, education, and support. This is particularly valuable for patients with anxiety about drug or dose changes because such anticipatory effects can lead to symptom exacerbation and complicate treatment decisions. Case 1 also demonstrates how simultaneous drug changes can complicate the application of pharmacogenetics and, as such, changes in medications should be made sequentially rather than simultaneously, whenever possible. Case 2, on the other hand, highlights how pharmacogenetic testing can be used to elucidate potential reasons for drug therapy failure, while also reducing the provision of unnecessary (e.g., electroconvulsive therapy) and costly interventions (e.g., multiple admissions). In both cases, pharmacogenetic testing was performed in a reactive fashion, but it is not

TABLE 7–2. Pharmacogenetic test results for clinical case 1

Gene	Genotype	Phenotype
CYP2D6	*1/*4	Intermediate metabolizer
CYP2C19	*1/*2	Intermediate metabolizer
CYP2C9	*1/*1	Normal metabolizer
CYP1A2	*1B/*1C	Normal metabolizer
CYP3A4	*1/*1	Normal metabolizer

difficult to imagine how both scenarios could have been mitigated or completely avoided if pharmacogenetic information was available at the commencement of therapy.

The Future of Pharmacogenetic Testing

Pharmacogenetic testing is likely to become standard practice in psychiatry, assuming barriers related to the cost/reimbursement and clinical integration of testing can be resolved. Pharmacogenetic testing will continue to evolve and will be integrated with important clinical (e.g., renal and hepatic functioning), personal (e.g., age, sex), and lifestyle (e.g., smoking, diet) information as well as emerging "omic" (e.g., microbiomic, polygenic risk scores) factors to further enhance precision psychiatry. In the meantime, the clinical use of current evidence-based pharmacogenetic testing tools is warranted and, as shown herein, can have significant impact on the provision of psychiatric drug treatment and most importantly on the well-being of the individuals receiving these therapies.

TABLE 7–3. Pharmacogenetic test results for clinical case 2

Gene	Genotype	Phenotype
CYP2D6	*2/*17	Normal metabolizer
CYP2C19	*1/*17	Rapid metabolizer

KEY POINTS

- Pharmacogenetic testing aligns well with the goals of precision psychiatry, because it provides an approach for addressing individual variability in drug efficacy and tolerability.

- The pharmacogenetic evidence base can be divided into drugs that affect pharmacokinetic, pharmacodynamic, and immune-related processes, with the first category having the most evidence of clinical relevance for psychiatric medications.

- Collectively, current pharmacogenetics knowledge supports the use of *CYP2C19, CYP2C9, CYP2D6, HLA-A,* and *HLA-B* genetic information to guide drug selection and dosing in psychiatry.

- Although pharmacogenetic testing may use a gatekeeper or direct-to-consumer model, the general consensus is that the involvement of a health care provider is essential for proper interpretation and implementation of pharmacogenetic testing results.

- Preemptive pharmacogenetic testing would likely have the greatest impact, but given that this approach has not been tested, point-of-care and reactive approaches are currently favored, with the latter being the most utilized approach in psychiatry.

References

American Society of Health-System Pharmacists: ASHP statement on the pharmacist's role in clinical pharmacogenomics. Am J Health Syst Pharm 72(7):579–581, 2015 25788513

Amstutz U, Shear NH, Rieder MJ, et al: Recommendations for HLA-B*15:02 and HLA-A*31:01 genetic testing to reduce the risk of carbamazepine-induced hypersensitivity reactions. Epilepsia 55(4):496–506, 2014 24597466

Association for Molecular Pathology: Association for Molecular Pathology position statement: best practices for clinical pharmacogenomic testing. September 4, 2019. Available at: www.amp.org/AMP/assets/File/position-statements/2019/Best_Practices_for_PGx_9_4_2019.pdf?pass=96. Accessed February 16, 2021.

Bousman CA, Dunlop BW: Genotype, phenotype, and medication recommendation agreement among commercial pharmacogenetic-based decision support tools. Pharmacogenomics J 18(5):613–622, 2018 29795409

Bousman CA, Hopwood M: Commercial pharmacogenetic-based decision-support tools in psychiatry. Lancet Psychiatry 3(6):585–590, 2016 27133546

Bousman CA, Jaksa P, Pantelis C: Systematic evaluation of commercial pharmacogenetic testing in psychiatry: a focus on CYP2D6 and CYP2C19 allele coverage and results reporting. Pharmacogenet Genomics 27(11):387–393, 2017 28777243

Bousman CA, Maruf AA, Müller DJ: Towards the integration of pharmacogenetics in psychiatry: a minimum, evidence-based genetic testing panel. Curr Opin Psychiatry 32(1):7–15, 2019a 30299306

Bousman CA, Zierhut H, Müller DJ: Navigating the labyrinth of pharmacogenetic testing: a guide to test selection. Clin Pharmacol Ther 106(2):309–312, 2019b 31004441

Bousman CA, Bengesser SA, Aitchison KJ, et al: Review and consensus on pharmacogenomic testing in psychiatry. Pharmacopsychiatry 54:5–17, 2021 33147643

Caudle KE, Rettie AE, Whirl-Carrillo M, et al: Clinical pharmacogenetics implementation consortium guidelines for CYP2C9 and HLA-B genotypes and phenytoin dosing. Clin Pharmacol Ther 96(5):542–548, 2014 25099164

Centers for Disease Control and Prevention: Therapeutic drug use. 2016. Available at: www.cdc.gov/nchs/fastats/drug-use-therapeutic.htm. Accessed February 16, 2021.

Chen P, Lin JJ, Lu CS, et al: Carbamazepine-induced toxic effects and HLA-B*1502 screening in Taiwan. N Engl J Med 364(12):1126–1133, 2011 21428768

Clinical Pharmacogenetics Implementation Consortium: Implementation. 2019. Available at: cpicpgx.org/implementation. Accessed February 16, 2021.

Crettol S, de Leon J, Hiemke C, et al: Pharmacogenomics in psychiatry: from therapeutic drug monitoring to genomic medicine. Clin Pharmacol Ther 95(3):254–257, 2014 24196844

Dean L: Phenytoin therapy and HLA-B*15: 02 and CYP2C9 genotypes, in Medical Genetics Summaries. Edited by Pratt VM, Scott SA, Pirmohamed M, et al. Bethesda, MD, National Center for Biotechnology Information, 2012

Fabbri C, Corponi F, Albani D, et al: Pleiotropic genes in psychiatry: calcium channels and the stress-related FKBP5 gene in antidepressant resistance. Prog Neuropsychopharmacol Biol Psychiatry 81:203–210, 2018 28989100

Fan M, Bousman CA: Commercial pharmacogenetic tests in psychiatry: do they facilitate the implementation of pharmacogenetic dosing guidelines? Pharmacopsychiatry 53(4):174–178, 2020 30900236

Gaedigk A, Simon SD, Pearce RE, et al: The CYP2D6 activity score: translating genotype information into a qualitative measure of phenotype. Clin Pharmacol Ther 83(2):234–242, 2008 17971818

Gaedigk A, Ingelman-Sundberg M, Miller NA, et al: The Pharmacogene Variation (PharmVar) Consortium: incorporation of the human cytochrome P450 (CYP) allele nomenclature database. Clin Pharmacol Ther 103(3):399–401, 2018 29134625

Haga SB, Kantor A: Horizon scan of clinical laboratories offering pharmacogenetic testing. Health Aff (Millwood) 37(5):717–723, 2018 29733708

Haga SB, O'Daniel JM, Tindall GM, et al: Survey of US public attitudes toward pharmacogenetic testing. Pharmacogenomics J 12(3):197–204, 2012 21321582

Hicks JK, Bishop JR, Sangkuhl K, et al: Clinical Pharmacogenetics Implementation Consortium (CPIC) guideline for CYP2D6 and CYP2C19 genotypes and dosing of selective serotonin reuptake inhibitors. Clin Pharmacol Ther 98(2):127–134, 2015 25974703

Hicks JK, Sangkuhl K, Swen JJ, et al: Clinical Pharmacogenetics Implementation Consortium guideline (CPIC) for CYP2D6 and CYP2C19 genotypes and dosing of tricyclic antidepressants: 2016 update. Clin Pharmacol Ther 102(1):37–44, 2017 27997040

Keeling NJ, Rosenthal MM, West-Strum D, et al: Preemptive pharmacogenetic testing: exploring the knowledge and perspectives of US payers. Genet Med 21(5):1224–1232, 2019 31048813

McKillip RP, Borden BA, Galecki P, et al: Patient perceptions of care as influenced by a large institutional pharmacogenomic implementation program. Clin Pharmacol Ther 102(1):106–114, 2017 27981566

Müller DJ, Kekin I, Kao AC, Brandl EJ: Towards the implementation of CYP2D6 and CYP2C19 genotypes in clinical practice: update and report from a pharmacogenetic service clinic. Int Rev Psychiatry 25(5):554–571, 2013 24151801

Phillips EJ, Sukasem C, Whirl-Carrillo M, et al: Clinical Pharmacogenetics Implementation Consortium guideline for HLA genotype and use of carbamazepine and oxcarbazepine: 2017 update. Clin Pharmacol Ther 103(4):574–581, 2018 29392710

Pratt VM, Del Tredici AL, Hachad H, et al: Recommendations for clinical CYP2C19 genotyping allele selection: a report of the Association for Molecular Pathology. J Mol Diagn 20(3):269–276, 2018 29474986

Pratt VM, Cavallari LH, Del Tredici AL, et al: Recommendations for clinical CYP2C9 genotyping allele selection: a joint recommendation of the Association for Molecular Pathology and College of American Pathologists. J Mol Diagn 21(5):746–755, 2019 31075510

Ramsey LB, Prows CA, Zhang K, et al: Implementation of pharmacogenetics at Cincinnati Children's Hospital Medical Center: lessons learned over 14 years of personalizing medicine. Clin Pharmacol Ther 105(1):49–52, 2019 30058217

Royal College of Pathologists of Australasia: Utilisation of pharmacogenetics in healthcare. July 2018. Available at: www.rcpa.edu.au/Library/College-Policies/Position-Statements/Utilisation-of-pharmacogenetics-in-health-care. Accessed February 16, 2021.

Schärfe CPI, Tremmel R, Schwab M, et al: Genetic variation in human drug-related genes. Genome Med 9(1):117, 2017 29273096

Stanek EJ, Sanders CL, Taber KA, et al: Adoption of pharmacogenomic testing by US physicians: results of a nationwide survey. Clin Pharmacol Ther 91(3):450–458, 2012 22278335

Sukasem C, Chantratita W: A success story in pharmacogenomics: genetic ID card for SJS/TEN. Pharmacogenomics 17(5):455–458, 2016 27027537

Swen JJ, Nijenhuis M, de Boer A, et al: Pharmacogenetics: from bench to byte—an update of guidelines. Clin Pharmacol Ther 89(5):662–673, 2011 21412232

Tangamornsuksan W, Chaiyakunapruk N, Somkrua R, et al: Relationship between the HLA-B*1502 allele and carbamazepine-induced Stevens-Johnson syndrome and toxic epidermal necrolysis: a systematic review and meta-analysis. JAMA Dermatol 149(9):1025–1032, 2013 23884208

Volpi S, Bult CJ, Chisholm RL, et al: Research directions in the clinical implementation of pharmacogenomics: an overview of US programs and projects. Clin Pharmacol Ther 103(5):778–786, 2018 29460415

Walden LM, Brandl EJ, Changasi A, et al: Physicians' opinions following pharmacogenetic testing for psychotropic medication. Psychiatry Res 229(3):913–918, 2015 26298505

Whirl-Carrillo M, McDonagh EM, Hebert JM, et al: Pharmacogenomics knowledge for personalized medicine. Clin Pharmacol Ther 92(4):414–417, 2012 22992668

Yip VL, Pirmohamed M: The HLA-A*31:01 allele: influence on carbamazepine treatment. Pharm Genomics Pers Med 10:29–38, 2017 28203102

Zhang JP, Lencz T, Zhang RX, et al: Pharmacogenetic associations of antipsychotic drug-related weight gain: a systematic review and meta-analysis. Schizophr Bull 42(6):1418–1437, 2016 27217270

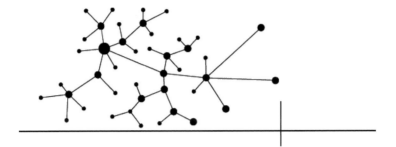

PART 4

TRANSLATIONAL NEUROBIOLOGICAL APPROACHES

PART 4

TRANSLATIONAL NEUROBIOLOGICAL
APPROACHES

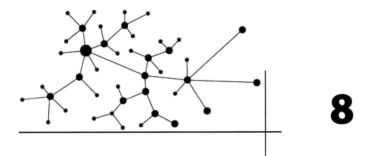

8

TREATMENT PREDICTION BIOMARKERS FOR MAJOR DEPRESSIVE DISORDER

Matthew D. Sacchet, Ph.D.

Christian A. Webb, Ph.D.

Diego A. Pizzagalli, Ph.D.

History

Among mental illnesses, major depressive disorder (MDD) is the leading contributor to the global burden of disease and is associated with a staggering loss of $210.5 billion per year from disability and impacted productivity (Greenberg et al. 2015). MDD is among the most prevalent of all mental

MDS was partially supported by the Rappaport Mental Health Research Fellowship from McLean Hospital. CAW was partially supported by K23 MH108752, R01 MH116969, and a NARSAD Young Investigator Grant from the Brain and Behavior Research Foundation. DAP was partially supported by R37 MH068376 and R01 MH101521 from the National Institute of Mental Health. The content is solely the responsibility of the authors and does not necessarily represent the official views of the funding agencies.

illnesses, with over 16 million Americans experiencing a depressive episode each year (Substance Abuse and Mental Health Services Administration 2013). MDD is highly recurrent, with approximately three out of four depressed individuals experiencing more than one depressive episode (Boland and Keller 2010; Kessler and Wang 2010; Wittchen et al. 2000). It is also difficult to treat, with only one out of three patients having their depression remit after initial treatment (Trivedi et al. 2006; Westen and Morrison 2001), and those in primary care having an even lower remission rate (one out of four) (Vuorilehto et al. 2009).

Understanding the biological mechanisms that underlie depressive pathophysiology and comprehending how treatments may influence these mechanisms are key topics for MDD research because they show promise for guiding the development and selection of interventions for improved clinical outcomes. Toward this goal, there has been a growing interest in understanding neural features that predict treatment outcome. The overarching goals of this chapter are to 1) highlight one of the most promising biological predictors of treatment outcome for MDD (pretreatment activity of the rostral anterior cingulate cortex [rACC]); 2) emphasize limitations in the current MDD treatment biomarker literature, including difficulties in predicting treatment-*specific* outcomes, the practicality of using neural biomarkers in clinical practice, and methodological concerns (e.g., small sample size) that have prevented clinical adoption; and 3) provide an overview of what we believe are promising future directions for brain-based prediction of treatment outcomes for MDD.

Current Knowledge and Approaches

ROSTRAL ANTERIOR CINGULATE CORTEX AND THE PREDICTION OF MDD TREATMENT RESPONSE

Individual studies have identified a number of clinical and demographic variables that predict relatively worse outcomes from pharmacological and behavioral treatments. These predictors include comorbid psychiatric illness (Carter et al. 2012), general medical conditions (Trivedi et al. 2006), higher levels of depressive symptoms (Trivedi et al. 2006), chronicity of depressive episodes (Souery et al. 2007), anxious depression (Fava et al. 2008), female gender (Trivedi et al. 2006), older age (Fournier et al. 2009), lower socioeconomic status (Jakubovski and Bloch 2014), non-Caucasian race (Trivedi et al. 2006), and less education (Trivedi et al. 2006). Major limitations of these predictors include the failure to replicate in subsequent studies and the limited information these predictors provide regarding the mechanisms of treatment response (Pizzagalli et al. 2018). Given these limitations, considerable research has focused on biological markers of treatment response.

A particularly promising marker of treatment outcome for MDD is baseline (pretreatment) activity levels within the rostral (i.e., pregenual) ACC (including Brodmann areas 24 and 32). Results from the first study of this marker were published in 1997 and showed that greater baseline (i.e., before pharmacological treatment) activity (as assessed using resting glucose metabolism via PET) within the rACC predicted better MDD treatment outcome (Mayberg et al. 1997). This finding has subsequently been replicated across assessment methods, including additional studies that used PET and studies that used single-photon emission computed tomography, source-localized electroencephalography (EEG), or functional MRI (fMRI). Moreover, this marker was found to predict treatment outcome across a range of treatment modalities for MDD, including antidepressant medication/pharmacology (e.g., selective serotonin reuptake inhibitors [SSRIs], atypical antidepressants, and ketamine), placebo, sleep deprivation, and brain stimulation, including transcranial magnetic stimulation (TMS) (Korb et al. 2011; Pizzagalli 2011; Sikora et al. 2016). While there have been failures to replicate this finding (e.g., Arns et al. 2015; Brody et al. 1999; Little et al. 2005; Teneback et al. 1999) and even reversed findings (predicting response from electroconvulsive therapy [McCormick et al. 2007] and cognitive-behavioral therapy [Konarski et al. 2009; Siegle et al. 2006]), further evidence for the robustness of using pretreatment rACC activity for treatment prediction stems from a quantitative meta-analysis of 23 studies which found that this effect was replicated 19 times, with a weighted effect size (Cohen's *d*) of 0.918 (Pizzagalli 2011). Moreover, a recent multisite study provided an additional replication of a link between increased pretreatment rACC activity and better treatment response, while addressing several limitations of prior studies, including small sample size. Specifically, by assessing 248 depressed outpatients from the Establishing Moderators and Biosignatures of Antidepressant Response for Clinical Care (EMBARC) study, we showed that rACC activity predicted response to an 8-week administration of sertraline or placebo even when controlling for clinical and demographic variables previously linked to treatment outcome. This provides evidence of the *incremental predictive validity* of rACC activity in a well-characterized large sample (Pizzagalli et al. 2018).

Despite robust evidence that rACC activity predicts outcome to antidepressant therapies, the mechanisms that underlie this predictive relationship are currently unknown. On the basis of a substantial literature that implicates 1) frontocingulate dysfunction in MDD and 2) the rACC as a core hub within the default mode brain system (Buckner et al. 2008), we have previously theorized that the predictive relationship between rACC activity and improved clinical response may be related to adaptive self-referential processing and improved cognitive control capacities that are related to the modulation of the default mode brain system (Pizzagalli 2011; Pizzagalli et al. 2018). Although speculative, based on evidence that the rACC is involved in inhibiting negative information (Eugène et al. 2010), emotion-related amygdalar activity (Etkin et al. 2006), and emotional biases (Blair et al. 2013), reduced resting rACC activity may index disrupted interplay between the default mode network and frontally mediated cognitive control networks; such disruption might underlie depression-related cognitive processes, including chronic repetitive negative self-referential thought (i.e., depressive rumination) and impaired ability to modulate negative emotions and attentional control (Pizzagalli 2011).

Taken together, there is considerable evidence indicating that pretreatment rACC activity, measured in a variety of ways, predicts outcomes across a range of treatment modalities. Although not treatment specific, rACC activity may still prove useful in clinical contexts. For example, one study found that pretreatment rACC activity can be enhanced via cognitive training, which in turn improves antidepressant response to TMS (Li et al. 2014). While promising, further research is necessary to definitively understand the mechanistic role of rACC activity in MDD and in predicting treatment response.

LIMITATIONS OF BRAIN-BASED TREATMENT PREDICTION FOR MDD

Pretreatment predictors of outcome can be classified as either "prognostic" or "prescriptive" predictors (the latter are also known as *moderators)* (Cohen and DeRubeis 2018). Prognostic predictors refer to a main effect of a predictor variable on treatment outcome. For example, in the EMBARC study described earlier, higher levels of resting rACC theta current density predicted greater depressive symptom improvement *across* treatment conditions (Pizzagalli et al. 2018). That is, there was a main effect of rACC theta power on outcome, but no treatment group–by–rACC theta interaction. In addition, studies have found that higher levels of rACC theta activity predict better treatment outcome with a variety of interventions (e.g., SSRI, sleep deprivation, and TMS). This further suggests that rACC activity is a general (treatment nonspecific) marker of depression prognosis.

In contrast, a pretreatment variable is considered to be a *prescriptive* predictor if levels of that variable *moderate* treatment group differences in a clinical outcome (i.e., a significant treatment group–by–pretreatment variable interaction). Thus, prescriptive variables are more informative for treatment *selection* than are prognostic variables (but see Lorenzo-Luaces et al. 2017). To date, several studies (albeit often using small samples) have provided initial evidence for prescriptive predictors, including behavioral (word fluency; Bruder et al. 2014), electrophysiological (loudness-dependent auditory-evoked potential; Juckel et al. 2007), and neuroimaging (glucose metabolism in the insula; McGrath et al. 2013) variables. While promising, it will be necessary to replicate and extend these findings before we integrate any of these behavioral, EEG, or neuroimaging markers into clinical care for the purpose of informing treatment selection for depressed patients.

Given their associated costs and assessment burden, it will be important to carefully consider the benefit of neuroimaging and/or electrophysiological approaches in real-world clinics. Moreover, additional studies are needed to demonstrate that a given neuroimaging or electrophysiological variable predicts treatment response *over* the contribution of much less expensive and more easily administered self-report and clinician-administered measures (e.g., clinical and demographic characteristics) (Kessler et al. 2017). It is also important to highlight that any single predictor variable may only account for a small amount of outcome variance (Pizzagalli et al. 2018). In this context, multivariable machine learning approaches can be used to incorporate large numbers of baseline variables to model predictive relationships to clinical outcomes. Indeed, several studies have used machine learning to model complex relationships among multivariate sets of prescriptive predictors for the purpose of informing optimal treatment selection (see, e.g., Cohen et al. 2020; DeRubeis et al. 2014; Huibers et al. 2015; Webb et al. 2019).

Sample size is another important consideration in treatment prediction. For example, a recent simulation study provided evidence that the sample size required for adequately powered tests of prescriptive predictors of depression treatment response is substantially larger than those of most published studies (i.e., >300 per treatment group) (Luedtke et al. 2019). It may be possible to increase sample size by pooling data across studies if there is sufficient overlap in predictor and outcome variables. An alternative study design is to leverage naturalistic (i.e., observational) treatment data sets, which may provide substantially larger sample sizes than those in randomized controlled trials (RCTs). In this context, naturalistic data sets must include sufficient baseline assessments of predictors in addition to relevant outcome measures. A major challenge associated with observational data sets is that patients are not randomly assigned to treatment conditions, as they are in RCTs. As a result, treatment groups may differ in baseline patient characteristics. Statistical approaches can be used to address this limitation by balancing treatment groups; for example, by using propensity score matching or weighting approaches (Hirshberg and Zubizarreta 2017; see Kessler et al. 2019).

Conclusion and Future Directions

MDD is associated with substantial personal and societal burden (Greenberg et al. 2015), and while there are a variety of treatment options, including pharmacological, psychological, and neurostimulation interventions, there are currently no empirically validated approaches for selecting the optimal treatment for individual depressed patients. Instead, treatment selection continues to be largely based on a trial-and-error approach, which typically introduces significant delays in the identification of effective treatments, is often associated with inadequately addressed symptoms (including increased suicidal behaviors), and may contribute to treatment dropout. In this context, the goals of the current chapter were to highlight the promise of neuroimaging-based treatment prediction for MDD and to note several limitations in the current literature, including the limited applicability of biomarkers for predicting which *specific* treatment is best suited for a given individual, the practicality of brain-based clinical approaches, and methodological considerations (e.g., small sample sizes leading to underpowered tests).

Before we can effectively integrate the neuroscience of MDD into clinical practice, it will be necessary to develop new approaches that enable the further incorporation of patient-specific information, which can ultimately be used for patient-specific clinical inference. Toward this objective, several approaches have been gaining momentum in the literature and promise to inform patient-specific psychiatry. For example, as mentioned above, machine learning methods may provide computational leverage by utilizing multiple complex sets of variables to make clinical inferences about specific patients. A growing literature shows that neuroimaging data can be used to differentiate depressed from healthy individuals (e.g., Fu et al. 2008; Mwangi et al. 2012; Sacchet et al. 2015a, 2015b; for review, see Kambeitz et al. 2017), and a similarly promising albeit smaller set of studies provide evidence that machine learning approaches may be useful for treatment prediction (Lee et al. 2018). Recent developments in human brain mapping that provide unprecedented person-specific information may also be useful for the clinical prediction of treatment outcomes in MDD. For example, several methods have been developed that enable the characterization of fMRI-based large-scale functional brain systems at the person-specific level (e.g., Gordon et al. 2017; Wang et al. 2015). Normative approaches are another new set of methodologies that promise to inform the advancement of empirical treatment prediction. In this context, Dr. Andre Marquand and colleagues have recently pioneered a normative method for the statistically meaningful brain mapping of person-specific features related to psychopathology (Marquand et al. 2016; Wolfers et al. 2018). Such approaches promise to unite patient-specific brain mapping and behavior with treatment selection. Finally, recent developments in "deep phenotyping" (including highly repeated assessments of single individuals) may prove useful for the development of person-specific treatment prediction in psychopathology (Fisher and Boswell 2016; Poldrack et al. 2015).

In conclusion, while brain-based treatment prediction for MDD requires further research, the continued development of increasingly advanced and nuanced brain-based treatment selection shows promise for improving clinical outcomes for the treatment of this burdensome condition.

KEY POINTS

- Major depressive disorder (MDD), among the most common of all mental disorders, is particularly difficult to treat, with only one-third of patients remitting after initial treatment. Thus, elucidating the neural mechanisms underlying depression is essential in order to guide improved development and selection of interventions.

- One of the most promising biological predictors of treatment outcome for MDD is pretreatment activity of the rostral anterior cingulate cortex, measured in numerous ways (e.g., functional MRI, source-localized electroencephalography) across various treatment modalities (e.g., selective serotonin reuptake inhibitors, transcranial magnetic stimulation, ketamine). However, the precise mechanisms that underlie this relationship are unknown.

- Limitations of MDD treatment biomarker literature includes numerous challenges related to the ability to predict which specific treatment is best suited for each individual, the feasibility of using neural biomarkers in clinical practice, the need for evidence to show that neural biomarkers better predict treatment response compared with less expensive measures, and methodological concerns (e.g., sample size).

- Future directions include developing novel approaches, including machine learning methods that may better help incorporate patient-specific information, in addition to the use of "deep phenotyping" for the development of person-specific treatment prediction in psychiatric illness.

References

Arns M, Etkin A, Hegerl U, et al: Frontal and rostral anterior cingulate (rACC) theta EEG in depression: implications for treatment outcome? Eur Neuropsychopharmacol 25(8):1190–1200, 2015 25936227

Blair KS, Otero M, Teng C, et al: Dissociable roles of ventromedial prefrontal cortex (vmPFC) and rostral anterior cingulate cortex (rACC) in value representation and optimistic bias. Neuroimage 78:103–110, 2013 23567883

Boland RJ, Keller MB: Course and outcome of depression, in Handbook of Depression, 2nd Edition. Edited by Gotlib IH, Hammen CL. New York, Cambridge University Press, 2010, pp 23–43

Brody AL, Saxena S, Silverman DH, et al: Brain metabolic changes in major depressive disorder from pre- to post-treatment with paroxetine. Psychiatry Res 91(3):127–139, 1999 10641577

Bruder GE, Alvarenga JE, Alschuler D, et al: Neurocognitive predictors of antidepressant clinical response. J Affect Disord 166:108–114, 2014 25012418

Buckner RL, Andrews-Hanna JR, Schacter DL: The brain's default network: anatomy, function, and relevance to disease. Ann N Y Acad Sci 1124(1):1–38, 2008 18400922

Carter GC, Cantrell RA, Victoria Zarotsky, et al: Comprehensive review of factors implicated in the heterogeneity of response in depression. Depress Anxiety 29(4):340–354, 2012 22511365

Cohen ZD, DeRubeis RJ: Treatment selection in depression. Annu Rev Clin Psychol 14(1):209–236, 2018 29494258

Cohen ZD, Kim TT, Van HL, et al: A demonstration of a multi-method variable selection approach for treatment selection: recommending cognitive-behavioral versus psychodynamic therapy for mild to moderate adult depression. Psychother Res 30(2):137–150, 2020 30632922

DeRubeis RJ, Cohen ZD, Forand NR, et al: The Personalized Advantage Index: translating research on prediction into individualized treatment recommendations. A demonstration. PLoS One 9(1):e83875, 2014 24416178

Etkin A, Egner T, Peraza DM, et al: Resolving emotional conflict: a role for the rostral anterior cingulate cortex in modulating activity in the amygdala. Neuron 51(6):871–882, 2006 16982430

Eugène F, Joormann J, Cooney RE, et al: Neural correlates of inhibitory deficits in depression. Psychiatry Res 181(1):30–35, 2010 19962859

Fava M, Rush AJ, Alpert JE, et al: Difference in treatment outcome in outpatients with anxious versus nonanxious depression: a STAR*D report. Am J Psychiatry 165(3):342–351, 2008 18172020

Fisher AJ, Boswell JF: Enhancing the personalization of psychotherapy with dynamic assessment and modeling. Assessment 23(4):496–506, 2016 26975466

Fournier JC, DeRubeis RJ, Shelton RC, et al: Prediction of response to medication and cognitive therapy in the treatment of moderate to severe depression. J Consult Clin Psychol 77(4):775–787, 2009 19634969

Fu CHY, Mourao-Miranda J, Costafreda SG, et al: Pattern classification of sad facial processing: toward the development of neurobiological markers in depression. Biol Psychiatry 63(7):656–662, 2008 17949689

Gordon EM, Laumann TO, Gilmore AW, et al: Precision functional mapping of individual human brains. Neuron 95(4):791–807.e7, 2017 28757305

Greenberg PE, Fournier A-A, Sisitsky T, et al: The economic burden of adults with major depressive disorder in the United States (2005 and 2010). J Clin Psychiatry 76(2):155–162, 2015 25742202

Hirshberg DA, Zubizarreta JR: On two approaches to weighting in causal inference. Epidemiology 28(6):812–816, 2017 28817467

Huibers MJH, Cohen ZD, Lemmens LHJM, et al: Predicting optimal outcomes in cognitive therapy or interpersonal psychotherapy for depressed individuals using the Personalized Advantage Index approach. PLoS One 10(11):e0140771, 2015 26554707

Jakubovski E, Bloch MH: Prognostic subgroups for citalopram response in the STAR*D trial. J Clin Psychiatry 75(7):738–747, 2014 24912106

Juckel G, Pogarell O, Augustin H, et al: Differential prediction of first clinical response to serotonergic and noradrenergic antidepressants using the loudness dependence of auditory evoked potentials in patients with major depressive disorder. J Clin Psychiatry 68(8):1206–1212, 2007 17854244

Kambeitz J, Cabral C, Sacchet MD, et al: Detecting neuroimaging biomarkers for depression: a meta-analysis of multivariate pattern recognition studies. Biol Psychiatry 82(5):330–338, 2017 28110823

Kessler RC, Wang PS: The epidemiology of depression, in Handbook of Depression, 2nd Edition. Edited by Gotlib IH, Hammen CL. New York, Cambridge University Press, 2010, pp 5–22

Kessler RC, van Loo HM, Wardenaar KJ, et al: Using patient self-reports to study heterogeneity of treatment effects in major depressive disorder. Epidemiol Psychiatr Sci 26(1):22–36, 2017 26810628

Kessler RC, Bossarte RM, Luedtke A, et al: Machine learning methods for developing precision treatment rules with observational data. Behav Res Ther 120:103412, 2019 31233922

Konarski JZ, Kennedy SH, Segal ZV, et al: Predictors of nonresponse to cognitive behavioural therapy or venlafaxine using glucose metabolism in major depressive disorder. J Psychiatry Neurosci 34(3):175–180, 2009 19448846

Korb AS, Hunter AM, Cook IA, et al: Rostral anterior cingulate cortex activity and early symptom improvement during treatment for major depressive disorder. Psychiatry Res 192(3):188–194, 2011 21546222

Lee Y, Ragguett R-M, Mansur RB, et al: Applications of machine learning algorithms to predict therapeutic outcomes in depression: a meta-analysis and systematic review. J Affect Disord 241:519–532, 2018 30153635

Li C-T, Hsieh J-C, Huang H-H, et al: Cognition-modulated frontal activity in prediction and augmentation of antidepressant efficacy: a randomized controlled pilot study. Cereb Cortex 26(1):202–210, 2014 25165064

Little JT, Ketter TA, Kimbrell TA, et al: Bupropion and venlafaxine responders differ in pretreatment regional cerebral metabolism in unipolar depression. Biol Psychiatry 57(3):220–228, 2005 15691522

Lorenzo-Luaces L, DeRubeis RJ, van Straten A, et al: A prognostic index (PI) as a moderator of outcomes in the treatment of depression: a proof of concept combining multiple variables to inform risk-stratified stepped care models. J Affect Disord 213:78–85, 2017 28199892

Luedtke A, Sadikova E, Kessler RC: Sample size requirements for multivariate models to predict between-patient differences in best treatments of major depressive disorder. Clin Psychol Sci 7(3):445–461, 2019

Marquand AF, Rezek I, Buitelaar J, et al: Understanding heterogeneity in clinical cohorts using normative models: beyond case-control studies. Biol Psychiatry 80(7):552–561, 2016 26927419

Mayberg HS, Brannan SK, Mahurin RK, et al: Cingulate function in depression: a potential predictor of treatment response. Neuroreport 8(4):1057–1061, 1997 9141092

McCormick LM, Boles Ponto LL, Pierson RK, et al: Metabolic correlates of antidepressant and antipsychotic response in patients with psychotic depression undergoing electroconvulsive therapy. J ECT 23(4):265–273, 2007 18090701

McGrath CL, Kelley ME, Holtzheimer PE, et al: Toward a neuroimaging treatment selection biomarker for major depressive disorder. JAMA Psychiatry 70(8):821–829, 2013 23760393

Mwangi B, Ebmeier KP, Matthews K, et al: Multi-centre diagnostic classification of individual structural neuroimaging scans from patients with major depressive disorder. Brain 135(Pt 5):1508–1521, 2012 22544901

Pizzagalli DA: Frontocingulate dysfunction in depression: toward biomarkers of treatment response. Neuropsychopharmacology 36(1):183–206, 2011 20861828

Pizzagalli DA, Webb CA, Dillon DG, et al: Pretreatment rostral anterior cingulate cortex theta activity in relation to symptom improvement in depression: a randomized clinical trial. JAMA Psychiatry 75(6):547–554, 2018 29641834

Poldrack RA, Laumann TO, Koyejo O, et al: Long-term neural and physiological phenotyping of a single human. Nat Commun 6:8885, 2015 26648521

Sacchet MD, Livermore EE, Iglesias JE, et al: Subcortical volumes differentiate major depressive disorder, bipolar disorder, and remitted major depressive disorder. J Psychiatr Res 68(C):91–98, 2015a 26228406

Sacchet MD, Prasad G, Foland-Ross LC, et al: Support vector machine classification of major depressive disorder using diffusion-weighted neuroimaging and graph theory. Front Psychiatry 6:21, 2015b 25762941

Siegle GJ, Carter CS, Thase ME: Use of FMRI to predict recovery from unipolar depression with cognitive behavior therapy. Am J Psychiatry 163(4):735–738, 2006 16585452

Sikora M, Heffernan J, Avery ET, et al: Salience network functional connectivity predicts placebo effects in major depression. Biol Psychiatry Cogn Neurosci Neuroimaging 1(1):68–76, 2016 26709390

Souery D, Oswald P, Massat I, et al: Clinical factors associated with treatment resistance in major depressive disorder: results from a European multicenter study. J Clin Psychiatry 68(7):1062–1070, 2007 17685743

Substance Abuse and Mental Health Services Administration: Results from the 2012 National Survey on Drug Use and Health: Mental Health Findings. 2013. Available at: www.samhsa.gov/data/sites/default/files/NSDUHmhfr2012/NSDUHmhfr2012.pdf. Accessed February 16, 2021.

Teneback CC, Nahas Z, Speer AM, et al: Changes in prefrontal cortex and paralimbic activity in depression following two weeks of daily left prefrontal TMS. J Neuropsychiatry Clin Neurosci 11(4):426–435, 1999 10570754

Trivedi MH, Rush AJ, Wisniewski SR, et al: Evaluation of outcomes with citalopram for depression using measurement-based care in STAR*D: implications for clinical practice. Am J Psychiatry 163(1):28–40, 2006 16390886

Vuorilehto MS, Melartin TK, Isometsä ET: Course and outcome of depressive disorders in primary care: a prospective 18-month study. Psychol Med 39(10):1697–1707, 2009 19250580

Wang D, Buckner RL, Fox MD, et al: Parcellating cortical functional networks in individuals. Nat Neurosci 18(12):1853–1860, 2015 26551545

Webb CA, Trivedi MH, Cohen ZD, et al: Personalized prediction of antidepressant v. placebo response: evidence from the EMBARC study. Psychol Med 49(7):1118–1127, 2019 29962359

Westen D, Morrison K: A multidimensional meta-analysis of treatments for depression, panic, and generalized anxiety disorder: an empirical examination of the status of empirically supported therapies. J Consult Clin Psychol 69(6):875–899, 2001 11777114

Wittchen HU, Carter RM, Pfister H, et al: Disabilities and quality of life in pure and comorbid generalized anxiety disorder and major depression in a national survey. Int Clin Psychopharmacol 15(6):319–328, 2000 11110007

Wolfers T, Doan NT, Kaufmann T, et al: Mapping the heterogeneous phenotype of schizophrenia and bipolar disorder using normative models. JAMA Psychiatry 75(11):1146–1155, 2018 30304337

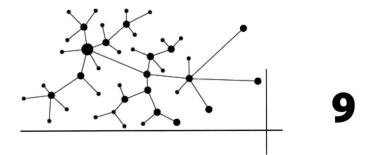

9

TRANSLATIONAL NEUROBIOLOGICAL APPROACHES TO PRECISION MEDICINE FOR FEAR AND PTSD

Nathaniel G. Harnett, Ph.D.
Antonia V. Seligowski, Ph.D.
Daniel Pine, Ph.D.
Kerry J. Ressler, M.D., Ph.D.

History

Trauma and stress-related disorders remain a major public health burden that contributes to severe emotional, social, and financial burdens for victims and their families. In particular, PTSD affects approximately 8% of the U.S. population (Kessler et al. 2005) and is accompanied by functionally debilitating symptoms that include intrusions (e.g., nightmares), avoidance of trauma-related stimuli, negative alterations in cognition and mood

The work was supported by NIH grants R01MH108665, R01MH094757, R21MH112956 and K00MH119603, the Frazier Foundation Grant for Mood and Anxiety Research, and NIMH Intramural Research Program project number ZIAMH002781.

(e.g., guilt, shame), and hyperarousal (e.g., exaggerated startle) (American Psychiatric Association 2013). The symptoms observed in PTSD are thought to be associated with dysregulated fear- and threat-related neural circuitry. Along with great advances in the neuroscience of fear and threat processing, the past several decades have seen a proliferation of research on the neurobiological underpinnings of PTSD.

Neurobiological investigations of PTSD have predominantly focused on neural circuitry that underlies threat learning and memory processes, and have fostered an important translational bridge between the basic understanding of threat-related circuitry and the clinical phenomenology of the disorder. Together, the prior work has implicated specific neural targets that may be prime candidates for precise translational therapeutics for modulating the dysfunctional threat circuitry in PTSD. Here, we discuss the basics of fear/threat learning processes that are important for modeling PTSD symptoms in both human and animal research. Further, we provide an overview of advances in our understanding of the neurobiological circuitry at the systems and molecular levels that are relevant to fear and PTSD. We then discuss current candidates for translational therapeutic approaches that bridge genetic, epigenetic, and intermediate biological phenotype approaches for PTSD and other trauma-related disorders.

Current Knowledge and Approaches

ADAPTIVE THREAT PROCESSING AND DYSFUNCTION IN PTSD

Pavlovian Threat Conditioning

PTSD symptoms are conceptualized as disruptions in natural learning processes that underlie fear and threat-related behaviors. Thus, to study individuals who have the disorder, PTSD researchers have often utilized Pavlovian threat conditioning, a behavioral paradigm in which individuals form a learned threat association. We note here a distinction between the traditional use of "fear" (i.e., the subjective sense of danger or harm) and the current use of "threat" (i.e., biobehavioral responses and circuitry activated in response to a stimulus) in the context of conditioning (LeDoux and Pine 2016). In this chapter, we refer to "threat" to describe the methodological processes and operationalized measures across humans and animals related to conditioned responses, and we use "fear" to describe the underlying cognitive-affective processes thought to be involved in PTSD. *Threat acquisition* is the successful development of an associative memory between a previously neutral cue and an external threat (i.e., learning of the cue-threat association). During threat acquisition, a previously innocuous stimulus (conditioned stimulus; CS) is paired with a biologically salient and aversive stimulus (unconditioned stimulus; UCS) that elicits an innate, reflexive response (unconditioned response; UCR). The associative memory is evidenced by expression of an anticipatory threat response to the CS (conditioned response; CR). *Threat expression* refers to the physical manifestations of the CR.

In humans, threat expression is indexed and quantified most typically by sympathetic activation of the autonomic nervous system. This includes skin conductance responses (i.e., change in sweat excretion in the palms), startle responses as seen in electromyography, and changes in heart rate in response to the CS (Lipp et al. 1994; Öhman and Soares 1993; Peri et al. 2000). Threat expression in response to the CS (i.e., the CR) is thought to reflect a preparatory, defensive mechanism that serves to diminish the magnitude of the subsequent UCR (Baxter 1966; Goodman et al. 2018; Wood et al. 2012). Although threat processing is used as a probe to understand PTSD circuitry, it should be stressed that the formation and expression of associative threat memories are normal and adaptive aspects of healthy function.

Once the CS and UCS are no longer paired, a threat response is no longer adaptive and in healthy physiology, one begins to suppress the CR to the CS (i.e., *threat extinction*). Following repeated presentations of the CS without the UCS, a separate, inhibitory extinction memory is formed which suppresses the previously learned threat memory (Bouton 1993; Craske et al. 2014). Thus, the prior cue no longer elicits the defensive response as no threat is likely to occur. However, the initial threat memory is not unlearned or forgotten, per se, but rather it is suppressed by the new context-dependent extinction or "safety" memory. The original threat memory can be subsequently re-expressed by re-exposure to the UCS following extinction within the extinction context (i.e., *threat reinstatement)* or if the CS is presented in the original acquisition context (i.e., *threat renewal)*. Thus, threat memories can be suppressed in safe contexts (i.e., during extinction) but are available when the danger may be more likely to reoccur.

Threat Learning Deficits in PTSD

Prior PTSD research has identified alterations in Pavlovian threat learning processes. While there can be important individual differences, in general, those with PTSD are able to acquire threat memories to danger cues and form extinction memories as do non-PTSD control participants (Diener et al. 2016; Garfinkel et al. 2014; Milad et al. 2009; Peri et al. 2000; Rabinak et al. 2017). However, individuals with PTSD display disruptions in these processes, in which threat expression during acquisition and extinction is greater than that seen in control subjects (Fani et al. 2012; Norrholm et al. 2011; Peri et al. 2000). Thus, individuals with PTSD appear to form stronger fear memories compared with control subjects.

Additionally, individuals with PTSD show a diminished ability to differentiate a CS that predicts a subsequent UCS presentation (i.e., a danger cue) from a non-UCS-related stimulus (i.e., a safety cue), such that the threat memory is expressed in response to non-threat-related stimuli (Jovanovic et al. 2009, 2010; Rabinak et al. 2017). These individuals show evidence of *threat generalization*, in which the learned threat association is inappropriately expressed in response to neutral or safe stimuli. Thus, individuals with PTSD have difficulty in differentiating danger-related stimuli from safety-related stimuli. In addition, although those with PTSD can sometimes successfully form an initial extinction memory, they often show difficulty in recalling the extinction memory in the nonthreatening context (i.e., reduced extinction recall) (Milad et al. 2008, 2009; Rougemont-Bücking et al. 2011). Further, these individuals show greater levels of threat renewal than do those without PTSD (Garfinkel et al. 2014). Therefore, although the extinction memory is formed in those with PTSD, it does not sufficiently inhibit the originally acquired fear memory.

TRANSLATIONAL INSIGHTS INTO THE NEURAL CIRCUITRY OF FEAR AND THREAT

Neurobiology of Threat Learning

Pavlovian threat conditioning is a highly translational model that allows for investigation of fear and PTSD-related phenomena at multiple translational levels (Figure 9–1). Pavlovian threat conditioning processes are supported by a core network of brain regions centered on the prefrontal cortex (PFC), hippocampus, and amygdala that are integral to threat learning and expression. Research in both animals and humans demonstrates that the amygdala is the central site of CS-UCS convergence and is critical for the formation of threat memories (Hitchcock and Davis 1986; Knight et al. 1999; LaBar et al. 1998; LeDoux et al. 1988, 1990). Specifically, sensory information about the CS and UCS is sent through the sensory cortices and thalamus to the basolateral nucleus of the amygdala (BLA), which encodes the CS-UCS association. The association is then sent to the central nucleus of the amygdala (CeA) to elicit threat memory expression via downstream projections to the autonomic nervous system (LeDoux et al. 1988, 1990; Romanski and LeDoux 1992, 1993). Further work in animals and humans suggests that the hippocampus augments the threat memory by supporting context-related processing such as information about the environment and

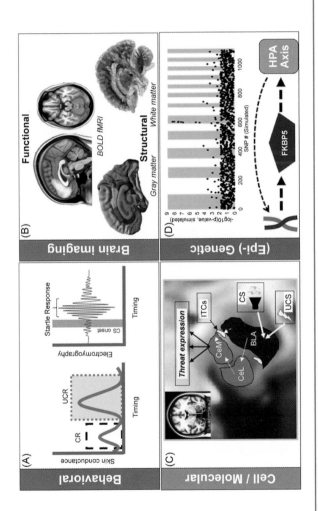

Figure 9–1.   Schematic overview of translational levels for understanding fear and threat.

To view this figure in color, see Plate 5 in Color Gallery.

(A) Behavioral correlates of the conditioned response (CR) and unconditioned response (UCR) can be probed through physiological recording. **(B)** Neural substrates that support fear and threat conditioning may be probed through both functional (to index neural activity) and structural (to index gray and white matter morphology) brain imaging. **(C)** Cell and molecular approaches allow for investigation of specific microcircuits, such as those within the amygdala, that support threat conditioning processes. **(D)** Insights from both genomic and epigenomic approaches can identify individual risk factors and potential physiological pathways that can modulate fear and threat processing. BLA=basolateral nucleus of the amygdala; CeL=lateral central amygdala; CeM=centromedial amygdala; CS=conditioned stimulus; fMRI=functional MRI; HPA=hypothalamic-pituitary-adrenal; ITCs=intercalated cells; SNP=single nucleotide polymorphism; UCS=unconditioned stimulus.

the timing of the CS and UCS (Czerniawski et al. 2012; Harnett et al. 2016; Selden et al. 1991). In addition, human cognitive neuroscience research suggests that components of the PFC, particularly the medial PFC (mPFC), play a key role in learning and memory processes. The dorsomedial PFC supports threat detection and monitoring processes, and upregulates CeA activation to enhance the fear response (Carter and van Veen 2007; Li and McNally 2014; Milad et al. 2007a; Wood et al. 2012).

Conversely, human neuroscience research demonstrates that the ventromedial PFC is critical for suppression of the threat response via inhibitory projections to the amygdala (Motzkin et al. 2015; Urry et al. 2006). Ventromedial PFC and hippocampal activation appear to be necessary to form the inhibitory extinction memory specific to the present context (Milad et al. 2007b). Specifically, the magnitude of ventromedial PFC and hippocampal activation, and the functional synchrony between these regions, are tied to the strength of the threat extinction memory (Kalisch et al. 2006; Milad et al. 2007b). Importantly, the brain regions that mediate threat acquisition also appear to underlie the generalization of the threat memory to different stimuli (Dunsmoor et al. 2011; Lissek et al. 2014). Further, prior work demonstrates that stress exposure potentiates threat generalization processes, and that disrupted neural activity may play a role in threat generalization in PTSD (Dunsmoor et al. 2017; Harnett et al. 2018; Kaczkurkin et al. 2017). Together, the extant literature suggests that Pavlovian threat conditioning processes are primarily supported by a PFC-hippocampus-amygdala network.

Human Neuroscience and PTSD

Prior work suggests that the neural circuitry that supports Pavlovian threat conditioning processes is altered in individuals with PTSD. Meta-analyses have consistently demonstrated heightened activation of the amygdala and dorsomedial PFC, and reduced activation of the ventromedial PFC, in those with PTSD compared with non-PTSD control subjects (Etkin and Wager 2007; Hayes et al. 2012; Patel et al. 2012). Several neuroimaging studies that utilized Pavlovian threat conditioning procedures in PTSD have demonstrated that these alterations in activity are related to disrupted threat learning processes. For example, individuals with PTSD show greater amygdala activation during threat acquisition compared with non-PTSD control subjects (Bremner et al. 2005). Additionally, individuals with PTSD show altered ventromedial PFC, hippocampal, and amygdala activation during threat memory extinction and extinction recall (Milad et al. 2009; Rougemont-Bücking et al. 2011).

The structural morphology of this neural circuit is also altered in PTSD. Early MRI studies of hippocampal morphology in PTSD noted reduced hippocampal volume in PTSD patients (Bremner et al. 1995, 1997). These findings have since been replicated in a recent, large-scale meta-analysis of structural MRI data (Logue et al. 2018). In addition, the cortical morphology of the PFC is different in PTSD, such that those with PTSD show reduced volume of the dorsomedial PFC and reduced thickness of the ventromedial PFC compared with non-PTSD control subjects (Bing et al. 2013; Bryant et al. 2008; Herringa et al. 2012; Li et al. 2014; Wrocklage et al. 2017). Several studies have also noted reductions in amygdala volume in individuals with and without PTSD who are exposed to trauma (Ganzel et al. 2008; Morey et al. 2012). Interestingly, reductions of amygdala volume in trauma-exposed individuals co-occur with heightened amygdala activations (Ganzel et al. 2008).

Further, differences in the white matter pathways that interconnect the PFC, hippocampus, and amygdala have also been observed such that the microstructure of the cingulum bundle, uncinate fasciculus, and fornix/stria terminalis have all been found to vary with PTSD symptom expression (Fani et al. 2016; Harnett et al. 2020; Olson et al. 2017; Sanjuan et al. 2013). Together, this research demonstrates that the PFC, hippocampus, and amygdala have clear roles in the pathology of PTSD.

CELLULAR, MOLECULAR, AND GENETIC MECHANISMS OF FEAR AND PTSD

Specific Cell Populations Within the Amygdala

Pavlovian threat conditioning research in animals has contributed to a rapidly growing understanding of cellular and molecular processes that underlie threat memories and hold relevance for PTSD. In particular, given its prominent role in the threat learning processes and dysfunction observed in PTSD, cellular characterization of the amygdala has received a great deal of attention and has led to the identification of cell-specific mechanisms of threat processes. Although the amygdala is composed of several nuclei, its principal subdivisions are the BLA and the CeA. The acquisition of threat memories is supported by local microcircuits within the BLA. Prior work has demonstrated that parvalbumin (PV) and somatostatin (SOM) GABAergic interneurons within the BLA bidirectionally gate threat learning, such that PV neuron activation during CS presentations and SOM activation during UCS presentations facilitate the formation of threat memories (Wolff et al. 2014).

In addition to its role in threat acquisition, the BLA is also important for the formation of extinction memories. Specifically, activation of Thy1-expressing pyramidal neurons in the BLA during extinction training contributes to greater threat memory extinction (Ciocchi et al. 2010; Herry et al. 2008; McCullough et al. 2018; Wolff et al. 2014). Neurons within the CeA regulate the expression of threat memories through downstream projections to subcortical and brain stem pathways, which in turn mediate the behavioral and physiological effectors of threat responses. The CeA appears to be gated by protein kinase C, delta-type neurons that inhibit output neurons of the CeA, which are themselves inhibited by SOM-expressing neurons (for review, see Fenster et al. 2018; Gafford and Ressler 2016). Corticotropin-releasing hormone (CRH)–expressing neurons within the medial CeA appear to support the expression of acquired threat memories, while CRH neurons within the lateral CeA appear to support threat memory extinction (Gafford and Ressler 2016; Gafford et al. 2012). Intercalated cells (ITCs) outside of the BLA and CeA have been found to inhibit CeA output neurons, and these ITCs receive input from sensory cortices and the BLA, which suggests another mechanism for extinction memory expression (Amano et al. 2010; Paré and Smith 1993).

Together, these cells within the amygdala form specific microcircuits that regulate the acquisition, expression, and extinction of threat memories. In particular, these specific microcircuits appear to support "fear on" and "fear off" aspects of amygdala function (Ciocchi et al. 2010; Haubensak et al. 2010; Herry et al. 2008). Critically, knowledge of these cell circuits can contribute to the targeting of specific cells for the modulation of threat-related behaviors. Given that prior work has demonstrated that behavior is changed by selective activation or inhibition of specific cells within the amygdala (Herry et al. 2008; Wolff et al. 2014), these microcircuits may be ideal pharmacological targets for the translational treatment of dysfunctional fear processes in humans.

Large-Scale Genetic Approaches to PTSD

In addition to the identification of cell-specific circuitry, recent studies have uncovered potential genetic and epigenetic mechanisms that are related to threat learning and PTSD. New technology has led to the development of genome-wide association studies (GWASs) that leverage large databases of genetic information from individuals to identify genetic loci that are associated with psychiatric disease. Several, likely underpowered, studies that examined GWAS approaches to PTSD have implicated several genes in the early development of large-scale PTSD genetics studies (Almli et al. 2015; Duncan et al. 2018; Kilaru et al. 2016; Logue et al. 2013; Stein et al. 2016; Wolf et al. 2014; Xie et al. 2013). A more recent gene-based GWAS found that neuroligin-1, a protein involved in the formation of neuron synapses, is involved in PTSD symptomatology (Almli et al. 2015; Kilaru et al. 2016).

PTSD-risk single nucleotide polymorphisms for these and other identified polymorphisms have been associated with altered neural activity in key threat learning regions such as the amygdala and dorsomedial PFC.

Findings from the largest GWAS of PTSD completed to date, incorporating data from 20,730 individuals, have been reported (Duncan et al. 2018). Although the GWAS did not replicate prior studies of risk alleles, it did find PTSD to be moderately heritable and to share significant genetic overlap with other psychiatric disorders (particularly schizophrenia). Interestingly, the heritability of PTSD appears to be much greater in females compared with males, which suggests important sex differences that should be considered when researching the neurobiological underpinnings of the disorder. Of note, recent GWASs of PTSD have not yet identified specific genetic loci across large, diverse populations. The lack of single genetic targets in PTSD from GWAS results may be partially due to the sheer number of genetic targets being tested, or to potential compound effects from some loci across different ancestries. However, based on findings of other very large-scale GWASs (e.g., schizophrenia, depression), it is expected that the expanded multisite consortia will deliver GWAS findings that are robust to ancestry and trauma type.

The Epigenome and PTSD

Gene expression, which is directly regulated by epigenetic processes, is important for threat learning and PTSD. *Epigenetic regulation* refers to molecular mechanisms that modify DNA properties without changing the underlying DNA sequence. Prior work has demonstrated that threat learning processes are dependent upon histone modification and DNA methylation of multiple genes related to learning, memory, and the function of cells in the amygdala, hippocampus and PFC. For example, the consolidation of threat memories is partially dependent on the epigenetic regulation of gene expression for proteins involved in neural plasticity such as brain-derived neurotrophic factor (Bredy et al. 2007; Lubin et al. 2008). A wealth of research has recently come to light on the epigenetic regulation of another protein that appears to be important for PTSD. Specifically, FK506 binding protein 51 (FKBP5) modulates glucocorticoid receptor sensitivity. As glucocorticoids are released as part of the stress response, FKBP5 is upregulated, and within the cell, FKBP5 suppresses glucocorticoid receptor translocation to the nucleus, thus diminishing the glucocorticoid receptor feedback (for review, see Binder 2009). Prior human studies have noted that adults with varying histories of childhood trauma show marked differences in expression of the FKBP5 gene (*FKBP5*) as adults (Klengel et al. 2013). Single-nucleotide polymorphisms that regulate *FKBP5* expression and

DNA methylation have been associated with functional and structural brain differences in those with PTSD (Fani et al. 2013, 2016). Further, it has recently been suggested that epigenetic modulation of FKBP5 is altered in parent-to-child transmission of risk, possibly related to the intergenerational epigenetic transmission of heritability for PTSD risk (Yehuda et al. 2016). Together, these findings suggest that there may be specific molecular targets that underscore susceptibility to PTSD and that these may be different across individuals, which necessitates a precision medicine approach to treatment stratification.

STRENGTHS AND LIMITATIONS OF PAVLOVIAN MODELING

Strengths

Pavlovian threat conditioning has served as a quantitative, robust, and reproducible approach to understanding individual differences in the physiology of PTSD because of the replicable findings of altered threat processing among those with PTSD compared with control subjects (e.g., extinction deficits). Another major strength of Pavlovian conditioning in PTSD is its immediate translational applicability. Associative learning is an important aspect of survival and is preserved across much of the animal kingdom. Pavlovian threat conditioning can thus be performed in multiple species and enables the investigation of PTSD-related phenomena that are not possible in humans (e.g., optogenetics) in order to understand the molecular underpinnings of threat-related processes. The translational nature of Pavlovian threat conditioning thus suggests that it may be an important tool for facilitating PTSD treatment and precision medicine approaches. It should also be noted that Pavlovian threat conditioning procedures are inherently of only minor discomfort to humans, are well tolerated, and can be completed with minimally aversive stimuli such as mild shocks, white-noise bursts, or short air-blasts. Thus, Pavlovian threat conditioning has several important strengths for modeling dysfunctional fear processes in PTSD.

Limitations

Despite the advantages of Pavlovian conditioning models of PTSD, there are several limitations that should be understood (Grupe and Heller 2016). Although threat learning is well preserved across species, there is significant individual variability in the acquisition, expression, and extinction of threat memories. For example, although the amygdala is known to be critical for threat learning, some healthy individuals may not show significant amygdala activation despite learning a threat association. A recent meta-analysis of threat learning studies in humans did not find significant amygdala activation, partially because of such variability (Fullana et al. 2016). In fact, recent research suggests that reduced amygdala activation is not necessarily a sign of an unacquired threat association, but may only reflect the lack of conditioned or unconditioned skin conductance responses (Marin et al. 2020). Thus, although multiple levels of investigation are available in threat conditioning (e.g., physiology, neural), the individual variability in these measures make it difficult to determine the most efficient level to focus on for precision medicine. Therefore, the lack of robust brain region activations or psychophysiological responses during threat learning may be a hindrance for developing generalizable neurophysiological biomarkers of PTSD. Other tasks, such as passive viewing of fearful faces, robustly activate the amygdala in both healthy individuals and those with PTSD (Hariri et al. 2003; Stevens et al. 2013). However, the individual variability in fear processing may also be associated with meaningful differences in individual pathophysiology. Understanding individual differences in fear processing will likely be crucial for the development of the next level of precision medicine in trauma- and stress-related disorders.

Another important consideration is that trauma-related disorders, such as PTSD, involve much more than disrupted fear processes. Individuals with PTSD also show reductions in positive affect, greater negative affect, disrupted social cognition, guilt and shame, and self-referential processing. Although traditional Pavlovian threat conditioning excels at testing certain aspects of PTSD pathology, other paradigms and procedures may better capture the neurobiology that mediates disruption in these other processes. Therefore, future research should more carefully explore these other approaches, as well as consider methods to expand on typical fear research methods to capture other aspects of PTSD phenomenology.

Future Directions

Currently, standard treatment approaches in PTSD include pharmacotherapy and trauma-focused cognitive-behavioral therapies that have achieved moderate success in diminishing PTSD symptoms for some individuals (Hoskins et al. 2015; Steenkamp et al. 2015). However, these treatments are not effective for all individuals, in part because of individual variability in fear- and threat-related processing. The development of personalized, precision medicine techniques will be necessary to effectively treat patients and reduce the public health burden of PTSD. Given the burgeoning research on the neurobiology of dysfunctional fear processing in PTSD, there are several potential avenues that may provide for effective prediction and treatment tools.

EARLY IDENTIFICATION AND PREDICTION

Individual variability in fear processing and treatment response suggests that PTSD may be composed of biological subtypes that are more or less responsive to different approaches. Recent work suggests that individual variability in PTSD risk can be identified early after trauma exposure. Several studies have identified psychophysiological (Hinrichs et al. 2017, 2019), brain function (Harnett et al. 2018; Stevens et al. 2017; van Rooij et al. 2018), and brain structure (Harnett et al. 2020) markers of PTSD risk in the early aftermath of trauma exposure. In addition to the prior research, ongoing GWASs are identifying more robust polygenic risk scores for PTSD. Rare-variant, epigenetic, and transcriptomic analyses provide additional insight into the molecular mechanisms of PTSD. Thus, current research demonstrates that there are systems-level and molecular markers that represent biological subtypes of posttraumatic susceptibility (e.g., at-risk versus resilient). Integrating information at these levels may therefore lead to improved identification of biological subtypes of PTSD, which would be valuable for precision medicine approaches to treatment.

TREATMENT TARGETING

A better understanding of the neurobiological basis of dysfunctional fear processing can provide important neural targets for personalized medicine for individuals with PTSD. Epigenetic mechanisms regulate the impact of stress on the formation of fear memories that are supported by identifiable and targetable microcircuitry in the brain. Modulation of these gene- and/or cell-specific pathways of fear processing may help to augment specific processes in individuals with PTSD. For example, the development of noninvasive methods for modifying extinction memory circuits may be used to improve extinction learning in those with PTSD, leading to greater responses to ongoing therapies. Targeting these molecular pathways may help to improve PTSD symptoms in previously unresponsive patients.

Conclusion

Significant progress has been made toward understanding differential risk factors as well as physiological, neural, and genetic mechanisms that are related to risk for PTSD in the aftermath of trauma. Of note, there is considerable individual variation, and precision medicine approaches will be critical for identifying and treating PTSD based on these underlying individual differences. Targeting specific aspects of fear, trauma, and stress dysregulation will depend upon knowledge of biomarkers and underlying neural circuits. Advances in quantifying (in a reproducible and reliable way) individual differences in physiology and behavior, combined with (epi)genetic markers of risk, will improve our ability to address specific aspects of PTSD across individuals. We hope that such approaches will lead to improved guidelines and methods for future clinical trials and clinical practice.

KEY POINTS

- PTSD, a major public health burden affecting approximately 8% of the U.S. population, is characterized by symptoms thought to be associated with dysregulated fear- and threat-related neural circuitry.

- Pavlovian threat conditioning, a behavioral paradigm in which individuals form a learned threat association, has served as a quantitative, robust, and reproducible approach to understanding individual differences in the physiology of PTSD because of the replicable findings of altered threat processing among those with PTSD compared with control subjects.

- Meta-analyses have consistently demonstrated heightened activation of the amygdala and dorsomedial prefrontal cortex (PFC), and reduced activation of the ventromedial PFC, in those with PTSD compared with non-PTSD control subjects. Both preclinical and human research demonstrates that the amygdala and its connections to the PFC and hippocampus are critical for threat detection, the formation of threat memories, and the fear response.

- Cells within the amygdala form specific microcircuits that regulate the acquisition, expression, and extinction of threat memories. Knowledge of these cell circuits can contribute to the targeting of specific cells for the modulation of threat-related behaviors.

- Recent genome-wide association studies (GWASs) of PTSD have not yet identified specific genetic loci across large, diverse populations; however, it is anticipated that the expanded multisite consortia will deliver GWAS findings that are robust to ancestry and trauma type.

- Threat learning processes are dependent on histone modification and DNA methylation of multiple genes related to learning, memory, and the function of cells in the amygdala, hippocampus, and PFC.

References

Almli LM, Stevens JS, Smith AK, et al: A genome-wide identified risk variant for PTSD is a methylation quantitative trait locus and confers decreased cortical activation to fearful faces. Am J Med Genet B Neuropsychiatr Genet 168B(5):327–336, 2015 25988933

Amano T, Unal CT, Paré D: Synaptic correlates of fear extinction in the amygdala. Nat Neurosci 13(4):489–494, 2010 20208529

American Psychiatric Association: Diagnostic and Statistical Manual of Mental Disorders, 5th Edition. Arlington, VA, American Psychiatric Association, 2013

Baxter R: Diminution and recovery of the UCR in delayed and trace classical GSR conditioning. J Exp Psychol 71(3):447–451, 1966 5908829

Binder EB: The role of FKBP5, a co-chaperone of the glucocorticoid receptor in the pathogenesis and therapy of affective and anxiety disorders. Psychoneuroendocrinology 34 (suppl 1):S186–S195, 2009 19560279

Bing X, Ming-Guo Q, Ye Z, et al: Alterations in the cortical thickness and the amplitude of low-frequency fluctuation in patients with post-traumatic stress disorder. Brain Res 1490:225–232, 2013 23122880

Bouton ME: Context, time, and memory retrieval in the interference paradigms of Pavlovian learning. Psychol Bull 114(1):80–99, 1993 8346330

Bredy TW, Wu H, Crego C, et al: Histone modifications around individual BDNF gene promoters in prefrontal cortex are associated with extinction of conditioned fear. Learn Mem 14(4):268–276, 2007 17522015

Bremner JD, Randall P, Scott TM, et al: MRI-based measurement of hippocampal volume in patients with combat-related posttraumatic stress disorder. Am J Psychiatry 152(7):973–981, 1995 7793467

Bremner JD, Randall P, Vermetten E, et al: Magnetic resonance imaging-based measurement of hippocampal volume in posttraumatic stress disorder related to childhood physical and sexual abuse—a preliminary report. Biol Psychiatry 41(1):23–32, 1997 8988792

Bremner JD, Vermetten E, Schmahl C, et al: Positron emission tomographic imaging of neural correlates of a fear acquisition and extinction paradigm in women with childhood sexual-abuse-related post-traumatic stress disorder. Psychol Med 35(6):791–806, 2005 15997600

Bryant RA, Felmingham K, Whitford TJ, et al: Rostral anterior cingulate volume predicts treatment response to cognitive-behavioural therapy for posttraumatic stress disorder. J Psychiatry Neurosci 33(2):142–146, 2008 18330460

Carter CS, van Veen V: Anterior cingulate cortex and conflict detection: an update of theory and data. Cogn Affect Behav Neurosci 7(4):367–379, 2007 18189010

Ciocchi S, Herry C, Grenier F, et al: Encoding of conditioned fear in central amygdala inhibitory circuits. Nature 468(7321):277–282, 2010 21068837

Craske MG, Treanor M, Conway CC, et al: Maximizing exposure therapy: an inhibitory learning approach. Behav Res Ther 58:10–23, 2014 24864005

Czerniawski J, Ree F, Chia C, et al: Dorsal versus ventral hippocampal contributions to trace and contextual conditioning: differential effects of regionally selective NMDA receptor antagonism on acquisition and expression. Hippocampus 22(7):1528–1539, 2012 22180082

Diener SJ, Nees F, Wessa M, et al: Reduced amygdala responsivity during conditioning to trauma-related stimuli in posttraumatic stress disorder. Psychophysiology 53(10):1460–1471, 2016 27412783

Duncan LE, Ratanatharathorn A, Aiello AE, et al: Largest GWAS of PTSD (N=20070) yields genetic overlap with schizophrenia and sex differences in heritability. Mol Psychiatry 23(3):666–673, 2018 28439101

Dunsmoor JE, Prince SE, Murty VP, et al: Neurobehavioral mechanisms of human fear generalization. Neuroimage 55(4):1878–1888, 2011 21256233

Dunsmoor JE, Otto AR, Phelps EA: Stress promotes generalization of older but not recent threat memories. Proc Natl Acad Sci USA 114(34):9218–9223, 2017 28784793

Etkin A, Wager TD: Functional neuroimaging of anxiety: a meta-analysis of emotional processing in PTSD, social anxiety disorder, and specific phobia. Am J Psychiatry 164(10):1476–1488, 2007 17898336

Fani N, Tone EB, Phifer J, et al: Attention bias toward threat is associated with exaggerated fear expression and impaired extinction in PTSD. Psychol Med 42(3):533–543, 2012 21854700

Fani N, Gutman D, Tone EB, et al: FKBP5 and attention bias for threat: associations with hippocampal function and shape. JAMA Psychiatry 70(4):392–400, 2013 23407841

Fani N, King TZ, Shin J, et al: Structural and functional connectivity in posttraumatic stress disorder: associations with FKBP5. Depress Anxiety 33(4):300–307, 2016 27038411

Fenster RJ, Lebois LAM, Ressler KJ, Suh J: Brain circuit dysfunction in posttraumatic stress disorder: from mouse to man. Nat Rev Neurosci 19(9):535–551, 2018 30054570

Fullana MA, Harrison BJ, Soriano-Mas C, et al: Neural signatures of human fear conditioning: an updated and extended meta-analysis of fMRI studies. Mol Psychiatry 21(4):500–508, 2016 26122585

Gafford GM, Ressler KJ: Mouse models of fear-related disorders: Cell-type-specific manipulations in amygdala. Neuroscience 321:108–120, 2016 26102004

Gafford GM, Guo J-D, Flandreau EI, et al: Cell-type specific deletion of GABA(A)α1 in corticotropin-releasing factor-containing neurons enhances anxiety and disrupts fear extinction. Proc Natl Acad Sci USA 109(40):16330–16335, 2012 22992651

Ganzel BL, Kim P, Glover GH, et al: Resilience after 9/11: multimodal neuroimaging evidence for stress-related change in the healthy adult brain. Neuroimage 40(2):788–795, 2008 18234524

Garfinkel SN, Abelson JL, King AP, et al: Impaired contextual modulation of memories in PTSD: an fMRI and psychophysiological study of extinction retention and fear renewal. J Neurosci 34(40):13435–13443, 2014 25274821

Goodman AM, Harnett NG, Knight DC: Pavlovian conditioned diminution of the neurobehavioral response to threat. Neurosci Biobehav Rev 84:218–224, 2018 29203422

Grupe DW, Heller AS: Brain imaging alterations in posttraumatic stress disorder. Psychiatr Ann 46(9):519–526, 2016

Hariri AR, Mattay VS, Tessitore A, et al: Neocortical modulation of the amygdala response to fearful stimuli. Biol Psychiatry 53(6):494–501, 2003 12644354

Harnett NG, Shumen JR, Wagle PA, et al: Neural mechanisms of human temporal fear conditioning. Neurobiol Learn Mem 136:97–104, 2016 27693343

Harnett NG, Ference EW III, Wood KH, et al: Trauma exposure acutely alters neural function during Pavlovian fear conditioning. Cortex 109:1–13, 2018 30265859

Harnett NG, Ference EW III, Knight AJ, et al: White matter microstructure varies with acute post-traumatic stress severity following medical trauma. Brain Imaging Behav 14(4):1012–1024, 2020 30519996

Haubensak W, Kunwar PS, Cai H, et al: Genetic dissection of an amygdala microcircuit that gates conditioned fear. Nature 468(7321):270–276, 2010 21068836

Hayes JP, Hayes SM, Mikedis AM: Quantitative meta-analysis of neural activity in posttraumatic stress disorder. Biol Mood Anxiety Disord 2(1):9, 2012 22738125

Herringa R, Phillips M, Almeida J, et al: Post-traumatic stress symptoms correlate with smaller subgenual cingulate, caudate, and insula volumes in unmedicated combat veterans. Psychiatry Res 203(2–3):139–145, 2012 23021615

Herry C, Ciocchi S, Senn V, et al: Switching on and off fear by distinct neuronal circuits. Nature 454(7204):600–606, 2008 18615015

Hinrichs R, Michopoulos V, Winters S, et al: Mobile assessment of heightened skin conductance in posttraumatic stress disorder. Depress Anxiety 34(6):502–507, 2017 28221710

Hinrichs R, van Rooij SJH, Michopoulos V, et al: Increased skin conductance response in the immediate aftermath of trauma predicts PTSD risk. Chronic Stress (Thousand Oaks) 3:2470547019844441, 2019 31179413

Hitchcock J, Davis M: Lesions of the amygdala, but not of the cerebellum or red nucleus, block conditioned fear as measured with the potentiated startle paradigm. Behav Neurosci 100(1):11–22, 1986 3954873

Hoskins M, Pearce J, Bethell A, et al: Pharmacotherapy for post-traumatic stress disorder: systematic review and meta-analysis. Br J Psychiatry 206(2):93–100, 2015 25644881

Jovanovic T, Norrholm SD, Fennell JE, et al: Posttraumatic stress disorder may be associated with impaired fear inhibition: relation to symptom severity. Psychiatry Res 167(1–2):151–160, 2009 19345420

Jovanovic T, Norrholm SD, Blanding NQ, et al: Impaired fear inhibition is a biomarker of PTSD but not depression. Depress Anxiety 27(3):244–251, 2010 20143428

Kaczkurkin AN, Burton PC, Chazin SM, et al: Neural substrates of overgeneralized conditioned fear in PTSD. Am J Psychiatry 174(2):125–134, 2017 27794690

Kalisch R, Korenfeld E, Stephan KE, et al: Context-dependent human extinction memory is mediated by a ventromedial prefrontal and hippocampal network. J Neurosci 26(37):9503–9511, 2006 16971534

Kessler RC, Chiu WT, Demler O, et al: Prevalence, severity, and comorbidity of 12-month DSM-IV disorders in the National Comorbidity Survey Replication. Arch Gen Psychiatry 62(6):617–627, 2005 15939839

Kilaru V, Iyer SV, Almli LM, et al: Genome-wide gene-based analysis suggests an association between neuroligin 1 (NLGN1) and post-traumatic stress disorder. Transl Psychiatry 6(5):e820, 2016 27219346

Klengel T, Mehta D, Anacker C, et al: Allele-specific FKBP5 DNA demethylation mediates gene-childhood trauma interactions. Nat Neurosci 16(1):33–41, 2013 23201972

Knight DC, Smith CN, Stein EA, et al: Functional MRI of human Pavlovian fear conditioning: patterns of activation as a function of learning. Neuroreport 10(17):3665–3670, 1999 10619663

LaBar KS, Gatenby JC, Gore JC, et al: Human amygdala activation during conditioned fear acquisition and extinction: a mixed-trial fMRI study. Neuron 20(5):937–945, 1998 9620698

LeDoux JE, Pine DS: Using neuroscience to help understand fear and anxiety: a two-system framework. Am J Psychiatry 173(11):1083–1093, 2016 27609244

LeDoux JE, Iwata J, Cicchetti P, et al: Different projections of the central amygdaloid nucleus mediate autonomic and behavioral correlates of conditioned fear. J Neurosci 8(7):2517–2529, 1988 2854842

LeDoux JE, Ciocchetti P, Xagoraris A, et al: The lateral amygdaloid nucleus: sensory interface of the amygdala in fear conditioning. J Neurosci 10(4):1062–1069, 1990 2329367

Li L, Wu M, Liao Y, et al: Grey matter reduction associated with posttraumatic stress disorder and traumatic stress. Neurosci Biobehav Rev 43:163–172, 2014 24769403

Li SS, McNally GP: The conditions that promote fear learning: prediction error and Pavlovian fear conditioning. Neurobiol Learn Mem 108:14–21, 2014 23684989

Lipp OV, Sheridan J, Siddle DAT: Human blink startle during aversive and nonaversive Pavlovian conditioning. J Exp Psychol Anim Behav Process 20(4):380–389, 1994 7964520

Lissek S, Bradford DE, Alvarez RP, et al: Neural substrates of classically conditioned fear-generalization in humans: a parametric fMRI study. Soc Cogn Affect Neurosci 9(8):1134–1142, 2014 23748500

Logue MW, Baldwin C, Guffanti G, et al: A genome-wide association study of post-traumatic stress disorder identifies the retinoid-related orphan receptor alpha (RORA) gene as a significant risk locus. Mol Psychiatry 18(8):937–942, 2013 22869035

Logue MW, van Rooij SJH, Dennis EL, et al: Smaller hippocampal volume in post-traumatic stress disorder: a multisite ENIGMA-PGC study: subcortical volumetry results from posttraumatic stress disorder consortia. Biol Psychiatry 83(3):244–253, 2018 29217296

Lubin FD, Roth TL, Sweatt JD: Epigenetic regulation of BDNF gene transcription in the consolidation of fear memory. J Neurosci 28(42):10576–10586, 2008 18923034

Marin MF, Barbey F, Rosenbaum BL, et al: Absence of conditioned responding in humans: a bad measure or individual differences? Psychophysiology 57(1):e13350, 2020 30758048

McCullough KM, Daskalakis NP, Gafford G, et al: Cell-type-specific interrogation of CeA Drd2 neurons to identify targets for pharmacological modulation of fear extinction. Transl Psychiatry 8(1):164, 2018 30135420

Milad MR, Quirk GJ, Pitman RK, et al: A role for the human dorsal anterior cingulate cortex in fear expression. Biol Psychiatry 62(10):1191–1194, 2007a 17707349

Milad MR, Wright CI, Orr SP, et al: Recall of fear extinction in humans activates the ventromedial prefrontal cortex and hippocampus in concert. Biol Psychiatry 62(5):446–454, 2007b 17217927

Milad MR, Orr SP, Lasko NB, et al: Presence and acquired origin of reduced recall for fear extinction in PTSD: results of a twin study. J Psychiatr Res 42(7):515–520, 2008 18313695

Milad MR, Pitman RK, Ellis CB, et al: Neurobiological basis of failure to recall extinction memory in posttraumatic stress disorder. Biol Psychiatry 66(12):1075–1082, 2009 19748076

Morey RA, Gold AL, LaBar KS, et al: Amygdala volume changes in posttraumatic stress disorder in a large case-controlled veterans group. Arch Gen Psychiatry 69(11):1169–1178, 2012 23117638

Motzkin JC, Philippi CL, Wolf RC, et al: Ventromedial prefrontal cortex is critical for the regulation of amygdala activity in humans. Biol Psychiatry 77(3):276–284, 2015 24673881

Norrholm SD, Jovanovic T, Olin IW, et al: Fear extinction in traumatized civilians with posttraumatic stress disorder: relation to symptom severity. Biol Psychiatry 69(6):556–563, 2011 21035787

Öhman A, Soares JJF: On the automatic nature of phobic fear: conditioned electrodermal responses to masked fear-relevant stimuli. J Abnorm Psychol 102(1):121–132, 1993 8436688

Olson EA, Cui J, Fukunaga R, et al: Disruption of white matter structural integrity and connectivity in posttraumatic stress disorder: a TBSS and tractography study. Depress Anxiety 34(5):437–445, 2017 28294462

Paré D, Smith Y: The intercalated cell masses project to the central and medial nuclei of the amygdala in cats. Neuroscience 57(4):1077–1090, 1993 8309544

Patel R, Spreng RN, Shin LM, et al: Neurocircuitry models of posttraumatic stress disorder and beyond: a meta-analysis of functional neuroimaging studies. Neurosci Biobehav Rev 36(9):2130–2142, 2012 22766141

Peri T, Ben-Shakhar G, Orr SP, et al: Psychophysiologic assessment of aversive conditioning in posttraumatic stress disorder. Biol Psychiatry 47(6):512–519, 2000 10715357

Rabinak CA, Mori S, Lyons M, et al: Acquisition of CS-US contingencies during Pavlovian fear conditioning and extinction in social anxiety disorder and post-traumatic stress disorder. J Affect Disord 207:76–85, 2017 27716541

Romanski LM, LeDoux JE: Equipotentiality of thalamo-amygdala and thalamo-cortico-amygdala circuits in auditory fear conditioning. J Neurosci 12(11):4501–4509, 1992 1331362

Romanski LM, LeDoux JE: Information cascade from primary auditory cortex to the amygdala: corticocortical and corticoamygdaloid projections of temporal cortex in the rat. Cereb Cortex 3(6):515–532, 1993 7511012

Rougemont-Bücking A, Linnman C, Zeffiro TA, et al: Altered processing of contextual information during fear extinction in PTSD: an fMRI study. CNS Neurosci Ther 17(4):227–236, 2011 20406268

Sanjuan PM, Thoma R, Claus ED, et al: Reduced white matter integrity in the cingulum and anterior corona radiata in posttraumatic stress disorder in male combat veterans: a diffusion tensor imaging study. Psychiatry Res 214(3):260–268, 2013 24074963

Selden NRW, Everitt BJ, Jarrard LE, et al: Complementary roles for the amygdala and hippocampus in aversive conditioning to explicit and contextual cues. Neuroscience 42(2):335–350, 1991 1832750

Steenkamp MM, Litz BT, Hoge CW, et al: Psychotherapy for military-related PTSD: a review of randomized clinical trials. JAMA 314(5):489–500, 2015 26241600

Stein MB, Chen CY, Ursano RJ, et al: Genome-wide association studies of post-traumatic stress disorder in 2 cohorts of US army soldiers. JAMA Psychiatry 73(7):695–704, 2016 27167565

Stevens JS, Jovanovic T, Fani N, et al: Disrupted amygdala-prefrontal functional connectivity in civilian women with posttraumatic stress disorder. J Psychiatr Res 47(10):1469–1478, 2013 23827769

Stevens JS, Kim YJ, Galatzer-Levy IR, et al: Amygdala reactivity and anterior cingulate habituation predict posttraumatic stress disorder symptom maintenance after acute civilian trauma. Biol Psychiatry 81(12):1023–1029, 2017 28117048

Urry HL, van Reekum CM, Johnstone T, et al: Amygdala and ventromedial prefrontal cortex are inversely coupled during regulation of negative affect and predict the diurnal pattern of cortisol secretion among older adults. J Neurosci 26(16):4415–4425, 2006 16624961

van Rooij SJH, Stevens JS, Ely TD, et al: The role of the hippocampus in predicting future posttraumatic stress disorder symptoms in recently traumatized civilians. Biol Psychiatry 84(2):106–115, 2018 29110899

Wolf EJ, Rasmusson AM, Mitchell KS, et al: A genome-wide association study of clinical symptoms of dissociation in a trauma-exposed sample. Depress Anxiety 31(4):352–360, 2014 24677629

Wolff SBE, Gründemann J, Tovote P, et al: Amygdala interneuron subtypes control fear learning through disinhibition. Nature 509(7501):453–458, 2014 24814341

Wood KH, Ver Hoef LW, Knight DC: Neural mechanisms underlying the conditioned diminution of the unconditioned fear response. Neuroimage 60(1):787–799, 2012 22227141

Wrocklage KM, Averill LA, Cobb Scott J, et al: Cortical thickness reduction in combat exposed U.S. veterans with and without PTSD. Eur Neuropsychopharmacol 27(5):515–525, 2017 28279623

Xie P, Kranzler HR, Yang C, et al: Genome-wide association study identifies new susceptibility loci for posttraumatic stress disorder. Biol Psychiatry 74(9):656–663, 2013 23726511

Yehuda R, Daskalakis NP, Bierer LM, et al: Holocaust exposure induced intergenerational effects on FKBP5 methylation. Biol Psychiatry 80(5):372–380, 2016 26410355

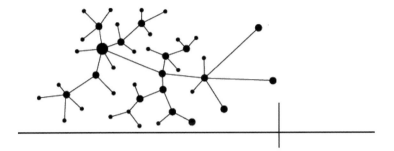

PART 5

New Approaches and Computational Models That Bridge Neuroscience Insights and Clinical Application

PART 5

NEW APPROACHES AND COMPUTATIONAL
MODELS THAT BRIDGE NEUROSCIENCE
INSIGHTS AND CLINICAL APPLICATION

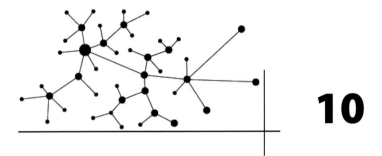

10

LATENT VARIABLE–BASED PREDICTIVE AND EXPLANATORY DISEASE MODELS

Martin P. Paulus, M.D.

History

Obtaining quantitative, reliable, and robust objective markers of disease is tantamount to the development of personalized interventions for individuals with mental health disorders. Yet, despite an ongoing search, objective markers in psychiatry have been elusive. In this chapter, we propose a pathway based on latent variable approaches to discover and develop objective markers in psychiatry.

Among the fundamental barriers is our limited understanding of the emergence of psychiatric disorders as a consequence of brain dysfunctions. The basic question that needs to be addressed is: of the measures that are not derived from patient self-assessment or assessment by a trained professional, which can be used to make more precise predictions about the individual's current state, future disease trajectory, or probability of response to a particular intervention? Finding the answer to this question will point programs of research in important directions that will greatly aid the patient, the mental health provider, the payer, and/or policy makers. Computational psychiatry

(Huys et al. 2016; Montague et al. 2012; Stephan and Mathys 2014) uses mathematical algorithmic approaches to advance a quantitative mechanistic understanding of the processes that underlie mental health and disease and aims to develop practical applications based on model-based analyses. Among these approaches is the use of unsupervised learning algorithms to discover the latent variable structure. We have previously proposed that there needs to be a fundamental shift in research focus, from seeking to find statistically significant differences between groups to seeking to develop predictive models that address real clinical needs (Paulus et al. 2016). Here, we examine the utility of one of the approaches for precision psychiatry.

An important first step toward a potential solution is to determine how computational psychiatry might improve our ability to make clinically meaningful predictions to delineate the current base rate of relationships among variables of interest or responses to intervention. A recent investigation of relationships focused on individual differences research based on 87 meta-analyses across six journals, yielding 708 meta-analytically derived correlations. The authors (Gignac and Szodorai 2016) reported a median correlation coefficient of 0.19. This means that, on average, having knowledge about an individual difference variable helps to explain about 3.6% of the variance in a dependent measure that we care to make predictions about. In comparison, a large study (Bosco et al. 2015) that examined 147,328 correlational effect sizes in applied psychology reported a median effect size of 0.16 (i.e., one measure explaining about 2.5% of the variance of the other measure). When it comes to interventions, a meta-synthesis of 62 meta-analyses of behavioral interventions that focused on health behavior change (Johnson et al. 2010) yielded Cohen's d effect sizes of 0.08 to 0.45. In other words, for these interventions, 53%–67% of the treatment group would be above the mean of the control group, between 82% and 97% of the two groups would overlap, and there would be a 52%–62% chance that a person picked at random from the treatment group would have a higher score than a person picked at random from the control group. These examples serve to remind us how modest our ability is to use variables from one level of analysis to explain another level, and how imprecisely we can forecast who will respond to a particular treatment.

What's more, there is not going to be a single or a small set of quantitative markers for a disease entity. Several investigators have emphasized that psychiatric disorders are "pluralistic," involve "multiple levels," and are "multicausal" (Kendler 2008)—in other words, it is likely that there are not going to be simple explanatory models in psychiatry. Moreover, psychiatric disorders must be explained across biological, psychological, and social-environmental domains with inherent "many to many" relationships (Kendler 2017a), a stipulation that challenges simplistic nosological frameworks.

There has been a split in the scientific community when it comes to explanatory models. On the one hand, some investigators have proposed to explain psychiatric disorders based on highly reduced basic neuroscience models, which are thought to provide novel targets for intervention. Others have suggested that explanations may not be possible because experiential signs and symptoms are emerging properties and cannot be reduced to underlying mechanistic dysfunctions. Fundamentally, explanatory models involve *mechanisms*, which in turn are tightly linked to *causation*. A mechanism is, roughly speaking, a set of entities and activities that are spatially, temporally, and causally organized in such a way that they exhibit the phenomenon to be explained (Menzies 2012). Causation can be defined as an antecedent event, condition, or characteristic that was necessary for the occurrence of the disease at the moment it occurred, given that other conditions are fixed (Rothman and Greenland 2005). Although it would be an important advance to have quantitative markers that also inform our understanding of mechanistic psychiatric disease models, it may be more reasonable to initially take a pragmatic stance—namely, to develop robust predictive objective markers.

One approach for a potential solution to reduce the complexity of multilevel mental health assessments is to determine whether there is a set of common latent variables that not only link levels of analyses but also help to reduce the number of variables. Latent variable approaches have a long history in psychology (Bollen 2002) and psychiatry (van Loo et al. 2012), although with some mixed success. In general, latent variables of symptoms have helped to develop reliable questionnaires (Watson et al. 2015) but have not provided strong evidence of subgroups among individuals with mood and anxiety disorders (van Loo et al. 2012). Recent developments in statistical learning (Hastie et al. 2001) have introduced sparsity constraints that aim to reduce the effect of noisy correlations on the underlying latent variable structure. Within the Bayesian framework, this approach has been termed *automated relevance detection* (Bunte et al. 2016).

Still, explanatory models are important for patients, providers and families who want to understand how psychiatric disorders emerge, how these disorders wax and wane, and how interventions improve these disorders or provide permanent cures. Psychiatric disorders are grounded in mental first-person experiences, are etiologically complex (Kendler 2005), and can be conceptualized as having a distinct course and characteristic symptoms (Kendler and Engstrom 2017). Thus, researchers must be able to provide empirically based explanatory models of psychiatric diseases that address these features and the stakeholders' concerns. However, it is also important not to substitute specific experiences and symptoms for the disorder but to merely take these elements as possible instantiation of an underlying latent process (Kendler 2017b). Yet, others have questioned whether the latent variable models are an appropriate conceptualization of psychiatric disorders (Zachar and Kendler 2017). A pragmatic view (Brendel 2003) is that explanatory models in psychiatry reflect what clinicians deem valuable in rendering people's behavior intelligible and thus help to guide treatment choices for mental illnesses. Taken together, there is a pragmatic need for developing evidence-based explanatory models in psychiatry that enable stakeholders to better understand these illnesses and adapt their lives accordingly.

Current Knowledge and Approaches

LATENT VARIABLES IN PSYCHIATRY

Latent variable models have been used extensively in psychology (Bollen 2002) and have been considered more recently in psychiatry as interest has grown in developing quantitative dimensions of psychopathology across different levels of analyses as proposed by the Research Domain Criteria approach (Cuthbert and Insel 2013; Insel et al. 2010). Latent variable theory considers a mental disorder as a latent variable that causes a constellation of symptoms (Cramer et al. 2010). This is in contrast to a discrete theory of psychiatric diagnoses. However, the distinction is more complex than is often presupposed, and some have suggested that the hypotheses of discrete versus continuum formulations are not mutually exclusive or exhaustive (Borsboom et al. 2016). These approaches have been used within the natural classification tradition iteratively as a way to offer different views about the criteria of validity (Zachar and Kendler 2017). One approach for integrating the discrete versus continuum distinction has been to use factor mixture modeling, which is a newer approach that represents a fusion of latent class analysis and factor analysis (Miettunen et al. 2016). There are a number of considerations when applying these types of models to psychiatry. For example, it is important to carefully select the times that form the basis of the data used to define latent variables in a health domain. Specifically, biases may be present and can affect the definition of the latent variable and the effects the latent variable has on other variables of interest (Palmer et al. 2002).

There have been various modifications of a simple latent variable model of mood and anxiety disorders. First, some researchers extended the latent variable model to include particular occasions and formed the latent variable trait-state-occasion model, finding that this approach provided the best fit for mood and anxiety disorders (Prenoveau et al. 2011). Second, others developed a *multiple indicator multiple cause* latent variable model that combines item reduction and validation (Halberstadt et al. 2012). Third, there has been an effort to simultaneously decompose depression heterogeneity on the person, symptom, and time levels, which yielded two symptom-level components ("cognitive," "somatic-affective"), two time-level components ("improving," "persisting"), and three person-level components characterized by different interaction patterns between the symptom and time components ("severe non-persisting," "somatic depression," and "cognitive depression") (Monden et al. 2015). There are conflicting views regarding whether these models adequately describe depression. For example, latent class techniques have not consistently identified specific symptom clusters in depression. Instead, identified latent variables consisted mostly of variables that quantify the symptoms of depressed mood and loss of interest (van Loo et al. 2012). Others have found that depression could best be described in terms of both qualitative differences between symptom categories and quantitative differences in severity (Ten Have et al. 2016).

As an alternative to latent variable models, network approaches have deviated from the common cause perspective and the associated latent variable model in which symptoms are seen only as effects of a common cause. However, some (Bringmann and Eronen 2018) have suggested that rather than focusing on this contrast, a more essential contrast to focus on would be that between the approaches of dynamic and static modeling, which can render a more useful framework for conceptualizing mental disorders. In general, there is a need to carefully evaluate the reliability and validity of traditional taxonomies with respect to boundaries between psychopathology and normality.

The Hierarchical Taxonomy of Psychopathology (HiTOP) model has emerged as a research effort to address these problems. It constructs psychopathological syndromes and their components/subtypes based on the observed covariation of symptoms, grouping related symptoms together and providing an effective way to summarize and convey information on risk factors, etiology, pathophysiology, phenomenology, illness course, and treatment response (Kotov et al. 2017). This approach has been based on the empirical observation that psychopathology is generally more dimensional than categorical (Conway et al. 2019). The goal of HiTOP is to empirically organize psychopathology, provide a connection between personality and psychopathology, develop a pragmatic set of latent variables for both research and the clinic, and develop novel models and assessment instruments for psychopathology constructs that are derived from an empirical approach (Krueger et al. 2018). HiTOP currently includes, at the highest level, a general factor of psychopathology. Further down are the five domains of detachment, antagonistic externalizing, disinhibited externalizing, thought disorder, and internalizing (along with a provisional sixth somatoform dimension) that align with maladaptive personality traits (Widiger et al. 2019). Others have highlighted the need to evaluate competing theories regarding their etiology of mood and anxiety disorders by integrating information from various domains, including latent variable models, neurobiology, and quasi-experimental data (Vaidyanathan et al. 2015).

Taken together, the development of latent variable models for psychiatry in general, and mood and anxiety disorders in particular, is a dynamic field that should provide important measures that may aid a clinician to quantitatively assess an individual and utilize these assessments for precision psychiatry.

MACHINE LEARNING AND PRECISION APPROACHES TO PSYCHIATRY

There is optimism regarding the use of machine learning tools with clinical data to generate individual-level predictions. However, at this stage, none of these approaches have been sufficiently well developed to be clinically actionable. At least three steps need to be taken to move this field forward. First, all future prediction studies should be preregistered with explicitly defined machine learning approaches, prespecified independent and dependent variables, and clearly specified populations. Second, all models generated by these tools need to be validated in a completely independent sample that has not been used to generate similar predictions. Third, the utility of the prediction model will need to be tested in a preregistered randomized controlled trial in which some of the individuals are used to generate predictions and some are not. Moreover, this information needs to be tied to clinical actions and outcome variables. Ultimately, a machine learning tool is only useful if it can be shown to save lives, improve patients faster and more completely, and save money.

Studies have been accumulating evidence of process dysfunctions that affect different aspects of behavior acquired via positive or negative reinforcement as well as Pavlovian conditioning. However, several shortcomings need to be considered. First, these studies often involve case-control designs, which have limited explanatory depth and often cannot resolve the specificity of the finding. Second, studies rarely compare models to determine whether alternative explanations can provide a better description of the data. Thus, there is some uncertainty as to whether the process dysfunction as proposed by the underlying model is the best possible explanation. Third, as pointed out earlier, it is very likely that psychiatric disorders are highly heterogeneous and that there is no uniform dysfunction. However, most studies use diagnostic labels or domain dysfunctions (e.g., anhedonia) as a monolithic label. Much larger studies will be needed to address these issues, and this has prompted some to propose a phased approach not unlike what has been used to develop new pharmacological agents (Paulus et al. 2016). Such a pipeline could be used to refine machine learning models and computational models, and to help move the field toward precision psychiatry.

Clinical Illustrations

Group factor analysis (GFA) is one latent variable approach that has been useful to link variables across units of analyses (e.g., to relate symptom changes to structural or functional neuroimaging characteristics) (Klami et al. 2015). This approach has several advantages. First, the Bayesian approach allows for a robust estimation of the latent variable structure even if the ratio of the number of variables to the number of cases is relatively small (i.e., of the order of one-tenth to one-half). Second, the GFA provides an estimation of the posterior distribution of factor scores, which enables one to quickly determine the statistical significance of the variables contributing to a factors. Third, sparse prior distributions across blocks of variables provide an efficient way of separating variables that contribute to the latent structure from those that do not.

Briefly, GFA uses a Bayesian approach and can be used to identify latent variables related to psychopathology, cognitive function, and neural circuit activation patterns. The goal of GFA is to find factors that separate relationships *within* groups of variables from those *between* groups. Thus, given a collection $X_1,..., X_M$ of M blocks (groups) of variables of dimension $D_1,..., D_M$, the task is to find $K<D_1+...+D_m$ factors that describe within-block associations as well as the dependencies between the blocks X_m. This is accomplished in a Bayesian inferential framework by placing an automatic relevance determination (ARD) prior on the structure of the factor solution, which assumes a low-rank representation (rank$<<$min(K,M)) of the factor loadings. The GFA solution thus differs from canonical correlation analysis or standard factor analysis by modeling the sparsity structure across multiple blocks based on the ARD prior (Tipping 2001). The main advantages of the model are that 1) it is conceptually very simple, essentially a regular Bayesian factor analysis model that appropriately differentiates within-block and between-block associations, and 2) it hence enables the tackling of factor analysis in scenarios with more than two blocks of data. The solution comprises a set of K factors that each contain a projection vector for each of the data sets that have a non-zero weight for that factor. Thus, this computational framework provides a useful approach in extracting objective markers across levels of analyses that can be used subsequently to make individual-level predictions.

Conclusions and Future Directions

In general, results from both machine learning and computational models in psychiatry point toward several recommendations for future investigations such that results from studies can be used to improve individual predictions or help to develop empirically guided, improved clinical decision making. First, there is a need for large, multisite studies that provide sufficient data to develop robust machine learning approaches or computational models that can be validated on sufficiently large samples that have not been used to train or test the models. Computational psychiatry is currently fragmented, and the clinical samples tend to be small. A consortium of investigators may help to advance the field (Paulus et al. 2016). Second, machine learning predictions are frequently evaluated based on their ability to correctly predict outcomes. However, they are rarely examined regarding whether they contribute to better decision making in a clinical context. For example, if a machine learning algorithm can predict improvement or non-improvement in a particular patient population, would this algorithm help to improve the number needed to treat if applied before the individuals undergo treatment? Currently, there are few studies that have taken this prospective approach (Kingslake et al. 2017). Third, computational models provide evidence-based explanations of behavior in disease populations, but most investigations do not actively compare alternative accounts of these explanations. Specifically, behavioral task performance could be explained by a reinforcement learning model or a belief-based updating model. These approaches provide complementary explanations of how the individual arrives at a decision. Nevertheless, these differences may be important for the development of process-specific behavioral interventions. Fourth, although many of the initial computational models were developed in animal models, there has been a surprising dearth of studies that use translational paradigms to examine computational dysfunctions in both humans and animals (for a possible exception, see Joyner et al. 2018). This would be particularly helpful in the development of novel pharmacological agents aimed at correcting some of these dysfunctions.

Taken together, computational psychiatry holds promise for both pragmatic and explanatory domains in psychiatry. However, the field is at an early stage, and discretion is the better part of valor when it comes to what impact the results will have on improving mental health assessment, prognosis, and treatment.

KEY POINTS

- To develop personalized interventions for psychiatric illnesses, we must acquire quantitative, reliable, and robust predictive objective markers.

- Although much of the prior psychiatric research has aimed to find statistically significant differences between groups, we propose instead to focus on developing predictive models using mathematical algorithmic approaches and unsupervised learning algorithms that address real clinical needs.

- There is a substantial demand for developing latent variable models to conceptualize psychiatric illness. Latent variable models, wherein the mental disorder is a latent variable that causes a collection of symptoms on a continuum, contrast with the current discrete classification of psychiatric disorders, and may better aid clinicians in quantitatively assessing and treating each individual patient.

- Machine learning methods can potentially generate individual-level predictions for psychiatry, but none of these approaches have been adequately developed to be clinically actionable.

- To advance psychiatric health assessment, prognosis, and treatment, there is a need for large multisite projects that provide enough data to develop robust machine learning approaches or computational models, and more investigations of computational models comparing evidenced-based explanations of behavior in psychiatric illness in addition to alternative accounts, as well as further use of translational paradigms to examine computational dysfunctions in humans and animals.

References

Bollen KA: Latent variables in psychology and the social sciences. Annu Rev Psychol 53:605–634, 2002 11752498

Borsboom D, Rhemtulla M, Cramer AO, et al: Kinds versus continua: a review of psychometric approaches to uncover the structure of psychiatric constructs. Psychol Med 46(8):1567–1579, 2016 26997244

Bosco FA, Aguinis H, Singh K, et al: Correlational effect size benchmarks. J Appl Psychol 100(2):431–449, 2015 25314367

Brendel DH: Reductionism, eclecticism, and pragmatism in psychiatry: the dialectic of clinical explanation. J Med Philos 28(5–6):563–580, 2003 14972761

Bringmann LF, Eronen MI: Don't blame the model: reconsidering the network approach to psychopathology. Psychol Rev 125(4):606–615, 2018 29952625

Bunte K, Leppäaho E, Saarinen I, et al: Sparse group factor analysis for biclustering of multiple data sources. Bioinformatics 32(16):2457–2463, 2016 27153643

Conway CC, Forbes MK, Forbush KT, et al: A hierarchical taxonomy of psychopathology can transform mental health research. Perspect Psychol Sci 14(3):419–436, 2019 30844330

Cramer AO, Waldorp LJ, van der Maas HL, et al: Comorbidity: a network perspective. Behav Brain Sci 33(2–3):137–150, discussion 150–193, 2010 20584369

Cuthbert BN, Insel TR: Toward the future of psychiatric diagnosis: the seven pillars of RDoC. BMC Med 11:126, 2013 23672542

Gignac GE, Szodorai ET: Effect size guidelines for individual differences researchers. Pers Individ Dif 102:74–78, 2016

Halberstadt SM, Schmitz KH, Sammel MD: A joint latent variable model approach to item reduction and validation. Biostatistics 13(1):48–60, 2012 21775486

Hastie T, Tibshirani R, Friedman JH: The Elements of Statistical Learning: Data Mining, Inference, and Prediction. New York, Springer, 2001

Huys QJ, Maia TV, Frank MJ: Computational psychiatry as a bridge from neuroscience to clinical applications. Nat Neurosci 19(3):404–413, 2016 26906507

Insel T, Cuthbert B, Garvey M, et al: Research domain criteria (RDoC): toward a new classification framework for research on mental disorders. Am J Psychiatry 167(7):748–751, 2010 20595427

Johnson BT, Scott-Sheldon LAJ, Carey MP: Meta-synthesis of health behavior change meta-analyses. Am J Public Health 100(11):2193–2198, 2010 20167901

Joyner MA, Gearhardt AN, Flagel SB: A translational model to assess sign-tracking and goal-tracking behavior in children. Neuropsychopharmacology 43(1):228–229, 2018 29192653

Kendler KS: Toward a philosophical structure for psychiatry. Am J Psychiatry 162(3):433–440, 2005 15741457

Kendler KS: Explanatory models for psychiatric illness. Am J Psychiatry 165(6):695–702, 2008 18483135

Kendler KS: David Skae and his nineteenth century etiologic psychiatric diagnostic system: looking forward by looking back. Mol Psychiatry 22(6):802–807, 2017a 28289276

Kendler KS: DSM disorders and their criteria: how should they inter-relate? Psychol Med 47(12):2054–2060, 2017b 28374657

Kendler KS, Engstrom EJ: Kahlbaum, Hecker, and Kraepelin and the transition from psychiatric symptom complexes to empirical disease forms. Am J Psychiatry 174(2):102–109, 2017 27523503

Kingslake J, Dias R, Dawson GR, et al: The effects of using the PReDicT Test to guide the antidepressant treatment of depressed patients: study protocol for a randomised controlled trial. Trials 18(1):558, 2017 29169399

Klami A, Virtanen S, Leppäaho E, et al: Group factor analysis. IEEE Trans Neural Netw Learn Syst 26(9):2136–2147, 2015 25532193

Kotov R, Krueger RF, Watson D, et al: The Hierarchical Taxonomy of Psychopathology (HiTOP): a dimensional alternative to traditional nosologies. J Abnorm Psychol 126(4):454–477, 2017 28333488

Krueger RF, Kotov R, Watson D, et al: Progress in achieving quantitative classification of psychopathology. World Psychiatry 17(3):282–293, 2018 30229571

Menzies P: The causal structure of mechanisms. Stud Hist Philos Biol Biomed Sci 43(4):796–805, 2012 22709915

Miettunen J, Nordström T, Kaakinen M, et al: Latent variable mixture modeling in psychiatric research—a review and application. Psychol Med 46(3):457–467, 2016 26526221

Monden R, Wardenaar KJ, Stegeman A, et al: Simultaneous decomposition of depression heterogeneity on the person-, symptom- and time-level: the use of three-mode principal component analysis. PLoS One 10(7):e0132765, 2015 26177365

Montague PR, Dolan RJ, Friston KJ, et al: Computational psychiatry. Trends Cogn Sci 16(1):72–80, 2012 22177032

Palmer RF, Graham JW, Taylor B, et al: Construct validity in health behavior research: interpreting latent variable models involving self-report and objective measures. J Behav Med 25(6):525–550, 2002 12462957

Paulus MP, Huys QJ, Maia TV: A roadmap for the development of applied computational psychiatry. Biol Psychiatry Cogn Neurosci Neuroimaging 1(5):386–392, 2016 28018986

Prenoveau JM, Craske MG, Zinbarg RE, et al: Are anxiety and depression just as stable as personality during late adolescence? Results from a three-year longitudinal latent variable study. J Abnorm Psychol 120(4):832–843, 2011 21604827

Rothman KJ, Greenland S: Causation and causal inference in epidemiology. Am J Public Health 95 (suppl 1):S144–S150, 2005 16030331

Stephan KE, Mathys C: Computational approaches to psychiatry. Curr Opin Neurobiol 25:85–92, 2014 24709605

Ten Have M, Lamers F, Wardenaar K, et al: The identification of symptom-based subtypes of depression: a nationally representative cohort study. J Affect Disord 190:395–406, 2016 26546775

Tipping ME: Sparse Bayesian learning and the relevance vector machine. J Mach Learn Res 1(3):211–244, 2001

Vaidyanathan U, Vrieze SI, Iacono WG: The power of theory, research design, and transdisciplinary integration in moving psychopathology forward. Psychol Inq 26(3):209–230, 2015 27030789

van Loo HM, de Jonge P, Romeijn JW, et al: Data-driven subtypes of major depressive disorder: a systematic review. BMC Med 10:156, 2012 23210727

Watson D, Stasik SM, Ellickson-Larew S, Stanton K: Extraversion and psychopathology: a facet-level analysis. J Abnorm Psychol 124(2):432–446, 2015 25751628

Widiger TA, Bach B, Chmielewski M, et al: Criterion A of the AMPD in HiTOP. J Pers Assess 101(4):345–355, 2019 29746190

Zachar P, Kendler KS: The philosophy of nosology. Annu Rev Clin Psychol 13:49–71, 2017 28482691

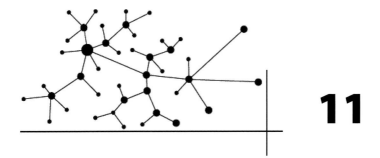

11

COMPUTATIONAL COGNITIVE METHODS FOR PRECISION PSYCHIATRY

Quentin J.M. Huys, M.D., Ph.D.

History

The burden of mental illnesses is large (World Health Organization 2017), and the treatment gap remains wide. While many different treatment approaches exist, it is often hard to predict who will respond to which treatment. Furthermore, a substantial fraction of those affected experience a relapsing or chronic course of illness (e.g., Angst et al. 2003). In this setting, it would clearly be useful if clinicians had the ability to target treatments more precisely.

Treatment precision has two facets. On the one hand, precise treatments remove the cause of the illness with minimal other effects. On the other hand, individuals differ and may react differently to the same treatment even if they suffer from the putatively same causative agent. Hence, an aim

The author would like to acknowledge support by the Max Planck UCL Centre for Computational Psychiatry and Ageing Research.

of precision treatment is for it to be personalized and to take constitutional or illness factors of individuals and their individual disease processes into account when refining the choice of treatment (Collins and Varmus 2015). Although this is a standard feature of many aspects of medicine, advances in molecular techniques have dramatically increased the scope of personalization and precision. A precision approach has arguably been most successful in the field of oncology, in which genomic signatures of individual cancers are used to guide treatment.

In psychiatry, parallel efforts have led to the use of genetic information regarding the effect of liver metabolic enzymes on the pharmacokinetic properties of medications, because ideal dosing will depend on the metabolism of the medication, and these tests are starting to enter standard clinical practice (Peterson et al. 2017). On a different level, personalization has long been woven tightly into the treatments of mental illnesses. For instance, cognitive-behavioral therapy aims to identify and then modify the individual's underlying core beliefs. The core beliefs that are the focus of the therapy are highly specific to the individual. A similar focus on the details of an individual's illness is a prominent feature of many psychotherapies. The understanding that mental illnesses are usually worsened by stress is reflected in the broad acceptance of the importance of holistic care—for example, in Engel's (1980) biopsychosocial model—and this in turn has facilitated specific social, financial, housing, and other support interventions, which certainly are "personalized." Precision psychiatry, as understood in this book, aims to leverage our recent advances in the understanding of the brain and the explosion in technological capacities to further improve how treatments are developed and targeted (Fernandes et al. 2017; Perna et al. 2018).

In this chapter I briefly outline the motivation for a computational approach to mental illness before focusing on the use of tasks to probe specific computational processes. A major hindrance to the translation of tasks into clinical practice is their apparent low reliability. Therefore, I examine possible causes of this in some detail.

Computational Psychiatry

When one is considering illnesses that arise from a particular organ, it is critically important to keep the main function of that organ in mind. For instance, many features of heart failure are only understandable when one is cognizant of the fact that the heart has a pumping function and is key to maintaining appropriate pressure gradients across the cardiovascular system. The same is true for the brain, the key function of which is to compute: storing information, deriving succinct summaries of it, and using that information to make predictions about the future. What sets the brain apart from all other organs is the fact that its ability to process information changes as a function of the information it has already processed and stored; in other words, it learns. Although other organs adapt, as do muscles, the changes in the brain's ability at a higher level are not just quantitative (such as more strength) but qualitative. Through learning, the brain can come to perform novel computations, and through its ability to compute, it can change how and what it learns. Just as the inability to meet pumping demands is the defining feature of heart disease, the inability to meet computing and storage demands shapes the signs and symptoms of brain disease (see "Computational Components of Depressive Symptoms" below for an example). While some computational demands have obvious consequences in terms of movement or sensory deficits, others are more subtle, affecting a brain's ability to solve abstract or complex social problems (i.e., to perform higher cognitive functions). An understanding of these dysfunctions is likely to require an understanding of the functions affected, and if these functions are primarily computational, then a computational approach might well be necessary.

COMPUTATIONAL COMPONENTS OF DEPRESSIVE SYMPTOMS

Computational processes are likely involved in both the etiology and the treatment of major depressive disorder, a syndrome with low mood, anhedonia. and low energy at its core (American Psychiatric Association 2013; Mitchell et al. 2009; World Health Organization 1990). The odds of having a first episode increase by a factor of nearly 10 after experiencing a major life event (Kendler et al. 2000). The causal link from experiences such as life events, which are external to the brain, to symptoms such as mood and energy must flow via some form of interpretation of the events and hence must involve a computational process and learning. Indeed, biases in information processing have long been established as risk factors for depression (Alloy et al. 1999). A similar argument can be made for psychotherapeutic treatments such as behavioral activation (Dimidjian et al. 2006; Jacobson et al. 1996). Although specific implementations of this therapy vary, they broadly involve teaching individuals to act from "outside in"—that is, to act according to their goals rather than their current emotional state, and supporting them in formulating specific, measurable, achievable, realistic, and temporally defined (SMART) goals. The aim is to increase the rate at which activities with positive consequences are performed, leading to an overall increased rate of experienced rewards and thereby a reduction in negative mood. While behavioral activation is a particularly clear example, the causal link of any psychotherapeutic intervention must at some point involve computational and learning processes because there are no direct influences on the brain systems that determine the symptoms. Interestingly, the original behavioral activation study found that response to the behavioral component appeared to relate to a change in cognitive features (attributional style) engendered by the intervention (Jacobson et al. 1996).

Computational psychiatry is a young field that is at the intersection of psychiatry, psychology, neuroscience, mathematics, statistics, and machine learning. It attempts to harness advances in theoretical and computational insights to address clinical issues in the realm of psychiatric illnesses (Huys et al. 2011, 2016b; Montague et al. 2012; Rutledge et al. 2019; Stephan and Mathys 2014; Stephan et al. 2016, 2017; Wang and Krystal 2014). The motivation for using mathematical and computational methods to approach subjective phenomena such as mood, paranoia, and trauma is, broadly speaking, twofold, reflecting the theoretical considerations about the nature of mental illnesses discussed above as well as data-analytic considerations (Bennett et al. 2019; Huys 2018; Huys et al. 2016b).

The data-analytic side itself has multiple aspects (Bzdok and Meyer-Lindenberg 2018; Stephan et al. 2017; Woo et al. 2017). First, testing computational theories about brain functions and their involvement in mental illness requires the use of advanced analytic methods. For instance, theories of learning are most thoroughly tested by building generative computational models and examining how well they explain data (Piray et al. 2019; Wetzels et al. 2010). Second, data of increasing richness, complexity, and volume are now being gathered routinely thanks to advances in neuroimaging, mobile devices, data storage, and online and computer technology (see, e.g., Gillan and Daw 2016). Researchers and clinicians are therefore increasingly faced with large data sets. Deriving insights from such data sets and correctly interpreting them requires familiarity with computational methods that range from programming to complex machine-learning. Large data sets also raise fundamental issues regarding the stability and validity of inference. Some inference problems—such as regression—become ill-posed when the dimensionality of the data (e.g., the number of data points per subject) is too high, and these problems require sophisticated methods such as regularization, dimensionality reduction, Bayesian model evidence estimation, cross-validation, or the training of deep neural networks.

An important contribution of data-analytic approaches is a renewed emphasis on cross-validation (Stone 1974). The term *prediction* has often been used to describe associations in correlational analyses (e.g., regressions), but such associations often do not generalize to novel data sets, and hence they represent instances of overfitting (Huys et al. 2016b). These instances can be addressed by validating them on a separate data set, and techniques such as cross-validation provide estimates of the likely generalizability of any findings. More generally, machine learning approaches enable the pragmatic discovery of potential signatures of illness or treatment response. This is becoming more attractive as the cost of acquiring vast data sets is reduced (Rutledge et al. 2019).

These arguments suggest why computational methods are likely to play an important role in the development of novel targets and treatments for mental illnesses (Maia et al. 2017; Wang and Krystal 2014). They also suggest that researchers in the area of mental health are likely to be faced with computational challenges, and thus it may be useful to ensure researcher literacy with computational methods through teaching programs.

Tasks to Measure Computational Functions

There are many ways in which computational tools can come to support precision psychiatry in everyday clinical practice. We have previously described a broad procedure for bringing computational tools into the clinic that is modeled on the drug developmental pipeline, with a large number of tools being examined preclinically, and the most promising ones being optimized for robustness prior to being put through randomized clinical trials (Paulus et al. 2016). Clearly, this is not a project to be fulfilled by a single lab; there is an urgent need for large-scale collaborations (Browning et al. 2020).

In this chapter, I focus on one important role that computational tools will likely assume in daily clinical practice: that of measurement using tasks. Measurements of relevant computational processes could have many different applications, such as diagnosis, treatment allocation, treatment monitoring, and risk assessment. Tasks are likely to play a key role in measurement because they represent the most direct approach to measuring specific learning and computational functions. There is now a large and rapidly growing wealth of tasks that activate, and thereby measure, increasingly complex and well-defined computational functions (Aylward et al. 2019; Berwian et al. 2020; Browning et al. 2015; Daw et al. 2011; Frank et al. 2004; Huys and Renz 2017; Huys et al. 2012, 2013; Mathews and MacLeod 2005; Mkrtchian et al. 2017; Pizzagalli et al. 2005; Rutledge et al. 2017). The recent increase in mobile devices and computers, coupled with the development of toolboxes for efficient task deployment in browsers or apps, has profoundly reduced barriers to the deployment of tasks as probes in clinical settings (Gillan and Daw 2016; Rutledge et al. 2019).

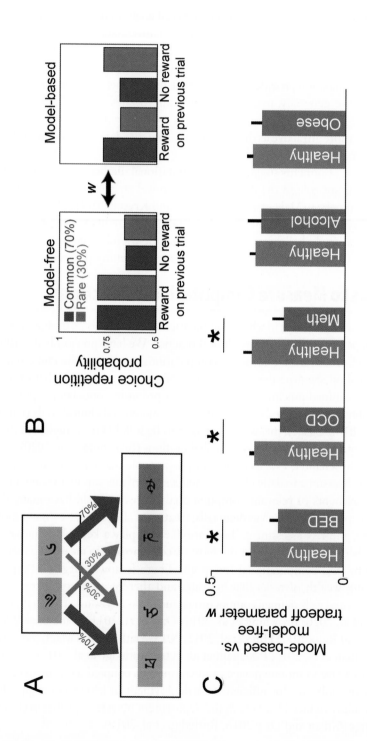

Figure 11–1. (*Opposite page*) Two-step task.

To view this figure in color, see Plate 6 in Color Gallery.

(A) Participants must first choose among two of the green stimuli. Each of the stimuli probabilistically leads to one of the second-stage stimulus sets with high probability, and to the other set with low probability. Participants then choose one of the two resulting second-stage stimuli and obtain a reward or not. **(B)** A model-free strategy here corresponds to repeating the first-stage (green) choice if the second-stage choice was rewarded, irrespective of the frequency of the transition observed. A model-based strategy takes the transition probability into account: after a rare transition, a reward leads to a switch at the first stage. Consider choosing the left green choice, but transitioning to the blue second stage and then obtaining a reward. In order to gain another reward from the same blue stimulus, the best strategy takes the transition probability into account and leads to a switch of the unchosen first-stage stimulus. Individuals typically use a mixture of these two strategies, which can be measured by the parameter w. **(C)** Patients who have binge-eating disorder (BED), obsessive-compulsive disorder (OCD), or methamphetamine dependence (Meth), but not obesity or alcohol dependence, show a reduction in the parameter w that trades off between these strategies (i.e., they show a shift toward mode-free decision making).

Source. Panels A and B adapted and redrawn from Daw et al. 2011. Panel C adapted and redrawn from Voon et al. 2015.

For instance, the widely used two-step task (Figure 11–1) attempts to capture an individual's tendency to learn and make decisions via one of two strategies: model-free or model-based (Daw et al. 2011). Model-free learning has been related to habitual decisions, and model-based learning to goal-directed behavior (Friedel et al. 2015). In model-free learning, individuals learn by summing up prediction errors over multiple repetitions. Model-free decisions that rely on these values hence change slowly over time. In contrast, model-based decisions require on-the-fly inference. While this approach to decision-making is computationally demanding, it is also able to more rapidly adjust to any new information. In large samples across multiple settings, patients with a variety of compulsive disorders—including obsessive-compulsive disorder, binge eating, and methamphetamine dependence—show a characteristic pattern on this and related tasks, with a bias toward model-free and away from model-based reasoning (Gillan et al. 2016, 2020; Patzelt et al. 2019; Voon et al. 2015). Patients with alcohol addiction do not show this pattern (Huys et al. 2016a; Nebe et al. 2018).

Another example task is the affective Go-NoGo task (Guitart-Masip et al. 2012) (Figure 11–2). Tasks that measure Pavlovian influences on instrumental choice have shown robust sensitivity to alcohol dependence (Garbusow et al. 2019), anxiety (Mkrtchian et al. 2017), trauma (Ousdal et al. 2018), and suicidality (Millner et al. 2019). The last-mentioned finding in particular is noteworthy. The authors modified the task so that individuals could learn to avoid or escape unpleasant sounds either through active (Go) or passive (NoGo) behavior. Patients with lifetime nonfatal suicidal thoughts and behaviors showed a selective increase in the tendency to actively escape from the aversive noise. Tasks such as these have great potential as structured probes for directly measuring—with high precision and at low cost—high-level processes that are not accessible to techniques such as self-report, observation, or biochemical or neuroimaging assays (Barch et al. 2008).

For the ideal clinical scenario, such tasks would result in task-derived measures (TDMs) of specific computational or learning processes that a) are mechanistically involved in causing illness and b) are amenable to interventions. The impact of a particular intervention might then be mediated by its impact on the TDMs (Figure 11–3A). In this situation, measuring the TDMs would have substantial value for precision psychiatry. The presence of a raised or reduced TDM would indicate the presence of the particular etiological process. This in turn would enable differential treatment allocation to those interventions known to impact this particular TDM. In the absence of any abnormalities in any TDMs, futile exposure to likely unhelpful treatment could be avoided.

The key steps toward these goals hinge on the notion of discovering and engaging mechanisms relevant to mental illnesses. First, tasks need to be designed that yield reliable, robust, and clinically deployable individual differences in a computational or learning process (Figure 11–3B). This area is currently in great need of development, and we will focus on it in the next section. Once such robust TDMs have been established, their relevance to particular symptoms or illnesses must be established, for instance, via traditional case-control or correlational dimensional studies. Here, the advent of online methods promises to greatly accelerate the examination of new probes (e.g., Gillan and Daw 2016; Gillan et al. 2016; Rouault et al. 2018). However, it is also worth pointing out the value of longitudinal studies. Although still correlational, the examination of how symptoms covary with a TDM within individuals over time avoids at least some of the more fundamental problems inherent in cross-sectional designs (Borsboom et al. 2009; Molenaar and Campbell 2009). We must then examine whether the TDMs can be engaged by interventions, and whether a change in the TDMs must mediate the improvement in symptoms due to targeted interventions. Clearly, this is a very high bar. Indeed, few tasks have been examined in all of these scenarios. One exception is the two-step task, which has not shown changes with clinical state after psychotherapy (Wheaton et al. 2019). Although negative, this finding may relate to the low reliability of the task (see next section), and such research is critical for the development of precision tools.

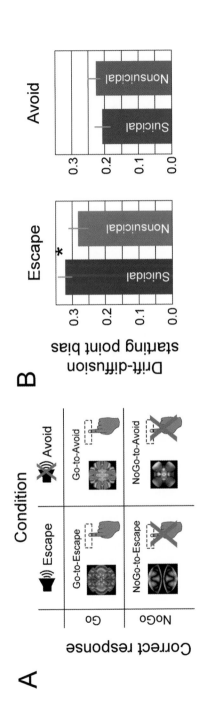

Figure 11–2. Affective Go-NoGo task.

To view this figure in color, see Plate 7 in Color Gallery.

(A) Individuals were taught to choose whether to Go or NoGo (respond on a button) for different stimuli. With some stimuli (fractals), an unpleasant tone could be escaped or entirely avoided by a Go response (*top row*). With other stimuli, the unpleasant tone could be escaped or avoided by a NoGo response (*bottom row*). (B) A computational model fitted to the data extracts a key parameter on which groups differed. Participants with a lifetime history of suicidal ideation showed a selective bias toward actively escaping, but did not show a bias in the avoid condition. The bias here was the starting point of a drift-diffusion model (Ratcliff and Smith 2004).

Source. Adapted from Millner et al. 2019.

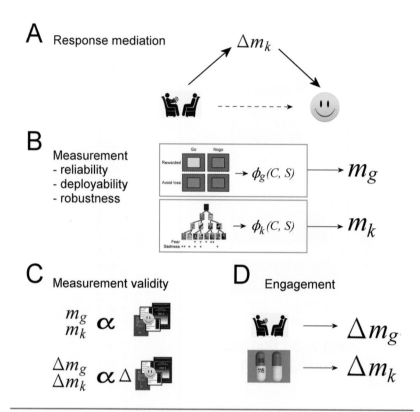

Figure I I–3. Measuring mechanisms for the clinic.

To view this figure in color, see Plate 8 in Color Gallery.

(A) For precision targeting, the measures derived from computational probes should mediate the effect of interventions. The measure m_k can be used to decide whether to apply intervention k if intervention k reduces measure m_k, and this measure m_k relates in a mechanistic or causal way to the illness. For instance, if antibiotics reduce certain bacterial cell counts, and these bacterial cell counts cause symptoms such as fever, then applying this antibiotic is likely to lead to an improvement in symptoms via its impact on the bacteria. **(B)** To be useful for precision targeting, computational probes, which might involve the results of a task being analyzed with some computational model and producing a measure m_k or m_g, must be reliable at the individual level. The probes must also be deployable in clinical settings and be robust to typical clinical situations. **(C)** Measurements derived from computational probes must be valid (i.e., changes in these measurements should covary with changes in other measures of illness within individuals over time and between individuals). **(D)** Treatments, be they novel or established, should impact the measurement.

Limitations of Current Task-Based Measurements

Computational probes that involve tasks must deliver reliable measurements if they are to be used clinically (Barch et al. 2008; Savitz et al. 2013). It has recently become clear that the reliability of many TDMs is still below the level of reliability deemed necessary for potential clinical utility (Barch et al. 2008; Savitz et al. 2013). Strikingly, this is even true for classical tasks that have stood the test of time. For instance, Hedge et al. (2018) examined tasks such as the Stroop, Eriksen flanker, and stop-signal tasks and found that although the effects at the group level were reliable, the effects at the individual level were not. Even the Stroop reaction time cost (i.e., the difference in reaction times to congruent and incongruent stimuli) only showed a test-retest intraclass correlation coefficient of 0.6. A meta-analysis of published test-retest reliability measurements and a large-scale online study suggest a reliability somewhere between 0.3 and 0.6 across a wide variety of tasks (Enkavi et al. 2019). Importantly, this value was substantially lower than the reliability of self-report surveys, which is around 0.6–0.7.

The causes for low reliability fall into four categories: time, strategy, noise, and research setting. First, if the underlying cognitive mechanism changes with time, the measure will appear less reliable. A variety of TDMs do show excellent split-half reliabilities or reliability when the task is repeated immediately, but this reliability drops when repetition occurs after a period of weeks to months (Ahn et al. 2020; Garbusow et al. 2014; Pooseh et al. 2018; Shahar et al. 2019). For instance, Ahn et al. (2020) reported reliabilities above 0.9 for immediate test-retest, but these fell to 0.8 within a month. A number of reports on the low test-retest reliability of tasks are based on the examination of reliability over delays of months or even years (Enkavi et al. 2019; Hedge et al. 2018). Although this may be the right timescale to examine cognitive processes that relate to stable personality factors, cognitive processes of relevance to the treatment of mental illnesses are expected to change on the same timescale as psychopathological states change and should be amenable to therapeutic interventions. As such, the aim should be the establishment of TDMs that are highly reliable over short periods, but sensitive to relevant psychopathological changes (Duff 2012) over a period of weeks.

Second, tasks may appear unreliable because the strategy an individual employs to solve the task changes. This will also reduce internal consistency (Hajcak et al. 2017). For example, through practice, individuals might discover shortcuts to solving a task, or engage less with demanding processes due to fatigue. The presence of such inconsistencies can be examined using measures such as split-half reliability. Their nature can be identified through computational modeling, enabling particular strategies to be formulated as generative models. These can then be run on the task and provide quantitative measures as to how well a particular strategy explains the behavior on a task (Berwian et al. 2020; Guitart-Masip et al. 2012; Huys et al. 2012, 2015; Schlagenhauf et al. 2014). Indeed, a change in strategy is likely to account for some of the changes seen with time, which have traditionally been ascribed to a change in the underlying cognitive mechanism.

Third, noise in a TDM will reduce the estimated reliability; this noise can sometimes be reduced by making tasks longer (Rouder and Haaf 2019), though this does not improve all TDMs equally (Enkavi et al. 2019). For instance, in learning tasks, early trials are informative about the learning process, but once a strategy has been selected and reached stability, additional trials no longer provide information about the learning process. Therefore, the best strategy to reduce noise in the estimation of a particular process depends on the specific process. Techniques such as active learning or adaptive design optimization provide principled ways of maximizing the amount of information acquired per trial (Chaloner and Verdinelli 1995; MacKay 1992; Myung et al. 2013; Paninski 2005). As an example, consider delay discounting (Ahn et al. 2020; Pooseh et al. 2018). In this, individuals must repeatedly choose between receiving a small monetary amount sooner (e.g., $7 now) or a larger amount later (e.g., $14 in 2 months). Traditional approaches ask a fixed set of questions. However, if the subject has already accepted waiting 2 months for $14, then they are very likely to also be willing to wait 2 months for $42, and hence this item will not add much information. An alternative is to choose an option in which the evidence gathered so far suggests equal probabilities for choosing the early and late option—an example of uncertainty sampling (Pooseh et al. 2018; Schulz et al. 2018; Settles 2012). Indeed, these ideas underlie adaptive testing in item response theory approaches (Embretson and Reise 2000) but have only rarely been exploited in the setting of tasks for mental health assessment (Aranovich et al. 2017).

Strong guarantees exist regarding the usefulness of information-guided adaptive optimization if the underlying process is static and does not interact with the process (Paninski 2005). However, human task strategies may change; in particular, a subject may respond to the presence of changes in the task with shifts in strategy. More global optimization problems are computationally challenging (Krause et al. 2008). But promising approaches include a combination of dynamic programming with adaptive design (Kim et al. 2017), and there is a dearth of optimization work that has explicitly attempted to avoid inducing changes in the underlying cognitive process, or indeed measured this.

Another important aspect of noise in TDMs is the reduction of estimated correlation with other processes of interest (Spearman 1987). This may lead to processes being deemed irrelevant when this is not the case (Rouder and Haaf 2019). One approach is to take uncertainty into account, either via computational models (Huys et al. 2012, 2013; Price et al. 2019; Shahar et al. 2019; Yang et al. 2020) or via hierarchical estimation procedures (Gelman et al. 2013; Huys et al. 2012, 2013; Piray et al. 2019; Rouder and Haaf 2019; Wetzels et al. 2010). Accounting for noise in the context of temporal reliability enables the estimation of a theoretical upper limit on reliability.

Tasks with higher theoretical reliability can in principle be lengthened or optimized to achieve this reliability, and hence may have clinical value. Taking uncertainty into account when examining covariation with other variables prevents the disregarding of potentially important processes.

Fourth, what exactly is viewed as "the same result" varies in different research settings (Borsboom et al. 2009; Cronbach 1957). In a traditional experimental psychology setting, a task is viewed as reliable if it produces an effect at the group level when repeated in a different sample. Variation between individuals hurts this notion of reliability. If individuals vary substantially, then the effect at the group level—usually measured by dividing the mean by the standard deviation—will necessarily be lower. On the other hand, in the context of the individual differences literature, a reliable measure is one that ranks individuals in the same order on repeated administrations. Here, variation between individuals—measured by correlation coefficients—generally increases reliability as the between-individual variability appears in the numerator (Hedge et al. 2018). Unlike questionnaires, tasks have generally been designed in the experimental psychology tradition, and hence are typically geared at maximizing group-level reliability. As such, the component of variability attributable to differences between individuals is generally lower (Enkavi et al. 2019; Hedge et al. 2018). This is one major reason for the comparatively low reliability of tasks compared with questionnaires and is a major hurdle for the translation of tasks into a clinical setting.

Conclusion and Future Directions

Computational approaches to mental health are motivated by the computational and learning functions of the brain, and by the complexity and quantity of data being acquired. Tasks are likely to be important for precision psychiatry because they enable the probing of specific learning and computational functions. However, tasks must be further developed to achieve the reliability and robustness necessary for clinical deployment. As described here, computational models are likely to play an important role in this because they can account for noise and strategy changes, and also facilitate adaptive sampling techniques. Once tasks have been designed that are both valid and reliable, researchers will need to shift their attention toward studies that ask whether the processes can be engaged by therapies, and whether they mediate therapeutic improvement. It might even be advantageous to consider such longitudinal studies early on (particularly in the setting of treatments).

Although the focus here has mainly been on tasks, similar arguments can be made for other techniques including, in particular, neuroimaging. Here, too, very reliable methods have not reached the reliabilities necessary for clinical deployment (Braun et al. 2012; Plichta et al. 2012; Savitz et al. 2013), and at least as far as they are to be used as measurements, similar arguments as for tasks can be made.

KEY POINTS

- When an organ is unable to meet the demands placed on it, illness can arise. The main functions of the brain are to compute and learn. Therefore, our understanding of mental illnesses will benefit from understanding the computational and learning functions the brain performs, and how these are affected in states of ill health.

- Measurement through a patient's performance of tasks enables us to probe highly specific computational and learning processes.

- For precision applications, measurement should be reliable, relate to the pathological process, and be engaged by therapeutic interventions.

- Identification of disease mechanisms via tasks can facilitate the development of targeted interventions and the targeted administration of therapies.

- The clinical use of tasks currently faces issues with regard to reliability and robustness, involving time, strategy, noise, and research setting, which are at least partially amenable to computational techniques.

References

Ahn W-Y, Gu H, Shen Y, et al: Rapid, precise, and reliable phenotyping of delay discounting using a Bayesian learning algorithm. Sci Rep 10(1):12091, 2020 32694654

Alloy LB, Abramson LY, Whitehouse WG, et al: Depressogenic cognitive styles: predictive validity, information processing and personality characteristics, and developmental origins. Behav Res Ther 37(6):503–531, 1999 10372466

American Psychiatric Association: Diagnostic and Statistical Manual of Mental Disorders, 5th Edition. Arlington, VA, American Psychiatric Association, 2013

Angst J, Gamma A, Sellaro R, et al: Recurrence of bipolar disorders and major depression. A life-long perspective. Eur Arch Psychiatry Clin Neurosci 253(5):236–240, 2003 14504992

Aranovich GJ, Cavagnaro DR, Pitt MA, et al: A model-based analysis of decision making under risk in obsessive-compulsive and hoarding disorders. J Psychiatr Res 90:126–132, 2017 28279877

Aylward J, Valton V, Ahn W-Y, et al: Altered learning under uncertainty in unmedicated mood and anxiety disorders. Nat Hum Behav 3(10):1116–1123, 2019 31209369

Barch DM, Carter CS, Committee CE: Measurement issues in the use of cognitive neuroscience tasks in drug development for impaired cognition in schizophrenia: a report of the second consensus building conference of the CNTRICS initiative. Schizophr Bull 34(4):613–618, 2008 18499705

Bennett D, Silverstein SM, Niv Y: The two cultures of computational psychiatry. JAMA Psychiatry 76(6):563–564, 2019 31017638

Berwian IM, Wenzel J, Collins AG, et al: Computational mechanisms of effort and reward decisions in depression and their relationship to relapse after antidepressant discontinuation. JAMA Psychiatry 77(5):513–522, 2020

Borsboom D, Kievit RA, Cervone D, et al: The two disciplines of scientific psychology, or: the disunity of psychology as a working hypothesis, in Dynamic Process Methodology in the Social and Developmental Sciences. Edited by Valsiner J, Molenaar PCM, Lyra MCDP, et al. New York, Springer, 2009, pp 67–98

Braun U, Plichta MM, Esslinger C, et al: Test-retest reliability of resting-state connectivity network characteristics using fMRI and graph theoretical measures. Neuroimage 59(2):1404–1412, 2012 21888983

Browning M, Behrens TE, Jocham G, et al: Anxious individuals have difficulty learning the causal statistics of aversive environments. Nat Neurosci 18(4):590–596, 2015 25730669

Browning M, Carter CS, Chatham C, et al: Realizing the clinical potential of computational psychiatry: report from the Banbury Center Meeting, February 2019. Biol Psychiatry 15(2):e5–e10, 2020 32113656

Bzdok D, Meyer-Lindenberg A: Machine learning for precision psychiatry: opportunities and challenges. Biol Psychiatry Cogn Neurosci Neuroimaging 3(3):223–230, 2018 29486863

Chaloner K, Verdinelli I: Bayesian experimental design: a review. Statistical Science 10(3):273–304, 1995

Collins FS, Varmus H: A new initiative on precision medicine. N Engl J Med 372(9):793–795, 2015 25635347

Cronbach LJ: The two disciplines of scientific psychology. American Psychologist 12(11):671–684, 1957

Daw ND, Gershman SJ, Seymour B, et al: Model-based influences on humans' choices and striatal prediction errors. Neuron 69(6):1204–1215, 2011 21435563

Dimidjian S, Hollon SD, Dobson KS, et al: Randomized trial of behavioral activation, cognitive therapy, and antidepressant medication in the acute treatment of adults with major depression. J Consult Clin Psychol 74(4):658–670, 2006 16881773

Duff K: Evidence-based indicators of neuropsychological change in the individual patient: relevant concepts and methods. Arch Clin Neuropsychol 27(3):248–261, 2012 22382384

Embretson SE, Reise SP: Item Response Theory for Psychologists. Mahway, NJ, Erlbaum, 2000

Engel GL: The clinical application of the biopsychosocial model. Am J Psychiatry 137(5):535–544, 1980 7369396

Enkavi AZ, Eisenberg IW, Bissett PG, et al: Large-scale analysis of test-retest reliabilities of self-regulation measures. Proc Natl Acad Sci USA 116(12):5472–5477, 2019 30842284

Fernandes BS, Williams LM, Steiner J, et al: The new field of "precision psychiatry." BMC Med 15(1):80, 2017 28403846

Frank MJ, Seeberger LC, O'reilly RC: By carrot or by stick: cognitive reinforcement learning in parkinsonism. Science 306(5703):1940–1943, 2004 15528409

Friedel E, Schlagenhauf F, Beck A, et al: The effects of life stress and neural learning signals on fluid intelligence. Eur Arch Psychiatry Clin Neurosci 265(1):35–43, 2015 25142177

Garbusow M, Schad DJ, Sommer C, et al: Pavlovian-to-instrumental transfer in alcohol dependence: a pilot study. Neuropsychobiology 70(2):111–121, 2014 25359491

Garbusow M, Nebe S, Sommer C, et al: Pavlovian-to-instrumental transfer and alcohol consumption in young male social drinkers: behavioral, neural and polygenic correlates. J Clin Med 8(8):E1188, 2019 31398853

Gelman A, Carlin J, Stern H, et al: Bayesian Data Analysis, 3rd Edition. Boca Raton, FL, Chapman & Hall/CRC Press, 2013

Gillan CM, Daw ND: Taking psychiatry research online. Neuron 91(1):19–23, 2016 27387647

Gillan CM, Kosinski M, Whelan R, et al: Characterizing a psychiatric symptom dimension related to deficits in goal-directed control. eLife 5:5, 2016 26928075

Gillan CM, Kalanthroff E, Evans M, et al: Comparison of the association between goal-directed planning and self-reported compulsivity vs obsessive-compulsive disorder diagnosis. JAMA Psychiatry 77(1):77–85, 2020 31596434

Guitart-Masip M, Huys QJM, Fuentemilla L, et al: Go and no-go learning in reward and punishment: interactions between affect and effect. Neuroimage 62(1):154–166, 2012 22548809

Hajcak G, Meyer A, Kotov R: Psychometrics and the neuroscience of individual differences: internal consistency limits between-subjects effects. J Abnorm Psychol 126(6):823–834, 2017 28447803

Hedge C, Powell G, Sumner P: The reliability paradox: why robust cognitive tasks do not produce reliable individual differences. Behav Res Methods 50(3):1166–1186, 2018 28726177

Huys QJM: Advancing clinical improvements for patients using the theory-driven and data-driven branches of computational psychiatry. JAMA Psychiatry 75(3):225–226, 2018 29344604

Huys QJM, Renz D: A formal valuation framework for emotions and their control. Biol Psychiatry 82(6):413–420, 2017 28838467

Huys QJM, Moutoussis M, Williams J: Are computational models of any use to psychiatry? Neural Netw 24(6):544–551, 2011 21459554

Huys QJM, Eshel N, O'Nions E, et al: Bonsai trees in your head: how the Pavlovian system sculpts goal-directed choices by pruning decision trees. PLOS Comput Biol 8(3):e1002410, 2012 22412360

Huys QJM, Pizzagalli DA, Bogdan R, et al: Mapping anhedonia onto reinforcement learning: a behavioural meta-analysis. Biol Mood Anxiety Disord 3(1):12, 2013 23782813

Huys QJM, Daw ND, Dayan P: Depression: a decision-theoretic analysis. Annu Rev Neurosci 38:1–23, 2015 25705929

Huys QJM, Deserno L, Obermayer K, et al: Model-free temporal-difference learning and dopamine in alcohol dependence: examining concepts from theory and animals in human imaging. Biol Psychiatry Cogn Neurosci Neuroimaging 1(5):401–410, 2016a 29560869

Huys QJM, Maia TV, Frank MJ: Computational psychiatry as a bridge from neuroscience to clinical applications. Nat Neurosci 19(3):404–413, 2016b 26906507

Jacobson NS, Dobson KS, Truax PA, et al: A component analysis of cognitive-behavioral treatment for depression. J Consult Clin Psychol 64(2):295–304, 1996 8871414

Kendler KS, Thornton LM, Gardner CO: Stressful life events and previous episodes in the etiology of major depression in women: an evaluation of the "kindling" hypothesis. Am J Psychiatry 157(8):1243–1251, 2000 10910786

Kim W, Pitt MA, Lu Z-L, Myung JI: Planning beyond the next trial in adaptive experiments: a dynamic programming approach. Cogn Sci (Hauppauge) 41(8):2234–2252, 2017 27988934

Krause A, Singh A, Guestrin C: Near-optimal sensor placements in gaussian processes: theory, efficient algorithms and empirical studies. J Mach Learn Res 9:235–284, 2008

MacKay DJC: Information-based objective functions for active data selection. Neural Comput 4:590–604, 1992

Maia TV, Huys QJM, Frank MJ: Theory-based computational psychiatry. Biol Psychiatry 82(6):382–384, 2017 28838466

Mathews A, MacLeod C: Cognitive vulnerability to emotional disorders. Annu Rev Clin Psychol 1:167–195, 2005 17716086

Millner AJ, den Ouden HEM, Gershman SJ, et al: Suicidal thoughts and behaviors are associated with an increased decision-making bias for active responses to escape aversive states. J Abnorm Psychol 128(2):106–118, 2019 30589305

Mitchell AJ, McGlinchey JB, Young D, et al: Accuracy of specific symptoms in the diagnosis of major depressive disorder in psychiatric out-patients: data from the MIDAS project. Psychol Med 39(7):1107–1116, 2009 19000337

Mkrtchian A, Aylward J, Dayan P, et al: Modeling avoidance in mood and anxiety disorders using reinforcement learning. Biol Psychiatry 82(7):532–539, 2017 28343697

Molenaar PC, Campbell CG: The new person-specific paradigm in psychology. Current Directions in Psychological Science 18(2):112–117, 2009

Montague PR, Dolan RJ, Friston KJ, et al: Computational psychiatry. Trends Cogn Sci 16(1):72–80, 2012 22177032

Myung JI, Cavagnaro DR, Pitt MA: A tutorial on adaptive design optimization. J Math Psychol 57(3–4):53–67, 2013 23997275

Nebe S, Kroemer NB, Schad DJ, et al: No association of goal-directed and habitual control with alcohol consumption in young adults. Addict Biol 23(1):379–393, 2018 28111829

Ousdal OT, Huys QJ, Milde AM, et al: The impact of traumatic stress on Pavlovian biases. Psychol Med 48(2):327–336, 2018 28641601

Paninski L: Asymptotic theory of information-theoretic experimental design. Neural Comput 17(7):1480–1507, 2005 15901405

Patzelt EH, Kool W, Millner AJ, et al: Incentives boost model-based control across a range of severity on several psychiatric constructs. Biol Psychiatry 85(5):425–433, 2019 30077331

Paulus MP, Huys QJM, Maia TV: A roadmap for the development of applied computational psychiatry. Biol Psychiatry Cogn Neurosci Neuroimaging 1(5):386–392, 2016 28018986

Perna G, Grassi M, Caldirola D, et al: The revolution of personalized psychiatry: will technology make it happen sooner? Psychol Med 48(5):705–713, 2018 28967349

Peterson K, Dieperink E, Anderson J, et al: Rapid evidence review of the comparative effectiveness, harms, and cost-effectiveness of pharmacogenomics-guided antidepressant treatment versus usual care for major depressive disorder. Psychopharmacology (Berl) 234(11):1649–1661, 2017 28456840

Piray P, Dezfouli A, Heskes T, et al: Hierarchical Bayesian inference for concurrent model fitting and comparison for group studies. PLOS Comput Biol 15(6):e1007043, 2019 31211783

Pizzagalli DA, Jahn AL, O'Shea JP: Toward an objective characterization of an anhedonic phenotype: a signal-detection approach. Biol Psychiatry 57(4):319–327, 2005 15705346

Plichta MM, Schwarz AJ, Grimm O, et al: Test-retest reliability of evoked BOLD signals from a cognitive-emotive fMRI test battery. Neuroimage 60(3):1746–1758, 2012 22330316

Pooseh S, Bernhardt N, Guevara A, et al: Value-based decision-making battery: a Bayesian adaptive approach to assess impulsive and risky behavior. Behav Res Methods 50(1):236–249, 2018 28289888

Price RB, Brown V, Siegle GJ: Computational modeling applied to the dot-probe task yields improved reliability and mechanistic insights. Biol Psychiatry 85(7):606–612, 2019 30449531

Ratcliff R, Smith PL: A comparison of sequential sampling models for two-choice reaction time. Psychol Rev 111(2):333–367, 2004 15065913

Rouault M, Seow T, Gillan CM, et al: Psychiatric symptom dimensions are associated with dissociable shifts in metacognition but not task performance. Biol Psychiatry 84(6):443–451, 2018 29458997

Rouder JN, Haaf JM: A psychometrics of individual differences in experimental tasks. Psychon Bull Rev 26(2):452–467, 2019 30911907

Rutledge RB, Moutoussis M, Smittenaar P, et al: Association of neural and emotional impacts of reward prediction errors with major depression. JAMA Psychiatry 74(8):790–797, 2017 28678984

Rutledge RB, Chekroud AM, Huys QJ: Machine learning and big data in psychiatry: toward clinical applications. Curr Opin Neurobiol 55:152–159, 2019 30999271

Savitz JB, Rauch SL, Drevets WC: Clinical application of brain imaging for the diagnosis of mood disorders: the current state of play. Mol Psychiatry 18(5):528–539, 2013 23546169

Schlagenhauf F, Huys QJM, Deserno L, et al: Striatal dysfunction during reversal learning in unmedicated schizophrenia patients. Neuroimage 89:171–180, 2014 24291614

Schulz E, Wu CM, Huys QJM, et al: Generalization and search in risky environments. Cogn Sci (Hauppauge) 42(8):2592–2620, 2018 30390325

Settles B: Active Learning. Williston, VT, Morgan & Claypool Publishers, 2012

Shahar N, Hauser TU, Moutoussis M, et al: Improving the reliability of model-based decision-making estimates in the two-stage decision task with reaction-times and drift-diffusion modeling. PLOS Comput Biol 15(2):e1006803, 2019 30759077

Spearman C: The proof and measurement of association between two things. By C. Spearman, 1904. Am J Psychol 100(3–4):441–471, 1987 3322052

Stephan KE, Mathys C: Computational approaches to psychiatry. Curr Opin Neurobiol 25:85–92, 2014 24709605

Stephan KE, Binder EB, Breakspear M, et al: Charting the landscape of priority problems in psychiatry, part 2: pathogenesis and aetiology. Lancet Psychiatry 3(1):84–90, 2016 26573969

Stephan KE, Schlagenhauf F, Huys QJM, et al: Computational neuroimaging strategies for single patient predictions. Neuroimage 145 (Pt B):180–199, 2017 27346545

Stone M: Cross-validation and multinomial prediction. Biometrika 61(3):509–515, 1974

Voon V, Derbyshire K, Rück C, et al: Disorders of compulsivity: a common bias towards learning habits. Mol Psychiatry 20(3):345–352, 2015 24840709

Wang X-J, Krystal JH: Computational psychiatry. Neuron 84(3):638–654, 2014 25442941

Wetzels R, Vandekerckhove J, Tuerlinckx F, et al: Bayesian parameter estimation in the expectancy valence model of the Iowa gambling task. J Math Psychol 54:14–27, 2010

Wheaton MG, Gillan CM, Simpson HB: Does cognitive-behavioral therapy affect goal-directed planning in obsessive-compulsive disorder? Psychiatry Res 273:94–99, 2019 30640057

Woo C-W, Chang LJ, Lindquist MA, et al: Building better biomarkers: brain models in translational neuroimaging. Nat Neurosci 20(3):365–377, 2017 28230847

World Health Organization: International Classification of Diseases, 10th Revision. Geneva, Switzerland, World Health Organization, 1990

World Health Organization: Depression and other common mental disorders: global health estimates. 2017. Available at: apps.who.int/iris/bitstream/handle/10665/254610/WHO-MSD-MER-2017.2-eng.pdf. Accessed February 18, 2021.

Yang J, Pitt MA, Ahn W-Y, et al: ADOpy: a python package for adaptive design optimization. Behav Res Methods September 8, 2020 [Epub ahead of print] 32901345

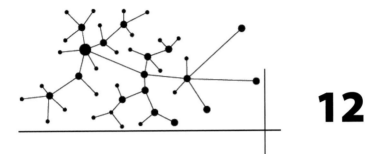

12

Toward Precision Cognitive-Behavioral Therapy via Reinforcement Learning Theory

Yael Niv, Ph.D.
Peter Hitchcock, Ph.D.
Isabel M. Berwian, Ph.D.
Gila Schoen, M.D.

Learning as a Basis for Mental Health Treatment

Cognitive-behavioral therapy (CBT) (Beck 1976, 2005), a leading method of psychotherapy, is a widely used treatment for many psychiatric conditions, including anxiety disorders, mood disorders, PTSD, obsessive-compulsive disorder (OCD), and substance abuse. The goal of CBT, in particular the second wave of CBT on which we will focus (Beck 2011), is to effect change in cognition, emotion, and behavior, understanding that changing any one of these affects change in the other two due to their interdependence. This is done by teaching patients new thought ("cognitive") and response ("behavioral") patterns with the aim of eventually, through repeated practice and generalization, displacing maladaptive automatic tendencies. A key CBT principle is that emotional responses (e.g., feeling scared, anxious, or sad) are not a direct consequence of external events, but rather are mediated by thoughts and internal schemas that filter external information and determine emotional and behavioral responses (see Appendix 2.1). By learning and practicing alternative interpretations and responses, we can gain control over our emotional wellbeing. CBT has been widely tested in randomized controlled trials and has a strong empirical evidence base (Butler et al. 2006; Hofmann et al. 2012).

Over the same time frame, research in cognitive neuroscience and psychology has converged on a theoretical framework called *reinforcement learning* (RL) (Sutton and Barto 2018) to explain trial-and-error learning, behavioral decision making, and their neural implementation. The key idea is that choices are based on learned *values* of available options. These values reflect the subjective reward value of expected outcomes (which could be negative for aversive outcomes) and are learned through trial and error, by comparing actual outcomes to expectations. The principle is that when we experience a "prediction error"—a discrepancy between what we expected and what actually happened—learning occurs and expectations (values) are updated.

RL theory has been widely tested in humans and animals, accumulating much support. Recent advances have extended the theory to explain multiple learning algorithms and their respective decision processes, which occur in parallel in the brain (in particular, habitual vs. goal-directed deliberative behavior; Daw et al. 2005), and to thinking about how learning is generalized or specialized to different scenarios (Gershman et al. 2015). This enhanced RL framework can be mapped relatively directly onto key concepts from CBT.

The goal of this chapter is to flesh out the links between second-wave CBT and RL.[1] Because RL theory is defined in computational terms (see next section), viewing CBT through the lens of RL can suggest ways to quantify the changes that a patient undergoes throughout treatment, and to potentially help determine which CBT intervention to employ at each stage of treatment. This highlights how developments in the growing field of computational psychiatry (Huys et al. 2016; Montague et al. 2012) could impact clinical practice.

---

[1]Because of space limitations, we forgo discussion of the links between CBT and Bayesian inference processes (which are strongly linked to RL), and refer the reader instead to an article by Moutoussis et al. (2018).

REINFORCEMENT LEARNING IN A NUTSHELL

RL arose as a theory of animal learning, specifically Pavlovian and instrumental conditioning (Sutton and Barto 1990). In *Pavlovian ("classical") conditioning*, a contingency between two events, one motivationally neutral and one motivationally relevant (e.g., the sound of a bell—a "conditional stimulus," or CS—followed by receipt of food, an "unconditional stimulus," or US) is experienced repeatedly. As a result, through learning, the CS comes to *predict* the occurrence of the US. This prediction is evidenced (and can be measured) by behavioral responses (e.g., salivation, quickening heart rate—a host of "conditioned responses") that automatically accompany said prediction. This type of learning is ubiquitous and can occur when a CS predicts the occurrence of a US (excitatory conditioning) or the absence of an otherwise available US (inhibitory conditioning). Importantly, learning may not enter awareness, and the automatic conditioned responses (which include emotions, increased heart rate, and sweating) are very hard to override.

This type of prediction learning is at the heart of RL theory. (For a more detailed overview of RL in the brain, see Niv 2009.) In RL, each stimulus (S) acquires a value $V(S)$ that reflects the subjective scalar value of the USs it predicts. For example, the first time the bell is heard, its value may be zero. If the tone is followed by a US, the US's reward value, R (positive values for appetitive USs like food, and negative values for aversive USs like pain), is compared with the prior expectation $V_{old}(S)$ to compute a prediction error, $PE = R - V_{old}(S)$. The new value of the stimulus is then updated based on the prediction error: $V_{new}(S) = V_{old}(S) + \alpha \cdot PE$, where α is a "learning rate" parameter between 0 and 1. This learning rule will update the value every time a prediction error is experienced, until the prediction error is zero (the prediction is correct). This model of trial-and-error prediction learning has one parameter, α, that can differ between individual learners or for different situations (see Appendix A1.1).

When the environment changes considerably (e.g., a tone CS that once reliably predicted a shock US is no longer followed by shock), instead of updating $V(S)$, the learner may infer that the current tone is not the same as the old one and thus initialize a completely new value, $V(S_2)$. The idea is that the learner makes inferences about the hidden (latent) causes of observed events and learns different values for different inferred latent causes. Rather than thinking of S as a stimulus, it denotes an inferred *state* of the world, corresponding to a latent cause (Gershman et al. 2010).

In *instrumental conditioning*, actions that the learner chooses can affect whether they will or will not receive reinforcement. For example, pressing a lever may be reinforced with food or with removal of an aversive sound. The learner must experiment with different actions and learn, through trial and error, which actions are effective in any given scenario. In RL terminology, the model for learning is similar to the prediction learning model; however, values are learned for each possible action a in each state (these values are called Q-values and denoted $Q(a \mid S)$, in contrast to the V-values for states, above). Again, learning proceeds based on prediction errors: after performing a chosen action in the current state, the outcome is used to compute a prediction error and update $Q(a \mid S)$.

This learning mechanism is only one way to compute values. Rather than storing and updating values after each experience, one can instead learn a *model of the environment:* how states follow one another given each action (the state "transition structure"), and what states are rewarding or punishing. Armed with this model, the learner can mentally simulate the consequences of different actions (or, in Pavlovian scenarios where actions are irrelevant, the unfolding of events over time) to calculate their value. This alternative algorithm has been termed *model-based learning*, in contrast to the "model-free" trial-and-error learning algorithm described above (Daw et al. 2005).

It appears that the brain uses both model-free and model-based methods for computing values and making decisions (Daw et al. 2005). The model-free system depends on dopaminergic prediction errors and a cortico–basal ganglia–thalamocortical loop involving the ventral and dorsolateral striatum and portions of the amygdala (see Appendix A1.2). It has been associated with *habitual* behavior—well-learned response patterns that require considerable experience with conflicting outcomes to learn new values and new actions. In contrast, the model-based system seems dopamine independent and relies on the hippocampus, frontal cortex, and a cortico–basal ganglia–thalamocortical loop involving the dorsomedial striatum. This system has been associated with deliberative, so-called goal-directed behavior, and is more flexible in its action selection because it can incorporate new information into the task model without extensive experience. However, simulating future outcomes requires mental effort, and there may be limits to how deeply one can search a tree of future options. Neural and behavioral evidence show that both systems operate in the brain in parallel; however, one or the other may be controlling behavior at any point in time. For example, you may use model-based RL to explicitly plan to go shopping on the way home from work. However, listening to the radio as you drive, your model-free system may take over and lead you to turn toward home habitually despite your plan otherwise.

In sum, RL theory suggests that to change behavioral responses, one can change the internal model of the task, which will affect deliberative planning (see also Moutoussis et al. 2018). However, since much of our behavior is habitual and relies on a lifetime of learning from trial and error, more permanent change may require experiencing prediction errors that will slowly change the values that our model-free system assigns to states and actions. Pharmacological treatments that affect dopamine (commonly used for a variety of mental health conditions) can affect this latter process because it depends on dopaminergic prediction errors. Moreover, if a situation changes too much, the learner may infer a new state rather than update an old state value. In psychotherapy, such new inferences may be helpful as long as future experience is ascribed to the newly inferred latent cause. Yet, because the mental representation of the old latent cause remains, quiescent but unchanged, an associated maladaptive judgment or behavior can reappear if the individual infers that this cause has returned. In the examples below, we will flesh out the implications of these ideas for psychotherapy.

COGNITIVE-BEHAVIORAL THERAPY IN A NUTSHELL

CBT is a problem-focused collaborative form of psychotherapy that aims to change maladaptive behavior and thought processes and improve emotional regulation (Beck 2011). A core premise of CBT is that external events do not cause us to feel and do things, but rather our cognitions offer a *subjective interpretation* of events that, in turn, causes feelings and actions. This interpretation is often automatic and implicit, building on a lifetime of previous experiences, and not a voluntary or conscious process. The profound implication is that we have some control over our emotional, cognitive, and behavioral responses. By changing our interpretations, we can avoid responding maladaptively (for an example, see Appendix A2.1).

How can interpretations be challenged and changed? Since emotions, thoughts, and actions are inextricably linked, the therapist can choose which avenue may be most amenable to change for each individual. For example, actions and emotional responses can result from thoughts. In the method of *cognitive restructuring*, these thoughts are challenged, their exaggerated or distorted nature is exposed, and alternatives are listed and practiced. This can help reduce the emotional response and enable alternative behavioral responses. Alternatively, being exposed to seemingly dangerous (but actually safe) situations and experiencing their neutral outcomes can help reduce maladaptive automatic emotional responses (such as the autonomic fear response) that arise as "false alarms." Once the emotional and bodily response is identified as a false alarm, one can additionally learn to turn off the alarm through relaxation and mindfulness techniques, or to wait it out knowing that there is no actual danger involved (for more detail, see Appendix A2.2). Moreover, reduction of the physiological stress itself enables increased flexibility of thought and action.

COGNITIVE-BEHAVIORAL THEORY IN REINFORCEMENT LEARNING TERMINOLOGY

The CBT framework for understanding and treating dysfunction can be mapped quite directly to core concepts from RL (for mapping to the related framework of Bayesian inference, see Moutoussis et al. 2018). In RL terms, idiosyncratic response patterns emanate from state and action values learned from direct experience (or from modeling by others, e.g., our parents) through model-free trial and error, or computed on the fly from a learned world model.

At a first pass, the *cognitive* aspects of CBT (e.g., cognitive restructuring) can be seen as targeting the *model-based* system. Cognitive distortions may manifest in or result from distortions in the learned (or assumed) model of the environment. For example, if one's estimated probability of transitioning from any state to a state accompanied by punishment is exaggerated, then every plan of action in this model may seem dangerous, leading to avoidance behavior. This mapping of model-based RL to the cognitive aspects of CBT suggests several avenues for change, each exploited in CBT: one can attempt to change the model of the environment, targeting the distorted transition estimates by challenging the validity of current assumptions, or by forcing oneself to execute a response plan that is estimated to produce negative outcomes and experiencing that these do not occur. This latter planned exposure will lead to changes both in the model of the environment and in learned action values used by the model-free system. In this way, both systems will promote healthier response patterns in the future.

Indeed, the *behavioral* component of CBT is strongly related to the *model-free* learning system: by orchestrating experiences and exposures that will lead to prediction errors, predictive values of states and actions can be retrained. Importantly, the model-free system may be (at least partly) inaccessible to cognitive methods—we cannot talk our amygdala and striatum into changing stored values without having experienced prediction errors. Indeed, a hallmark of model-free learning is that avoidance of relevant training experiences serves to maintain old values. Thus, after experiencing a traumatic event (e.g., a car accident), the more one avoids similar scenarios (e.g., by not driving), the longer the negative expected values will be maintained. They may even become ingrained over time, and potentially generalized to other (no longer experienced) scenarios (although RL theory does not currently model this phenomenon). This may explain why exposure-based methods are critical for CBT, and cognitive restructuring cannot usually stand alone. For an RL account of why exposure methods work, see Appendix A2.3.

Of note, RL theory and experimental findings suggest that model-based and model-free RL can occur even without direct experience, for example, by watching others behave and through mental simulation of internal models or replay of memories of previous experiences (Burke et al. 2010; Shohamy and Daw 2015). This may be a mechanism for runaway exaggerated values. Counterfactual learning from imaginary "what if" scenarios based on extreme and erroneous beliefs could lead to vastly distorted values, whereas real-world experience would better ground values in reality.

In this sense, the model at the heart of model-based learning (and related training of model-free values using internal simulations) may be the main source of value distortions—this system relies more directly on sampling from episodic memory, where outlier (e.g., traumatic) events are strongly encoded and preferentially retrieved (Brown and Kulik 1977; Madan et al. 2014; Rouhani and Niv 2019). This could lead to a distorted model that must be corrected through direct experience tied to the actual statistics of events in the environment, rather than their distorted representation in memory.

From Theory to Practice

CBT practice provides different protocols for different diagnoses and underlying pathologies. Here we briefly discuss two examples to illustrate the link to RL theory and point out how theoretical work in RL can further our understanding of the mechanisms of CBT treatment and development of better protocols (see Craske et al. 2014 for a similar approach using animal learning theory). We then discuss the implications of these links to precision psychiatry, and how quantification of an individual's learning and decision-making parameters can help tailor the therapeutic approach to each specific patient.

EXAMPLE: PROLONGED EXPOSURE FOR TREATMENT OF PTSD

One of the best-tested and most effective CBT methods for treating PTSD is *prolonged exposure* (Foa 2011). In prolonged exposure, during *imaginal exposures*, the patient retells the story of the traumatic event in the first person and in present tense, and in as much detail as possible (mentioning all senses—vision, smell, etc.) in the safety of the clinic. The story is recorded, and the patient listens to it daily. In each of six to eight therapy sessions, the patient retells the story (sometimes uncovering previously forgotten details) and receives the recording to listen to at home. Over time, putatively through a combination of desensitization/habituation and reorganization of the memory through retelling, the traumatic memory becomes less potent and the patient recovers function: trauma-related thoughts become less intrusive, the patient no longer feels under constant threat, and, aided by in vivo exposures, behaviors that had been avoided after the trauma are resumed.

The theory behind prolonged exposure suggests that for the protocol to be successful, two important conditions must be met: the retelling of the trauma has to gain access to the original fear construct (i.e., the original fear memory) and disconfirming evidence then has to be introduced (Foa and Kozak 1986). Although developed separately (with prolonged exposure far predating the relevant RL theory; Gershman et al. 2017), this method is extremely well aligned with the RL playbook: disconfirming experiences of safety generate prediction errors, and access to the original fear construct ensures that new learning is applied to the original state and not to a new state. Indeed, the protocol can cause much distress in the beginning—the patient is requested to revisit in detail memories that they have (unsuccessfully) tried to suppress for months and years, and to do so in an immersive way. If they are willing to do this, however, the method is very effective (Powers et al. 2010).

The precise and quantitative nature of formal RL theory may help us improve exposure therapy, especially where current recommendations are in conflict with experimental and theoretical work in RL. For example, building on inhibitory learning theory, Craske et al. (2014) recommend maximizing "expectancy violation" (the discrepancy between a patient's predicted and actual experience, i.e., the prediction error) during exposure to maximize learning of new safety associations that will compete with old trauma-related associations. However, the existence of multiple learning systems (model-based and model-free) suggests a more nuanced interpretation of some of their empirical results, and alternative methods for treatments. For example, one can modify the old association, that is, update previously learned values. Here, recent research suggests that large prediction errors can cause a learner to impute a new experience to a wholly different state, instead of revaluing an old state, thus leaving the original state value intact (Gershman et al. 2014, 2015). Indeed, experiments in rodents have shown that in the long-term, gradual extinction of a fear memory is more effective in modifying conditioned fear responding than abrupt extinction (Gershman et al. 2013), which suggests that moderate prediction errors are more effective than large ones. The use of RL theory to understand the principles that underlie when prediction errors maximally overwrite existing learning versus are relegated to new states, along with the measurement of individual differences in such thresholds using behavioral tasks (see "Conclusion" section), may eventually help us predict what type of exposure will be most effective for each patient.

An important caveat is that Pavlovian fear conditioning—the dominant animal model for PTSD and the experimental paradigm discussed above—assumes that learning is of a simple association between stimuli and an unavoidable aversive outcome. A traumatic memory is clearly more complex than a simple CS-US association, and more research is needed regarding how emotional events influence the organization of episodic memories (Cohen and Kahana 2019; Talmi et al. 2019). Similarly, our understanding of PTSD could be increased through measuring individual differences in learning from positive versus negative prediction errors (Arkadir et al. 2016) and work on generalization, and specifically why negative memories tend to be stronger and generalize more widely than positive memories. More generally, understanding how boundaries between different situations (states) are drawn by the brain, and how these change over time (with and without experience of similar states), would be especially informative for treating PTSD.

EXAMPLE: EXPOSURE AND RESPONSE PREVENTION IN OBSESSIVE-COMPULSIVE DISORDER

OCD is characterized by obsessions (thoughts, e.g., "there are deadly germs on my hands that may make me very ill") that increase subjective distress and anxiety, and compulsive actions that are performed to reduce this distress (e.g., washing hands, sometimes repeatedly). A prominent CBT treatment of OCD is *exposure and response prevention* (EXRP) (Abramowitz 1996; Meyer 1966), wherein the patient is guided through a series of exposures to sources of distress while avoiding the action that would reduce the distress. The goal is for the patient to learn that 1) the distress subsides over time even without performing the compulsion (so they can forgo the compulsion), and 2) the terrible outcome that they thought would happen if the compulsion is not performed does not occur (they don't die of a deadly disease).

From an RL perspective, one can conceptualize OCD in terms of Q-values—the values of different actions in different states. In OCD, the values of many states become negative *unless* a specific action is executed. So while the Q-value for a = "washing hands" is zero for many states, the Q-value of doing nothing in these states is presumably very negative. Performance of the obsession confirms the zero Q-value of the obsessive action (as nothing bad happens), yet prevents experiencing the outcome of not performing the obsession, so the value of other alternatives can remain erroneously negative. EXRP provides these learning experiences, which, through prediction errors, can retrain the negative values to zero. Moreover, because the value of a = "doing nothing" may generalize more widely to the value of the state in general, this training may generalize and prevent other obsessive actions (research on generalization in RL is, however, still in its infancy).

The EXRP protocol also includes imaginal exposures, in which the patient is asked to imagine and write down the worst-case scenario outcome of not performing the obsession. This challenges traditional extinction-based theories of OCD treatment, because there is no expectancy violation in this method. Rather, the patient is asked to imagine exactly what they fear will happen. RL theory may help explain why this is helpful: being forced to explicitly state the contingencies leading to the worst-case outcome may elaborate an otherwise sparsely represented world model such that the exact series of events will be clearly represented, together with their low transition probabilities. This explicitly thought-through representation may thereby decrease the estimated probability of feared outcomes.

Conclusion: Precision Psychotherapy—How Can Reinforcement Learning Theory Help?

CBT has its roots in behaviorism and decades of experiments on animal learning. Harnessing ideas from the contemporary version of this rich body of knowledge—reinforcement learning theory—can help develop even more effective treatment protocols. For example, RL experiments have shown that people have a higher learning rate for actions they choose freely compared with those they are forced to execute (Cockburn et al. 2014). This suggests that offering several options for actions in each situation may speed skill learning in CBT and may explain why it is beneficial to involve patients in the planning of exposures.

The quantitative nature of RL may also benefit precision psychiatry. RL theory defines the dynamics of learning as a set of equations and therefore allows quantification of individual parameters of the learning process using simple computerized decision-making tasks (Daw 2011). Indeed, fitting RL models to trial-by-trial choices in simple laboratory tasks is a means of measuring parameters such as an individual's learning rate (Niv et al. 2012), how this learning rate adapts to change in the environment (Behrens et al. 2007), differences in the rate of learning from positive versus negative prediction errors (Arkadir et al. 2016), the initial value ascribed to new choice options (Wittmann et al. 2008), and the tendency to use model-free versus model-based values in decision making (Gillan et al. 2016). Much current research in the field of computational psychiatry attempts to relate these parameters to psychopathologies and to discover individual differences that may be transdiagnostically linked to mental illness (Bennett et al. 2019; Huys et al. 2016; Montague et al. 2012). The hope is that measuring quantities that relate to the mechanisms underlying psychiatric illnesses in an objective way that does not rely on self-report will allow more precise treatment predictions.

Applied to CBT, this approach can also assist in measuring individual parameters of learning that can help a therapist better target the treatment methods, and track progress over time. For example, knowing that a patient's model-free learning is slower than their model-based learning can help set the pace for exposures relative to cognitive restructuring methods, or assist in determining which method would be more effective. Moreover, overall impaired trial-and-error learning can suggest that CBT will not be an effective method for this patient, and perhaps pharmacological treatment should be the first line of action. In this way, we may make progress on the long-sought-after goal of assigning patients to the most effective treatment (Cohen 2018).

Finally, parameters from RL models may be useful for measuring the effects of psychotherapy. As examples, a decrease in the tendency to assign negative values to novel stimuli (Wittmann et al. 2008) may reflect reduction in overgeneralizing negative prior knowledge, and increased flexibility in making choices (i.e., how willing a person is to explore options that do not have the highest value; Wilson et al. 2014) may track improvement due to treatment. Arguably, the goal of CBT is to provide patients with more flexible response options. By tracking flexibility using a simple computerized task administered repeatedly throughout the course of treatment, one can potentially determine when improvements have reached asymptote. In this way, RL theory—together with the set of tasks used to measure parameters of the learning process—can help develop *precision psychotherapy*, a therapeutic approach that uses objectively measurable indices of learning to most effectively help an individual.

Appendix 1: Reinforcement Learning

A1.1—UNDERSTANDING LEARNING RATES IN REINFORCEMENT LEARNING

Another way to write the RL update equation $V_{new}(S) = V_{old}(S) + \alpha \cdot (R - V_{old}(S))$ is $V_{new}(S) = V_{old}(S) \cdot (1 - \alpha) + \alpha \cdot R$. The latter highlights that learning is a weighted average between old knowledge $V_{old}(S)$ and new experience R, with the learning rate α determining the weighting of old and new information: high learning rates prioritize new experiences and cause the effects of old events to be "forgotten," whereas low learning rates allow values to reflect the effect of more past events. We emphasize that there is no single "correct" learning rate: in a stable but noisy environment it is advantageous to average over many events, whereas following an abrupt change it makes sense to learn quickly from new events (Yu and Dayan 2005). Indeed, experiments show that humans adjust their learning rate across tasks, and even within a task, in response to volatility as well as other factors (McGuire et al. 2014; Nassar et al. 2012). Therefore, even this extremely simplified one-parameter model can be used to describe interesting behavior that (normatively) adapts to task demands, and may potentially be disrupted due to mental illness.

A1.2—A CIRCUIT FOR MODEL-FREE REINFORCEMENT LEARNING

Neurally, dopamine signaling is widely believed to correspond to RL prediction errors (Barto 1995; Montague et al. 1996; Schultz et al. 1997). Numerous studies have shown that phasic dopamine bursts or pauses appear at times in a task where, in theory, the animal should be experiencing a prediction error. In humans, functional neuroimaging studies have identified a similar signal in the blood oxygenation activity recorded in the ventral striatum (Hare et al. 2008)—an area that receives dense dopaminergic projections. Indeed, the striatum, which receives widespread projections from sensory, motor and associative cortical areas, is thought to be the area representing the values of states and actions. Learning in corticostriatal synapses is modulated by dopamine, with dopamine concentration determining whether long-term changes in synapses will strengthen the synapse (long-term potentiation; when there is a surge of dopamine above baseline) or weaken it (long-term depression; when there is a dip in dopamine concentration below baseline) (Reynolds et al. 2001). This mechanism can easily implement the trial-and-error learning algorithm described in the section "Reinforcement Learning in a Nutshell" earlier in this chapter, because positive prediction errors signaled by phasic increases in dopamine concentration would lead to more firing of striatal neurons in the presence of the state or the state and action in the future (signaling the now-higher expected value) and vice-versa for negative prediction errors (dips in dopamine firing).

Appendix 2: Cognitive-Behavioral Therapy

A2.1—EXAMPLE APPLICATION OF CBT PRINCIPLES TO AN EVENT

Imagine someone interrupts you in a discussion. This event can raise different thoughts and interpretations, ranging from "How annoying, X is always so inconsiderate" to "What I was saying was probably not interesting...I bet everyone was relieved when he changed the topic." Each will lead to a different emotional response (e.g., feeling anger, insult, self-doubt) and different behavioral responses (e.g., try to speak over the interrupter; fall silent and speak less in this group in the future). According to CBT theory, individuals have internal *schemas*—ingrained beliefs that "filter" incoming information, biasing its subjective interpretation. For example, the schema "I am not good at anything" will favor the interpretation that one's contribution was boring or incorrect, whereas the schema "the world is against me" may favor the interpretation that an aggressive work environment has fostered a culture of interruption that must be fought.

A2.2—EXPOSURE-BASED METHODS

Recognizing that maladaptive thought, emotion, and behavior patterns that reach clinical significance are usually long entrained, the focus of CBT is to have repeated new learning experiences in which the patient can practice skills acquired in therapy until they have been perfected. For example, a socially anxious patient may first practice skills during planned exposures with a warm and encouraging fellow therapist from their therapist's practice. In this low-stakes interaction, the patient can practice tolerating distress, inhibiting the urge to escape or to deploy safety behaviors, and redirecting attention outward when it turns to negative self-judgments. The patient can then generalize these skills by performing them in more difficult situations, such as with a fellow-therapist confederate who now acts impassively or hostilely, and in less controlled settings, such as with a boss or with strangers. Through repeated exposure and practice (ideally, every day), fears will typically decrease and skills will become habitual. These skills then serve as a resource the patient can draw upon if fear later returns or if a life situation elicits heightened concern about negative judgment.

In practice, to plan the exposures, first the patient and therapist will create a scale, usually from 0 to 10, where 0 is no distress and 10 is the most distress possible. This scale will be populated with events at different levels: perhaps for a patient who suffers from social anxiety, watching TV at home is a 0, talking to the cashier at the supermarket is a 3, asking a stranger for directions on the street is a 5, making small-talk with a taxi driver is a 7, and going to a party where they don't know anyone is a 10. Exposures are then planned from level 3 or so and are gradually increased: first, the patient will practice going to the supermarket and saying "hello" to the cashier each time. When this has ceased to be threatening, perhaps they will purchase a small item at a kiosk where they have to ask the attendant for the item, climbing to level 4. After each set of exposures, the scale can be reevaluated for all events (some might now be less threatening than they were in the past) and the patient, with the therapist's guidance, chooses the next level/action that they find feasible to expose themselves to, and plans a new set of exposures. Depending on the diagnosis and the individual's learning propensities (e.g., whether they learn best model based or model free, and what their individual learning rate is), each exposure may need to be repeated a few or more times.

A2.3—EXPOSURES AND REINFORCEMENT LEARNING PREDICTION ERRORS

One reason for the gradual nature of exposures is obvious: the patient will not agree to do something too distressing, and even if they do it, they may decide to terminate the therapy due to the high level of distress. However, RL theory suggests at least two more reasons that gradual exposure is more effective. First, rewards and punishments are not merely external: if a socially anxious patient goes to a party on their own for their first exposure, their high subjective level of distress will function as an outcome for the action. If their initial estimate of the value of the action of "going to a party" was very low, this severe distress outcome will only confirm this prediction. As a result, there will be no prediction error, and no new learning. The exposure will have failed. Instead, a well-planned exposure at a low level of predicted distress (level 3) can lead to learning to the extent that the exposure is planned so well that the patient experiences less distress than expected. This can be achieved by discussing all possible outcomes and their cognitive appraisal, and planning for how to mitigate any distress that arises. The goal is for the patient to experience that the event that they predicted would lead to level 3 distress is not as bad as they thought, and distress may even dissipate to level 0 over time without escaping the situation. This will cause a prediction error that will result in learning.

A second advantage of gradual exposure is that prediction errors are not too large. Research suggests that large prediction errors prompt the creation of a new state (Gershman et al. 2010). This new state will then be updated with the new information, but the old value will remain unchanged. According to RL theory, to unlearn old maladaptive state and action values, one should experience prediction errors that are not too small (otherwise there will be no learning) and not too large (because they will cause state-splitting). CBT exposures seem tailored to deliver exactly such prediction errors.

KEY POINTS

- The goal of cognitive-behavioral therapy (CBT), a widely used method for many psychiatric conditions with a strong empirical evidence base, is to effect change in cognition, emotion, and behavior.

- Concomitant with the development of CBT, cognitive neuroscientists and psychologists converged on a theoretical framework called reinforcement learning (RL) to explain trial-and-error learning, behavioral decision making, and their neural implementation. RL suggests that learning occurs and expectations (values) are updated when we experience a "prediction error"—a discrepancy between what we expected and what actually happened.

- Humans employ both model-free and model-based decision-making mechanisms. The former depends on dopaminergic prediction error–based learning; involves the ventral and dorsolateral striatum and portions of the amygdala; and reflects ingrained, less flexible, habitual behavior. The latter seems dopamine independent; relies on the hippocampus, frontal cortex, and the dorsomedial striatum; and reflects flexible, prospective goal-directed planning.

- The CBT framework can be mapped directly to core concepts from RL. The cognitive aspects of CBT may be seen as targeting the model-based system, while the behavioral component of CBT is strongly related to the model-free learning system.

- RL may aid in improving CBT through the development of more effective treatment protocols, quantification of individual parameters of the learning process to help better tailor CBT, and measurement of the effects of psychotherapy.

References

Abramowitz JS: Variants of exposure and response prevention in the treatment of obsessive-compulsive disorder: a meta-analysis. Behavior Therapy 27(4):583–600, 1996

Arkadir D, Radulescu A, Raymond D, et al: DYT1 dystonia increases risk taking in humans. Elife 5:e14155, 2016 27249418

Barto AG: Adaptive critic and the basal ganglia, in Models of Information Processing in the Basal Ganglia. Edited by Houk JC, Davis JL, Beiser DG. Cambridge, MA, MIT Press, 1995, pp 215–232

Beck AT: Cognitive Therapy and the Emotional Disorders. New York, New American Library, 1976

Beck AT: The current state of cognitive therapy: a 40-year retrospective. Arch Gen Psychiatry 62(9):953–959, 2005 16143727

Beck JS: Cognitive Behavior Therapy: Basics and Beyond. New York, Guilford, 2011

Behrens TE, Woolrich MW, Walton ME, et al: Learning the value of information in an uncertain world. Nat Neurosci 10(9):1214–1221, 2007 17676057

Bennett D, Silverstein SM, Niv Y: The two cultures of computational psychiatry. JAMA Psychiatry 76(6):563–564, 2019 31017638

Brown R, Kulik J: Flashbulb memories. Cognition 5(1):73–99, 1977

Burke CJ, Tobler PN, Baddeley M, et al: Neural mechanisms of observational learning. Proc Natl Acad Sci USA 107(32):14431–14436, 2010 20660717

Butler AC, Chapman JE, Forman EM, et al: The empirical status of cognitive-behavioral therapy: a review of meta-analyses. Clin Psychol Rev 26(1):17–31, 2006 16199119

Cockburn J, Collins AG, Frank MJ: A reinforcement learning mechanism responsible for the valuation of free choice. Neuron 83(3):551–557, 2014 25066083

Cohen RT, Kahana MJ: Retrieved-context theory of memory in emotional disorders. bioRxiv, 2019. Available at: www.biorxiv.org/content/10.1101/817486v4. Accessed February 19, 2021.

Cohen ZD: Treatment selection: understanding what works for whom in mental health. Publicly Accessible Penn Dissertations, 2932, 2018. Available at: repository.upenn.edu/cgi/viewcontent.cgi?article=4718&context=edissertations. Accessed February 19, 2021.

Craske MG, Treanor M, Conway CC, et al: Maximizing exposure therapy: an inhibitory learning approach. Behav Res Ther 58:10–23, 2014 24864005

Daw ND: Trial by trial data analysis using computational models, in Decision Making, Affect, and Learning: Attention and Performance XXIII. Edited by Delgado MR, Phelps EA, Robbins TW. New York, Oxford University Press, 2011

Daw ND, Niv Y, Dayan P: Uncertainty-based competition between prefrontal and dorsolateral striatal systems for behavioral control. Nat Neurosci 8(12):1704–1711, 2005 16286932

Foa EB: Prolonged exposure therapy: past, present, and future. Depress Anxiety 28(12):1043–1047, 2011 22134957

Foa EB, Kozak MJ: Emotional processing of fear: exposure to corrective information. Psychol Bull 99(1):20–35, 1986 2871574

Gershman SJ, Blei DM, Niv Y: Context, learning, and extinction. Psychol Rev 117(1):197–209, 2010 20063968

Gershman SJ, Jones CE, Norman KA, et al: Gradual extinction prevents the return of fear: implications for the discovery of state. Front Behav Neurosci 7:164, 2013 24302899

Gershman SJ, Radulescu A, Norman KA, et al: Statistical computations underlying the dynamics of memory updating. PLOS Comput Biol 10(11):e1003939, 2014 25375816

Gershman SJ, Norman KA, Niv Y: Discovering latent causes in reinforcement learning. Curr Opin Behav Sci 5:43–50, 2015

Gershman SJ, Monfils M-H, Norman KA, et al: The computational nature of memory modification. Elife 6:e23763, 2017 28530550

Gillan CM, Kosinski M, Whelan R, et al: Characterizing a psychiatric symptom dimension related to deficits in goal-directed control. Elife 5:e11305, 2016 26928075

Hare TA, O'Doherty J, Camerer CF, et al: Dissociating the role of the orbitofrontal cortex and the striatum in the computation of goal values and prediction errors. J Neurosci 28(22):5623–5630, 2008 18509023

Hofmann SG, Asnaani A, Vonk IJ, et al: The efficacy of cognitive behavioral therapy: a review of meta-analyses. Cognit Ther Res 36(5):427–440, 2012 23459093

Huys QJ, Maia TV, Frank MJ: Computational psychiatry as a bridge from neuroscience to clinical applications. Nat Neurosci 19(3):404–413, 2016 26906507

Madan CR, Ludvig EA, Spetch ML: Remembering the best and worst of times: memories for extreme outcomes bias risky decisions. Psychon Bull Rev 21(3):629–636, 2014 24189991

McGuire JT, Nassar MR, Gold JI, et al: Functionally dissociable influences on learning rate in a dynamic environment. Neuron 84(4):870–881, 2014 25459409

Meyer V: Modification of expectations in cases with obsessional rituals. Behav Res Ther 4(4):273–280, 1966 5978682

Montague PR, Dayan P, Sejnowski TJ: A framework for mesencephalic dopamine systems based on predictive Hebbian learning. J Neurosci 16(5):1936–1947, 1996 8774460

Montague PR, Dolan RJ, Friston KJ, et al: Computational psychiatry. Trends Cogn Sci 16(1):72–80, 2012 22177032

Moutoussis M, Shahar N, Hauser TU, et al: Computation in psychotherapy, or how computational psychiatry can aid learning-based psychological therapies. Comput Psychiatr 2:50–73, 2018 30090862

Nassar MR, Rumsey KM, Wilson RC, et al: Rational regulation of learning dynamics by pupil-linked arousal systems. Nat Neurosci 15(7):1040–1046, 2012 22660479

Niv Y: Reinforcement learning in the brain. J Math Psychol 53(3):139–154, 2009

Niv Y, Edlund JA, Dayan P, et al: Neural prediction errors reveal a risk-sensitive reinforcement-learning process in the human brain. J Neurosci 32(2):551–562, 2012 22238090

Powers MB, Halpern JM, Ferenschak MP, et al: A meta-analytic review of prolonged exposure for posttraumatic stress disorder. Clin Psychol Rev 30(6):635–641, 2010 20546985

Reynolds JN, Hyland BI, Wickens JR: A cellular mechanism of reward-related learning. Nature 413(6851):67–70, 2001 11544526

Rouhani N, Niv Y: Depressive symptoms bias the prediction-error enhancement of memory towards negative events in reinforcement learning. Psychopharmacology (Berl) 236(8):2425–2435, 2019 31346654

Schultz W, Dayan P, Montague PR: A neural substrate of prediction and reward. Science 275(5306):1593–1599, 1997 9054347

Shohamy D, Daw ND: Integrating memories to guide decisions. Curr Opin Behav Sci 5:85–90, 2015

Sutton RS, Barto AG: Time-derivative models of Pavlovian reinforcement, in Learning and Computational Neuroscience: Foundations of Adaptive Networks. Edited by Gabriel M, Moore J. Cambridge, MA, MIT Press, 1990, pp 497–537

Sutton RS, Barto AG: Reinforcement Learning: An Introduction. Cambridge, MA, MIT Press, 2018

Talmi D, Lohnas LJ, Daw ND: A retrieved context model of the emotional modulation of memory. Psychol Rev 126(4):455–485, 2019 30973247

Wilson RC, Geana A, White JM, et al: Humans use directed and random exploration to solve the explore-exploit dilemma. J Exp Psychol Gen 143(6):2074–2081, 2014 25347535

Wittmann BC, Daw ND, Seymour B, et al: Striatal activity underlies novelty-based choice in humans. Neuron 58(6):967–973, 2008 18579085

Yu AJ, Dayan P: Uncertainty, neuromodulation, and attention. Neuron 46(4):681–692, 2005 15944135

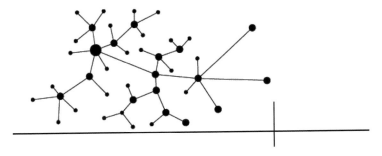

PART 6

DEVELOPING THE ACADEMIC DISCIPLINE OF PRECISION PSYCHIATRY

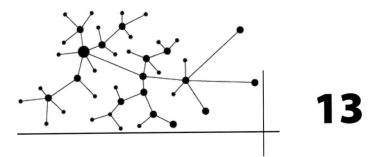

13

MOVING FROM PRECISION TO PERSONALIZED PSYCHIATRY

Clinical Perspectives on the New Era

Giampaolo Perna, M.D., Ph.D.
Charles B. Nemeroff, M.D., Ph.D.

History

THE UNMET NEEDS OF PSYCHIATRY

The percentage of the population experiencing mental health disorders has risen significantly since 2010, yet many adults with severe mental illness remain undiagnosed and untreated, which heavily affects their quality of life and relationships (Balon and Morreale 2019; McAllister-Williams et al. 2016; Wang et al. 2007). Even when these individuals are recognized and treated, and despite having therapeutic options, clinical outcomes are often unsatisfactory (Caldirola and Perna 2019; McAllister-Williams et al. 2020; Patterson and Van Ameringen 2016; Perna et al. 2020). The rising global economic burden of mental health–related disability and therapeutic treatments currently contributes to 32.4% of the years lived with disability and an annual global expenditure of $2.5 trillion, and the mental health care budget does not match actual costs (Kohn et al. 2018; Rehm and Shield 2019; Trautmann et al. 2016; Vigo et al. 2016, 2019). Further, the standard psychiatric "assessment and treatment" approach—grounded in clinicians' personal experience and evidence-based national/international guidelines—has highlighted controversy and inadequacies (McAllister-Williams et al. 2016; Perna and Nemeroff 2018). Reliable methods for determining the most effective treatment for each individual patient remain elusive.

A NEW AND REVOLUTIONARY APPROACH TO PSYCHIATRY

Precision medicine is an innovative approach for identifying distinctive characteristics of an individual related to health and disease in order to select appropriate and effective therapy to maximize the likelihood of favorable response and minimize adverse effects (National Research Council 2011; Personalized Medicine Coalition 2017; Sugeir and Naylor 2018). These characteristics encompass clinical, neurobiological, and lifestyle factors (Di Sanzo et al. 2017; Goetz and Schork 2018; König et al. 2017). Medical fields that use precision medicine—notably oncology and infectious disease—are seeing positive effects on the longitudinal course and outcomes of several illnesses (Johnson 2017; Le Tourneau et al. 2018; Ozomaro et al. 2013).

Precision medicine has a central role in worldwide initiatives in psychiatry and the neurosciences, including the Precision Medicine Initiative (White House, Office of the Press Secretary 2015a, 2015b), the Research Domain Criteria project (Insel 2014; Insel et al. 2010; Stein and Reed 2019), and the Brain Research through Advancing Innovative Neurotechnologies initiative (Insel et al. 2013; National Institutes of Health 2019).

Within the umbrella concept of precision approaches to psychiatry, we define *personalized medicine in psychiatry* (PMP) more narrowly as tailoring treatment to the individual characteristics of each patient. PMP's potential usefulness is evident (Fernandes et al. 2017; Perna and Nemeroff 2018). Tailoring mental health care to each patient's unique characteristics will likely improve diagnostic certainty and psychiatric disorder outcomes and thereby address the staggering disease burden of these disorders (World Federation for Mental Health 2012). However, PMP is far from being applied in everyday clinical practice (Perna et al. 2018a).

In this chapter, we review the opportunities and challenges associated with PMP, paying particular attention to its application in tailoring treatment for mood and anxiety disorders. We hope that the advances we discuss regarding "precision" medicine will result in improved patient outcomes via the application of "personalized" medicine.

Current Knowledge and Approaches

THE FUTURE OF PRECISION MEDICINE IN PSYCHIATRY

Developing a precision approach in psychiatry is a slow and challenging process because psychiatric disorders are highly complex and multifactorial conditions. Each psychiatric diagnosis is heterogeneous in many aspects, including clinical symptoms and neurobiological features (Fanous and Kendler 2005; Hodgson et al. 2017; Stephan et al. 2016). Therefore, large amounts of collectable information will be needed to support the development of innovative precision diagnostic and therapeutic strategies. Further steps will be needed to gather clinical, neurobiological, genetic, and individual information and translate it into reliable workable tools that can help clinicians in the diagnostic and therapeutic process (Ozomaro et al. 2013; Perna and Nemeroff 2018; Perna et al. 2018b). The multidimensional complexity of big data "requires a change of perspective, infrastructure, and methods for data collection, sharing and analyses" (Baro et al. 2015) in medicine that takes into account an innovative yet ethical vision of this evolution (Abbott et al. 2020; Ball et al. 2020; Evers 2009; Hays 2017; Perna and Nemeroff 2018).

Early theoretical papers and proof-of-concept studies have shown promise, but their applicability to current clinical practice has been overestimated (Cearns et al. 2019; Lydiard and Nemeroff 2019). For example, several *combinatorial pharmacogenetic tests* to support drug selection in psychiatric patients have recently become available (e.g.,the FDA-approved AmpliChip CYP450 Test from Roche; GeneSight from Assurex Health; Neuropharmagen, AB-Biotics), but they have different testing approaches and levels of evidence supporting their clinical utility. Recent meta-analytic results suggest that the clinical outcomes of patients with major depressive disorder (MDD) were significantly improved when care was guided by some of these tests compared with unguided care (Brown et al. 2020; Vilches et al. 2019). However, in the view of this chapter's authors, the real clinical utility and cost-effectiveness of this PMP strategy is still in doubt. Indeed, the largest randomized clinical trial of pharmacogenomics to predict antidepressant efficacy, the Genomics Used to Improve DEpression Decisions (GUIDED) study, failed to meet its primary efficacy outcome measure and failed to predict side effect liability (Greden et al. 2019). Obviously, the clinical effects of antidepressants or antipsychotics are not due solely to their rate of metabolism by cytochrome P450 enzymes (Bousman and Eyre 2020; Bousman and Hopwood 2016; Ozomaro et al. 2013; Rosenblat et al. 2017; Zeier et al. 2018).

Companies that market these tests often do not declare which specific genetic variants are included or the precise pharmacogenetic algorithms that lead to their reports (Zeier et al. 2018). Also, the limited sample sizes and low methodological rigor of many studies—which were funded by the companies that market the tests—may have undermined the reliability of available results (Cearns et al. 2019; Lydiard and Nemeroff 2019). As such, while pharmacogenetics-based tools may presently be helpful in some clinical situations, there are insufficient data to support their widespread use in clinical practice, and rigorous large-scale studies are warranted (Cearns et al. 2019; Goldberg and Nemeroff, in press; Hoehe and Morris-Rosendahl 2018; Krebs and Milani 2019; Lydiard and Nemeroff 2019; Majchrzak-Celinska and Baer-Dubowska 2017; Sullivan et al. 2018; Zeier et al. 2018).

BIG DATA

Very large-scale data collection (i.e., "big data") is crucial to enabling reliable individualized predictions in PMP. Big data collection has been aided by recent technological advances, such as the increased use of electronic medical records (EMRs) in hospitals and office-based health care (Castro et al. 2015; Hsiao and Hing 2014), which generates huge amounts of data that are easily collected and inexpensive to store and analyze. Clearly, EMR-collected information has limitations, especially when records are being pulled from different clinical centers. For example, data sets may be nonhomogeneous with several missing values, clinical information may be disorganized and unstandardized, different methods may be used for data collection, and some information may be coded in formats not immediately suitable for analysis.

However, there are promising examples of how appropriate analyses can successfully obtain clinical insights from EMRs, albeit not yet in relation to tailoring of treatment. A highly predictive model of suicidal behavior was built through the application of a probability-based machine learning algorithm on a large-scale health care database (longitudinal EMRs of approximately 1.7 million patients, spanning 15 years) (Barak-Corren et al. 2017). Also, the application of a natural language processing technique to EMR data from a U.S healthcare system (more than 4.2 million patients, spanning more than 20 years) provided a highly accurate diagnostic algorithm for bipolar disorder (Castro et al. 2015). Similarly, the application of bioinformatics tools to EMRs of multiple large hospitals enabled the correct classification of current mood state and definition of longitudinal outcomes in patients with MDD (Perlis et al. 2012).

Clearly, improvements are needed (e.g., the standardization and alignment of information collected in different centers and the use of common or mergeable platforms), and great attention must be payed to ethical and legal issues and patient privacy. However, the extensive use of EMRs, along with the application of new computational resources such as machine learning techniques, is expected to contribute to personalized diagnoses and treatment decisions in the near future (Adkins 2017).

REAL-TIME DATA COLLECTION THROUGH SMART WEARABLE DEVICES

Another promising contributor to PMP is the widespread development of digital technology tools, especially "wearables," which are particularly suitable for collecting highly personalized data using flexible approaches. *Wearable technology* refers to accessories and clothing that incorporate computer technologies—including smartphones, smart watches, fitness trackers, smart clothing, and ear-worn devices—which are increasingly used because they are minimally intrusive and can be worn continuously without affecting daily activities (Perna et al. 2018b). Personal digital technologies can regularly record patients' subjective and objective data, and can be linked to smart health information systems, thus enabling extensive data collection in large groups of interest for both enhanced clinical care and longer-term research. Such technology-based approaches enable researchers/clinicians to track multiple dimensions concurrently, in real time, in great detail and at scale (Bauer et al. 2020; Faurholt-Jepsen et al. 2019; Harvey et al. 2020; Perna et al. 2018b; Qian and Long 2017; Seppälä et al. 2019; Xu et al. 2014).

While such devices have been adopted in other medical fields, such as cardiology (Fung et al. 2015; Lobodzinski 2013), oncology (Gresham et al. 2018), and endocrinology (Ontario Health [Quality] 2019; Umpierrez and Klonoff 2018), their use in psychiatry is still relatively limited (Roberts et al. 2018). However, with the widespread use of internet-connected devices (Ashton 2009), researchers and clinicians will soon be able to evaluate and analyze, in real time, data received from each device (Bauer et al. 2020; Ben-Zeev et al. 2015; Glenn and Monteith 2014; Magee et al. 2018). Such analysis will improve diagnostic accuracy, increase the capability of monitoring each patient from subjective and objective points of view, and enable prompt and direct communication with patients in case of emergency or to encourage their greater involvement with their own treatment and prevention process (Bauer et al. 2020; Cheung et al. 2018; de la Torre Díez et al. 2018; Hernandez et al. 2015; Magee et al. 2018; Van Ameringen et al. 2017). Nonadherence is one of the main causes of treatment failure in psychiatry, but these new devices can improve the doctor-patient relationship and build trust in psychiatric therapies (Ben-Zeev et al. 2015; Lopez et al. 2019; Paik and Kim 2019; Perna et al. 2018b; Torous and Roberts 2017).

When combined with other powerful design strategies (e.g., genetic, neuroimaging, neurobiological, and clinical intervention studies) and applied to multiple groups of interest (e.g., clinical, "at high risk," and epidemiological populations), digital technology tools may help to increase our understanding of psychiatric disorders and improve personalized interventions. Research is being conducted in the remote monitoring of patients and the gathering of specific parameters and biomarkers to identify depression or anxiety disorders and improve therapeutic outcomes (Bauer et al. 2020; Faurholt-Jepsen et al. 2019; Seppälä et al. 2019). Although no definitive conclusions can yet be drawn concerning the clinical utility and cost-effectiveness of these new strategies, the ongoing research provides encouraging results, and we present some examples in the following section. However, planning for and using these devices in clinical practice requires a concrete evaluation of each patient's needs and the establishment of a privacy "code of conduct" to ensure that patients accept and easily integrate these tools into their everyday life (Ball et al. 2020; Bauer et al. 2020; Chan et al. 2012; Haghi et al. 2017; Kappeler-Setz et al. 2013; Perna et al. 2018b).

MACHINE LEARNING

Collecting large amounts of data over long periods of time is relatively easy to do. However, accurate prediction will require complex models that translate the information and link it to the clinical outcome. *Machine learning*, a subset of artificial intelligence, can successfully help automate the data analysis process and make predictions using statistical techniques to increase our understanding of relationships among the collected variables (Bzdok and Meyer-Lindenberg 2018; Cearns et al. 2019; Dwyer et al. 2018; Rutledge et al. 2019; Tai et al. 2019; Vu et al. 2018). The application of machine learning techniques has recently expanded in e-commerce, search engine results, financial services, automatic transport, social media, virtual assistants, and health care (Bzdok and Meyer-Lindenberg 2018; Cearns et al. 2019; Dwyer et al. 2018; Rutledge et al. 2019).

Machine learning is expected to revolutionize how we diagnose, treat, and monitor psychiatric disorders. The current aim is to build well-structured predictive models of diagnosis and outcomes (Bzdok and Meyer-Lindenberg 2018; Cearns et al. 2019; Dwyer et al. 2018; Perna et al. 2018b; Rutledge et al. 2019). For example, using machine learning in psychiatry could help predict patient response to pharmacological and nonpharmacological treatments and aid early identification of patients at high risk of adverse events. However, before these tools can be integrated, further research must identify relevant predictors. Though the research moves forward, the overall pace of development in detecting, defining, and treating psychiatric disorders is disappointing (Bzdok and Meyer-Lindenberg 2018; Cearns et al. 2019; Dwyer et al. 2018; Perna et al. 2018b; Rutledge et al. 2019).

Clinical Illustrations

PMP APPLICATION IN MOOD DISORDERS

Crucial aspects of PMP include more precise prediction of disease susceptibility, early diagnosis of disease, and personalized therapies, all of which are aimed at decreasing the morbidity and mortality associated with mental illnesses (Prendes-Alvarez and Nemeroff 2018). In this context, progress has been made in mood disorders (MDD and bipolar disorder).

In terms of *therapeutic outcomes* of mood disorders, a crucial aim is to increase the rate of favorable treatment responses. Of patients with MDD, 40%–60% obtain suboptimal responses to first-line treatment, of whom only about 35% obtain remission after switching to a second-line treatment, and 34%–48% of patients have treatment-resistant depression (Perna et al. 2020). Similarly, treatment-resistant bipolar depression is considered the major contributor to the large burden of bipolar disorder–associated disease. The prediction of which mood stabilizer is best for each individual patient with bipolar disorder is a major challenge in clinical practice (e.g., only one-third of lithium-treated patients obtain a complete clinical response) (McAllister-Williams et al. 2020).

In recent years, promising attempts have been made to develop outcome-predictive models. Two main strategies have been followed, namely, the application of innovative computational methods (e.g., machine learning) to "pure" clinical data to increase the predictive power of variables that are easily collected in clinical practice, and the enrichment of predictive models through the inclusion of multimodal individual variables such as genetic, biological, and neuroimaging information, and/or biomarkers. For example, the recent application of machine learning techniques to clinical data previously collected in the Sequenced Treatment Alternatives to Relieve Depression (STAR*D) (Phase 1) and Combining Medications to Enhance Depression Outcomes (CO-MED) studies provided a model capable of significantly predicting clinical remission to citalopram, escitalopram, and escitalopram-bupropion treatment, but not to venlafaxine-mirtazapine treatment, which suggests the model's specificity to identifying patients with MDD who are likely to respond to a specific antidepressant (Chekroud et al. 2016, 2017). Similarly, a combination of demographic and clinical variables, obtained using an machine learning approach on previous data from the Genome-Based Therapeutic Drugs for Depression study, significantly contributed to predicting MDD response and remission treatment with escitalopram, but not with nortriptyline, which suggests a potential for individualized prescription of escitalopram (Iniesta et al. 2016). However, a significant improvement to the model's performance, yielding significant drug-specific predictions of remission for both escitalopram and nortriptyline, was obtained through a subsequent reanalysis of the same sample's data using statistical learning on a larger number of factors, including common genetic variants and clinical variables (Iniesta et al. 2018). One recent report proposed using preliminary, potentially clinically relevant machine learning models for predicting lithium response in patients with bipolar disorder using only clinical data (Kim et al. 2019), even though higher prediction accuracy was found in a preliminary study that included neuroimaging data (Fleck et al. 2017). Because the bipolar disorder studies on this topic are limited and present considerable methodological heterogeneity, more research will be needed to draw any firm conclusion.

The inclusion of multiple variables in predictive models of treatment response is considered to be the most promising strategy for significantly increasing the accuracy of the predictions, because patients classified as having the same psychiatric disorder show considerable phenomenological and biological heterogeneity. Consistent with this, an ensemble learning model, which integrated imaging, genetic, and clinical information for individualized baseline prediction of early response to antidepressants in MDD, achieved a better performance (accuracy=0.86) than models that included only functional MRI (fMRI) or genetic data (Pei et al. 2020). In line with this idea, a recent meta-analysis on bipolar or unipolar depression found that machine learning classification algorithms predicted therapeutic outcomes with an overall accuracy of 0.82, but pooled estimates of classification accuracy were significantly greater in models informed by multiple data types, including neuroimaging, genetic, and clinical data predictors (Lee et al. 2018).

Recent preliminary studies suggest that other innovative variables might also enrich machine learning models. Pretreatment gene expression biomarkers (i.e., peripheral messenger RNA levels of genes selected from genome-wide transcriptome data) reached 0.76 accuracy in predicting nonremission after 8 weeks of citalopram treatment in patients with MDD, which suggests that these biomarkers might add considerable improvement to predictions when integrated into larger machine learning models (Guilloux et al. 2015). A "learning-augmented clinical assessment" workflow with "multi-omics," in which clinical assessment was enriched with a wide range of biological measures (e.g., metabolites, genetic data, metabolomic concentrations), demonstrated a significant improvement in prediction accuracy for antidepressant treatment outcomes in patients with MDD from 35% to 80% individualized by patient, compared with a model using only clinical predictors (Athreya et al. 2018). A very large study—including patients with MDD from the Mayo Clinic Pharmacogenomics Research Network Antidepressant Medication Pharmacogenomic Study, the International Selective Serotonin Reuptake Inhibitor (SSRI) Pharmacogenomics Consortium trials, and the STAR*D trial—found that machine learning can achieve accurate and replicable prediction of SSRI therapy response using total baseline depression severity combined with pharmacogenomic biomarkers (Athreya et al. 2019). Although these results have not yet definitively changed the way mood disorders are treated and how treatment outcomes are predicted, they seem to indicate a promising perspective.

PMP APPLICATION IN ANXIETY DISORDERS

In the field of anxiety disorders, the body of PMP research is more limited and less informative than that in mood disorders. This is disappointing given that anxiety disorders are among the most common mental disorders (lifetime prevalence is approximately 33.7% and 14.5% of the U.S. and European adult populations, respectively [Alonso et al. 2007; Bandelow and Michaelis 2015; Kessler et al. 2012]) and are associated with severe disability, impairment in quality of life, high psychiatric/medical comorbidity, and significant economic burden on society (Gustavsson et al. 2011; Nager and Atkinson 2016). Response rates to recommended first-line anxiety disorder treatments—such as SSRIs, serotonin-norepinephrine reuptake inhibitors, and cognitive-behavioral therapy (CBT)—are often below expectation, with 40%–60% of patients continuing to have residual and impairing symptoms (Bandelow 2020; Bandelow et al. 2017; Bokma et al. 2019; Koen and Stein 2011; Patterson and Van Ameringen 2016). In the following paragraphs, we provide examples of precision medicine application in anxiety disorders, mainly focused on personalized therapy for panic disorder (PD).

Our group recently proposed preliminary considerations toward a personalized approach for PD, with an attempt to define some homogeneous phenomenological profiles of PD, which may be relevant to therapeutic management (Caldirola and Perna 2019). We considered respiratory, cardiac, vestibular, and derealization/depersonalization profiles, based on individual clinical symptoms and biological patterns, with related implications for treatment (Caldirola and Perna 2019). Behavioral/respiratory hypersensitivity to hypercapnia—which is present in approximately 50%–70% of patients with PD and runs in families—is a reliable biomarker of vulnerability to PD. Some findings showed that an early decrease in hypersensitivity to hypercapnia—measured through the 35% carbon dioxide (CO_2)-inhalation laboratory test—after the first week of treatment significantly predicted good clinical outcome after a 1-month treatment with SSRIs, imipramine, or clomipramine, which suggests that CO_2 reactivity can be a useful objective predictor of short-term clinical outcome in patients with PD (Perna et al. 2002). Further, patients with PD displayed several pretreatment respiratory abnormalities (Perna and Caldirola 2018), including higher variability in baseline respiratory parameters and hematic indicators of chronic hyperventilation (Grassi et al. 2014). Preliminary findings showed that successful antipanic pharmacological treatments were associated with the normalization of some baseline respiratory parameters, such as blood pH and HCO_3^-/PO_4^-, which suggests that respiratory variables are worthy of future larger investigations as potential outcome predictors (Caldirola and Perna 2019). Finally, preliminary results suggested that low pretreatment end-tidal CO_2 may predict dropout or poorer outcomes from CBT (Davies and Craske 2014; Tolin et al. 2017), because patients with PD who had reduced pretreatment heart rate variability were more likely to show residual symptoms after completion of exposure therapy (Wendt et al. 2018). These are promising results, though confirmations are needed.

Only a few studies of genetic/epigenetic putative predictors are available in PD. Although they present heterogeneous methods and results, these studies suggest a potential role of genetic polymorphisms involving the serotonergic system and COMT (catechol O-methyltransferase), an enzyme involved in monoamine catabolism, in predicting responses to antipanic medication or CBT (Caldirola and Perna 2015; Lonsdorf et al. 2010), while recent preliminary findings proposed polymorphism of the orexin receptor 1 as a predictor of post-CBT improvement (Gottschalk et al. 2019). Reversibility of pretreatment monoamine oxidase A hypomethylation was suggested as a potential epigenetic correlate of response to CBT in patients with PD (Perna et al. 2016). A recent longitudinal epigenome-wide association study and pilot data in PD demonstrated the involvement of dynamic methylation of multiple genes in CBT outcomes (Ziegler et al. 2019).

A few brain imaging studies have investigated neural substrates that are potentially predictive of treatment response to CBT in patients with PD. Preliminary findings showed associations between pretreatment activation patterns—mainly involving anterior cingulate cortex–amygdala coupling during fear-conditioning and extinction tasks—and favorable response (Lueken et al. 2013). A subsequent attempt to integrate brain imaging and genetic data revealed that the above-described findings were driven by CBT responders with the L/L genotype of the 5-HTTLPR polymorphism (Lueken et al. 2015). More recently, a study that applied a machine learning approach to pre-CBT brain imaging data found that no single brain region was predictive of treatment response, while good predictive performance was achieved by integrating regional classifiers based on data from the acquisition and the extinction phases of a fear-conditioning task for the whole brain (Hahn et al. 2015). In contrast, support vector machine analysis of fMRI data acquired during a pretreatment interoception paradigm was not able to reliably predict individual response to CBT (Sundermann et al. 2017).

Clearly, progress toward a personalized therapy for PD—and for anxiety disorders in general—is inadequate. Large-scale data collection is lacking, and there are insufficient studies that attempt to combine multiple data levels to identify patterns with the highest predictive capacity and accuracy. A few studies displayed a preliminary potential, such as the attempt to quantify anxiety disorder risk in preschool children through application of a machine learning approach to diagnostic parent-report interviews (Carpenter et al. 2016), or to separate generalized anxiety disorder from MDD using a multimodal machine learning approach that integrated clinical, hormonal, and structural MRI data (Hilbert et al. 2017). Support vector machine analysis using neural correlates of social signals of threat suggested that neural activity across large-scale systems may aid in the diagnosis of social anxiety disorder (Xing et al. 2020). Pretreatment cortical hyperactivity to social threat signals may serve as a prognostic indicator of CBT success in social anxiety disorder (Klumpp et al. 2013). Finally, an ongoing randomized controlled study is examining multilevel prediction of response to behavioral activation and exposure-based therapy in generalized anxiety disorder (Santiago et al. 2020). However, more work will be required to draw reliable conclusions, and a number of methodological refinements and specific challenges must be addressed to improve diagnostic tools and treatment outcome in anxiety disorders (Lueken et al. 2016).

Conclusion and Future Directions

A groundbreaking change in data collection and analysis will be necessary to acquire valid predictive models for psychiatric disorders. At this point, the first question that clinicians and researchers should ask themselves is, "What is our goal now?" (Fernandes et al. 2017; Ozomaro 2013; Perna and Nemeroff 2018; Perna et al. 2018b).

The World Health Organization (2020) defines *health* as "a state of complete physical, mental and social well-being and not merely the absence of disease or infirmity," which means that mental health implies more than the lack of mental disorders. Hence, the goal of successful treatment is to achieve the highest possible quality of life for patients. In these terms, personalized psychiatry can be a turning point in the way mental illnesses are addressed and treated. If tech devices become part of integrated clinical systems, all types of data will be integrated into the global process of redefining diagnoses and treatment (Perna et al. 2018b). Artificial intelligence will assist experts in the medical decision-making process, with the aim to facilitate mental health care.

Now, several years after the introduction of precision medicine, progress in psychiatry has yet to produce tangible effects on the population. To realize the dream of precision medicine in clinical psychiatry, a change of direction is needed. The next steps will require both a structural and a procedural change in research and practice.

Clinicians should have an active role in the development of precision medicine (e.g., collecting data and guiding patients and family through the new systems). Indeed, artificial intelligence cannot replace one of most important assets in the healing and recovery process: the patient-clinician relationship.

Researchers should always take into account the actualization of the knowledge gained through studies, namely, considering to what extent results are applicable to clinical practice. A stronger cooperation between academic research and industry is also essential to accumulate the requisite strong evidence of the efficacy and cost-effectiveness of the developed tools. Governments and policy makers have the responsibility to promulgate new public health policies, provide strategic direction and funds, and regulate commercial medical devices and new pharmacological compounds.

Personalized psychiatry will require consideration beyond the "biological features" of psychiatric disorders. The data from "-omics" (e.g., genomics, epigenomics, proteomics, metabolomics, pharmacogenomics) and other techniques (i.e., neuroimaging, behavioral and neuropsychological assessment, and brain electrical activity) are necessary but not sufficient. Personalized psychiatry offers the idea of combining biological and clinical data with specific environmental, spiritual, and personal aspects relevant for each individual patient (Saveanu and Nemeroff 2012). Using information gained from patients' psychosocial situation, personal preferences, health beliefs, values, and goals enables clinicians to tailor a treatment intervention on the unique features of each patient.

PMP has the potential to change the way we conceptualize, identify, and treat mental health disorders, and this change should not be delayed any longer. To help realize this goal, the World Psychiatric Association has recently founded the Personalized Psychiatry section, whose mission is to secure, spread, and adopt the precision medicine approach in psychiatry. Not a palpable dream or a theoretical illusion, but a realistic approach.

KEY POINTS

- Given unsatisfactory clinical outcomes with our current approach to mental health assessment and treatment, a new approach is urgently needed. Personalized medicine in psychiatry (PMP) has emerged as an innovative approach for identifying distinctive features of an individual related to health and disease in order to select appropriate and effective therapy. More narrowly, PMP is focused on tailoring treatment.

- Because psychiatric disorders are highly heterogeneous both clinically and neurobiologically, it is likely that a large amount of multimodal data will be needed to reliably boost the development of innovative precision diagnostic and therapeutic strategies.

- Combinatoral pharmacogenetic tests, big data, and wearable technology are all sources of multimodal data that, while they each have limitations, show promise in improving classification and tailoring treatment in psychiatry.

- Promising progress has been made in PMP in developing models for mood disorders in order to predict their development and response to therapy, particularly when using variables from multiple sources. However, these results have yet to change the way psychiatry is practiced.

- PMP has the potential to change the way we conceptualize, identify, and treat mental health disorders. Realizing this goal will require support and cooperation from academic research, industry, governments, and policy makers, as well as consideration of both biological and clinical data, including patients' psychosocial situation, personal preferences, health beliefs, values, and goals.

References

Abbott R, Chang DD, Eyre HA: Ethical, policy, and research considerations for personalized psychiatry, in Personalized Psychiatry. Edited by Baune BT. London, Elsevier, 2020, pp 549–556

Adkins DE: Machine learning and electronic health records: a paradigm shift. Am J Psychiatry 174(2):93–94, 2017 28142275

Alonso J, Lépine J-P; ESEMeD/MHEDEA 2000 Scientific Committee: Overview of key data from the European Study of the Epidemiology of Mental Disorders (ESEMeD). J Clin Psychiatry 68 (suppl 2):3–9, 2007 17288501

Ashton K: That "Internet of things" thing. RFID Journal, 2009. Available at: www.rfidjournal.com/that-internet-of-things-thing. Accessed February 19, 2021.

Athreya A, Iyer R, Neavin D, et al: Augmentation of physician assessments with multi-omics enhances predictability of drug response: a case study of major depressive disorder. IEEE Comput Intell Mag 13(3):20–31, 2018 30467458

Athreya AP, Neavin D, Carrillo-Roa T, et al: Pharmacogenomics-driven prediction of antidepressant treatment outcomes: a machine-learning approach with multi-trial replication. Clin Pharmacol Ther 106(4):855–865, 2019 31012492

Ball TM, Kalinowski A, Williams LM: Ethical implementation of precision psychiatry. Personalized Medicine in Psychiatry 19–20:(2020):100046, 2020

Balon R, Morreale MK: Stigma of mental illness and us. Ann Clin Psychiatry 31(3):161–162, 2019 31369654

Bandelow B: Current and novel psychopharmacological drugs for anxiety disorders. Adv Exp Med Biol 1191:347–365, 2020 32002937

Bandelow B, Michaelis S: Epidemiology of anxiety disorders in the 21st century. Dialogues Clin Neurosci 17(3):327–335, 2015 26487813

Bandelow B, Michaelis S, Wedekind D: Treatment of anxiety disorders. Dialogues Clin Neurosci 19(2):93–107, 2017 28867934

Barak-Corren Y, Castro VM, Javitt S, et al: Predicting suicidal behavior from longitudinal electronic health records. Am J Psychiatry 174(2):154–162, 2017 27609239

Baro E, Degoul S, Beuscart R, et al: Toward a literature-driven definition of big data in healthcare. BioMed Res Int 2015:639021, 2015 26137488

Bauer M, Glenn T, Geddes J, et al: Smartphones in mental health: a critical review of background issues, current status and future concerns. Int J Bipolar Disord 8(1):2, 2020 31919635

Ben-Zeev D, Scherer EA, Wang R, et al: Next-generation psychiatric assessment: using smartphone sensors to monitor behavior and mental health. Psychiatr Rehabil J 38(3):218–226, 2015 25844912

Bokma WA, Wetzer GAAM, Gehrels JB, et al: Aligning the many definitions of treatment resistance in anxiety disorders: a systematic review. Depress Anxiety 36(9):801–812, 2019 31231925

Bousman CA, Eyre HA: "Black box" pharmacogenetic decision-support tools in psychiatry. Br J Psychiatry 42(2):113–115, 2020 31994639

Bousman CA, Hopwood M: Commercial pharmacogenetic-based decision-support tools in psychiatry. Lancet Psychiatry 3(6):585–590, 2016 27133546

Brown L, Vranjkovic O, Li J, et al: The clinical utility of combinatorial pharmacogenomic testing for patients with depression: a meta-analysis. Pharmacogenomics 21(8):559–569, 2020 32301649

Bzdok D, Meyer-Lindenberg A: Machine learning for precision psychiatry: opportunities and challenges. Biol Psychiatry Cogn Neurosci Neuroimaging 3(3):223–230, 2018 29486863

Caldirola D, Perna G: Is there a role for pharmacogenetics in the treatment of panic disorder? Pharmacogenomics 16(8):771–774, 2015 26083015

Caldirola D, Perna G: Toward a personalized therapy for panic disorder: preliminary considerations from a work in progress. Neuropsychiatr Dis Treat 15:1957–1970, 2019 31371969

Carpenter KLH, Sprechmann P, Calderbank R, et al: Quantifying risk for anxiety disorders in preschool children: a machine learning approach. PLoS One 11(11):e0165524, 2016 27880812

Castro VM, Minnier J, Murphy SN, et al: Validation of electronic health record phenotyping of bipolar disorder cases and controls. Am J Psychiatry 172(4):363–372, 2015 25827034

Cearns M, Hahn T, Baune BT: Recommendations and future directions for supervised machine learning in psychiatry. Transl Psychiatry 9(1):271, 2019 31641106

Chan M, Estève D, Fourniols JY, et al: Smart wearable systems: current status and future challenges. Artif Intell Med 56(3):137–156, 2012 23122689

Chekroud AM, Zotti RJ, Shehzad Z, et al: Cross-trial prediction of treatment outcome in depression: a machine learning approach. Lancet Psychiatry 3(3):243–250, 2016 26803397

Chekroud AM, Gueorguieva R, Krumholz HM, et al: Reevaluating the efficacy and predictability of antidepressant treatments: a symptom clustering approach. JAMA Psychiatry 74(4):370–378, 2017 28241180

Cheung K, Ling W, Karr CJ, et al: Evaluation of a recommender app for apps for the treatment of depression and anxiety: an analysis of longitudinal user engagement. J Am Med Inform Assoc 25(8):955–962, 2018 29659857

Davies CD, Craske MG: Low baseline pCO2 predicts poorer outcome from behavioral treatment: evidence from a mixed anxiety disorders sample. Psychiatry Res 219(2):311–315, 2014 24953422

de la Torre Díez I, Alonso SG, Hamrioui S, et al: IoT-based services and applications for mental health in the literature. J Med Syst 43(1):11, 2018 30519972

Di Sanzo M, Cipolloni L, Borro M, et al: Clinical applications of personalized medicine: a new paradigm and challenge. Curr Pharm Biotechnol 18(3):194–203, 2017 28240172

Dwyer DB, Falkai P, Koutsouleris N: Machine learning approaches for clinical psychology and psychiatry. Annu Rev Clin Psychol 14(1):91–118, 2018 29401044

Evers K: Personalized medicine in psychiatry: ethical challenges and opportunities. Dialogues Clin Neurosci 11(4):427–434, 2009 20135900

Fanous AH, Kendler KS: Genetic heterogeneity, modifier genes, and quantitative phenotypes in psychiatric illness: searching for a framework. Mol Psychiatry 10(1):6–13, 2005 15618952

Faurholt-Jepsen M, Geddes JR, Goodwin GM, et al: Reporting guidelines on remotely collected electronic mood data in mood disorder (eMOOD)—recommendations. Transl Psychiatry 9(1):162, 2019 31175283

Fernandes BS, Williams LM, Steiner J, et al: The new field of "precision psychiatry." BMC Med 15(1):80, 2017 28403846

Fleck DE, Ernest N, Adler CM, et al: Prediction of lithium response in first-episode mania using the LITHium Intelligent Agent (LITHIA): pilot data and proof-of-concept. Bipolar Disord 19(4):259–272, 2017 28574156

Fung E, Järvelin MR, Doshi RN, et al: Electrocardiographic patch devices and contemporary wireless cardiac monitoring. Front Physiol 6:149, 2015 26074823

Glenn T, Monteith S: New measures of mental state and behavior based on data collected from sensors, smartphones, and the Internet. Curr Psychiatry Rep 16(12):523, 2014 25308392

Goetz LH, Schork NJ: Personalized medicine: motivation, challenges, and progress. Fertil Steril 109(6):952–963, 2018 29935653

Goldberg JF, Nemeroff CB: Pharmacogenomics and antidepressants: efficacy and adverse drug reactions, in Psychiatric Genomics. Edited by Tsermpine E, Petrinos GP, Alde M. New York, Academic Press (in press)

Gottschalk MG, Richter J, Ziegler C, et al: Orexin in the anxiety spectrum: association of a HCRTR1 polymorphism with panic disorder/agoraphobia, CBT treatment response and fear-related intermediate phenotypes. Transl Psychiatry 9(1):75, 2019 30718541

Grassi M, Caldirola D, Di Chiaro NV, et al: Are respiratory abnormalities specific for panic disorder? A meta-analysis. Neuropsychobiology 70(1):52–60, 2014 25247676

Greden JF, Parikh SV, Rothschild AJ, et al: Impact of pharmacogenomics on clinical outcomes in major depressive disorder in the GUIDED trial: a large, patient- and rater-blinded, randomized, controlled study. J Psychiatr Res 111:59–67, 2019 30677646

Gresham G, Schrack J, Gresham LM, et al: Wearable activity monitors in oncology trials: current use of an emerging technology. Contemp Clin Trials 64:13–21, 2018 29129704

Guilloux JP, Bassi S, Ding Y, et al: Testing the predictive value of peripheral gene expression for nonremission following citalopram treatment for major depression. Neuropsychopharmacology 40(3):701–710, 2015 25176167

Gustavsson A, Svensson M, Jacobi F, et al: Cost of disorders of the brain in Europe 2010. Eur Neuropsychopharmacol 21(10):718–779, 2011 21924589

Haghi M, Thurow K, Stoll R: Wearable devices in medical internet of things: scientific research and commercially available devices. Healthc Inform Res 23(1):4–15, 2017 28261526

Hahn T, Kircher T, Straube B, et al: Predicting treatment response to cognitive behavioral therapy in panic disorder with agoraphobia by integrating local neural information. JAMA Psychiatry 72(1):68–74, 2015 25409415

Harvey P, Pendergrass C, Nemeroff C: Challenges in assessment of daytime sleepiness in cognitively impaired populations can be bypassed through use of ecological momentary assessment. 2020. Available at: www.researchgate.net/publication. Accessed February 19, 2021.

Hays P: Advancing Healthcare Through Personalized Medicine. New York, CRC Press, 2017

Hernandez J, McDuff DJ, Picard RW: Biophone: physiology monitoring from peripheral smartphone motions. Annu Int Conf IEEE Eng Med Biol Soc 2015:7180–7183, 2015 26737948

Hilbert K, Lueken U, Muehlhan M, et al: Separating generalized anxiety disorder from major depression using clinical, hormonal, and structural MRI data: a multimodal machine learning study. Brain Behav 7(3):e00633, 2017 28293473

Hodgson K, McGuffin P, Lewis CM: Advancing psychiatric genetics through dissecting heterogeneity. Hum Mol Genet 26(R2):R160–R165, 2017 28977440

Hoehe MR, Morris-Rosendahl DJ: The role of genetics and genomics in clinical psychiatry. Dialogues Clin Neurosci 20(3):169–177, 2018 30581286

Hsiao CJ, Hing E: Use and characteristics of electronic health record systems among office-based physician practices: United States, 2001–2012, in Electronic Health Records: Selected Analyses on Use and Incentive Payments. Edited by Eastman S. New York, Nova Science Publishers, 2014, pp 77–88

Iniesta R, Malki K, Maier W, et al: Combining clinical variables to optimize prediction of antidepressant treatment outcomes. J Psychiatr Res 78:94–102, 2016 27089522

Iniesta R, Hodgson K, Stahl D, et al: Antidepressant drug-specific prediction of depression treatment outcomes from genetic and clinical variables. Sci Rep 8(1):5530, 2018 29615645

Insel TR: The NIMH Research Domain Criteria (RDoC) project: precision medicine for psychiatry. Am J Psychiatry 171(4):395–397, 2014 24687194

Insel TR, Cuthbert B, Garvey M, et al: Research domain criteria (RDoC): toward a new classification framework for research on mental disorders. Am J Psychiatry 167(7):748–751, 2010 20595427

Insel TR, Landis SC, Collins FS, et al: Research priorities. Science 340(6133):687–688, 2013 23661744

Johnson TM: Perspective on precision medicine in oncology. Pharmacotherapy 37(9):988–989, 2017 28632968

Kappeler-Setz C, Gravenhorst F, Schumm J, et al: Towards long term monitoring of electrodermal activity in daily life. Pers Ubiquitous Comput 17(2):261–271, 2013

Kessler RC, Petukhova M, Sampson NA, et al: Twelve-month and lifetime prevalence and lifetime morbid risk of anxiety and mood disorders in the United States. Int J Methods Psychiatr Res 21(3):169–184, 2012 22865617

Kim TT, Dufour S, Xu C, et al: Predictive modeling for response to lithium and quetiapine in bipolar disorder. Bipolar Disord 21(5):428–436, 2019 30729637

Klumpp H, Fitzgerald DA, Phan KL: Neural predictors and mechanisms of cognitive behavioral therapy on threat processing in social anxiety disorder. Prog Neuropsychopharmacol Biol Psychiatry 45:83–91, 2013 23665375

Koen N, Stein DJ: Pharmacotherapy of anxiety disorders: a critical review. Dialogues Clin Neurosci 13(4):423–437, 2011 22275848

Kohn R, Ali AA, Puac-Polanco V, et al: Mental health in the Americas: an overview of the treatment gap. Rev Panam Salud Publica 42:e165, 2018 31093193

König IR, Fuchs O, Hansen G, et al: What is precision medicine? Eur Respir J 50(4):1700391, 2017 29051268

Krebs K, Milani L: Translating pharmacogenomics into clinical decisions: do not let the perfect be the enemy of the good. Hum Genomics 13(1):39, 2019 31455423

Le Tourneau C, Kamal M, Bièche I: Precision medicine in oncology: what is it exactly and where are we? Per Med 15(5):351–353, 2018 30260312

Lee Y, Ragguett RM, Mansur RB, et al: Applications of machine learning algorithms to predict therapeutic outcomes in depression: a meta-analysis and systematic review. J Affect Disord 241:519–532, 2018 30153635

Lobodzinski SS: ECG patch monitors for assessment of cardiac rhythm abnormalities. Prog Cardiovasc Dis 56(2):224–229, 2013 24215754

Lonsdorf TB, Rück C, Bergström J, et al: The COMTval158met polymorphism is associated with symptom relief during exposure-based cognitive-behavioral treatment in panic disorder. BMC Psychiatry 10:99, 2010 21110842

Lopez A, Schwenk S, Schneck CD, et al: Technology-based mental health treatment and the impact on the therapeutic alliance. Curr Psychiatry Rep 21(8):76, 2019 31286280

Lueken U, Straube B, Konrad C, et al: Neural substrates of treatment response to cognitive-behavioral therapy in panic disorder with agoraphobia. Am J Psychiatry 170(11):1345–1355, 2013 23982225

Lueken U, Straube B, Wittchen H-UU, et al: Therapygenetics: anterior cingulate cortex-amygdala coupling is associated with 5-HTTLPR and treatment response in panic disorder with agoraphobia. J Neural Transm (Vienna) 122(1):135–144, 2015 25223844

Lueken U, Zierhut KC, Hahn T, et al: Neurobiological markers predicting treatment response in anxiety disorders: a systematic review and implications for clinical application. Neurosci Biobehav Rev 66:143–162, 2016 27168345

Lydiard J, Nemeroff CB: Biomarker-guided tailored therapy. Adv Exp Med Biol 1192:199–224, 2019 31705496

Magee JC, Adut S, Brazill K, et al: Mobile app tools for identifying and managing mental health disorders in primary care. Curr Treat Options Psychiatry 5(3):345–362, 2018 30397577

Majchrzak-Celinska A, Baer-Dubowska W: Pharmacoepigenetics: an element of personalized therapy? Expert Opin Drug Metab Toxicol 13(4):387–398, 2017 27860490

McAllister-Williams RH, Cousins D, Lunn B: Clinical assessment and investigation in psychiatry. Medicine (United Kingdom) 44(11):630–637, 2016

McAllister-Williams RH, Sousa S, Kumar A, et al: The effects of vagus nerve stimulation on the course and outcomes of patients with bipolar disorder in a treatment-resistant depressive episode: a 5-year prospective registry. Int J Bipolar Disord 8(1):13, 2020 32358769

Nager AB, Atkinson RD: A Trillion-Dollar Opportunity: How Brain Research Can Drive Health and Prosperity. Information Technology & Innovation Foundation, Washington, DC, July 11, 2016

National Institutes of Health: Brain Research through Advancing Innovative Neurotechnologies (BRAIN) Working Group. Advisory committee to the NIH Director interim report. 2019. Available at: braininitiative.nih.gov. Accessed February 19, 2021.

National Research Council: Toward Precision Medicine: Building a Knowledge Network for Biomedical Research and a New Taxonomy of Disease. Washington, DC, National Academies Press, 2011

Ontario Health (Quality): Flash glucose monitoring system for people with type 1 or type 2 diabetes: a health technology assessment. Ont Health Technol Assess Ser 19(8):1–108, 2019 31942227

Ozomaro U: Personalized medicine and psychiatry: dream or reality? Psychiatric Times, October 9, 2013. Available at: www.psychiatrictimes.com/view/personalized-medicine-and-psychiatry-dream-or-reality. Accessed February 19, 2021.

Ozomaro U, Wahlestedt C, Nemeroff CB: Personalized medicine in psychiatry: problems and promises. BMC Med 11(1):132, 2013 23680237

Paik SH, Kim DJ: Smart healthcare systems and precision medicine. Adv Exp Med Biol 1192:263–279, 2019 31705499

Patterson B, Van Ameringen M: Augmentation strategies for treatment-resistant anxiety disorders: a systematic review and meta-analysis. Depress Anxiety 33(8):728–736, 2016 27175543

Pei C, Sun Y, Zhu J, et al: Ensemble learning for early-response prediction of antidepressant treatment in major depressive disorder. J Magn Reson Imaging 52(1):161–171, 2020 31859419

Perlis RH, Iosifescu DV, Castro VM, et al: Using electronic medical records to enable large-scale studies in psychiatry: treatment resistant depression as a model. Psychol Med 42(1):41–50, 2012 21682950

Perna G, Caldirola D: Is panic disorder a disorder of physical fitness? A heuristic proposal. F1000 Res 7:294, 2018 29623195

Perna G, Nemeroff CB: Personalized medicine in psychiatry: back to the future. Personalized Medicine in Psychiatry 1–2(Jan):1, 2018

Perna G, Bertani A, Caldirola D, et al: Antipanic drug modulation of 35% CO_2 hyperreactivity and short-term treatment outcome. J Clin Psychopharmacol 22(3):300–308, 2002 12006901

Perna G, Iannone G, Alciati A, et al: Are anxiety disorders associated with accelerated aging? A focus on neuroprogression. Neural Plast 2016:8457612, 2016 26881136

Perna G, Balletta R, Nemeroff C: Precision psychiatry: personalized clinical approach to depression, in Understanding Depression, Vol 1. Biological and Neurological Background. Edited by Yong-Ku K. New York, Springer, 2018a, pp 245–261

Perna G, Grassi M, Caldirola D, et al: The revolution of personalized psychiatry: will technology make it happen sooner? Psychol Med 48(5):705–713, 2018b 28967349

Perna G, Alciati A, Daccò S, et al: Personalized psychiatry and depression: the role of sociodemographic and clinical variables. Psychiatry Investig 17(3):193–206, 2020 32160691

Personalized Medicine Coalition: The Personalized Medicine Report: Opportunity, Challenges, and the Future. Washington, DC, Personalized Medicine Coalition, 2017. Available at: www.personalizedmedicinecoalition.org/ Userfiles/PMC-Corporate/file/ PMC_The_Personalized_Medicine_Report_Opportunity_Challenges_and_the_ Future.pdf. Accessed February 19, 2021.

Prendes-Alvarez S, Nemeroff CB: Personalized medicine: prediction of disease vulnerability in mood disorders. Neurosci Lett 669:10–13, 2018 27746310

Qian RC, Long YT: Wearable chemosensors: a review of recent progress. ChemistryOpen 7(2):118–130, 2017 29435397

Rehm J, Shield KD: Global burden of disease and the impact of mental and addictive disorders. Curr Psychiatry Rep 21(2):10, 2019 30729322

Roberts LW, Chan S, Torous J: New tests, new tools: mobile and connected technologies in advancing psychiatric diagnosis. NPJ Digit Med 1(1):20176, 2018 31304350

Rosenblat JD, Lee Y, McIntyre RS: Does pharmacogenomic testing improve clinical outcomes for major depressive disorder? A systematic review of clinical trials and cost-effectiveness studies. J Clin Psychiatry 78(6):720–729, 2017 28068459

Rutledge RB, Chekroud AM, Huys QJ: Machine learning and big data in psychiatry: toward clinical applications. Curr Opin Neurobiol 55:152–159, 2019 30999271

Santiago J, Akeman E, Kirlic N, et al: Protocol for a randomized controlled trial examining multilevel prediction of response to behavioral activation and exposure-based therapy for generalized anxiety disorder. Trials 21(1):17, 2020 31907032

Saveanu RV, Nemeroff CB: Etiology of depression: genetic and environmental factors. Psychiatr Clin North Am 35(1):51–71, 2012 22370490

Seppälä J, De Vita I, Jämsä T, et al: Mobile phone and wearable sensor-based mHealth approach for psychiatric disorders and symptoms: systematic review and link to the M-REsist project. JMIR Ment Health 6(2):e9819, 2019 30785404

Steiger A, Kimura M: Wake and sleep EEG provide biomarkers in depression. J Psychiatr Res 44(4):242–252, 2010 19762038

Stein DJ, Reed GM: Global mental health and psychiatric nosology: DSM-5, ICD-11, and RDoC. Br J Psychiatry 41(1):2, 2019 30672968

Stephan KE, Bach DR, Fletcher PC, et al: Charting the landscape of priority problems in psychiatry, part 1: classification and diagnosis. Lancet Psychiatry 3(1):77–83, 2016 26573970

Sugeir S, Naylor S: Critical care and personalized or precision medicine: who needs whom? J Crit Care 43:401–405, 2018 29174462

Sullivan PF, Agrawal A, Bulik CM, et al: Psychiatric genomics: an update and an agenda. Am J Psychiatry 175(1):15–27, 2018 28969442

Sundermann B, Bode J, Lueken U, et al: Support vector machine analysis of functional magnetic resonance imaging of interoception does not reliably predict individual outcomes of cognitive behavioral therapy in panic disorder with agoraphobia. Front Psychiatry 8:99, 2017 28649205

Tai AMY, Albuquerque A, Carmona NE, et al: Machine learning and big data: implications for disease modeling and therapeutic discovery in psychiatry. Artif Intell Med 99:101704, 2019 31606109

Tolin DF, Billingsley AL, Hallion LS, et al: Low pre-treatment end-tidal CO2 predicts dropout from cognitive-behavioral therapy for anxiety and related disorders. Behav Res Ther 90:32–40, 2017 27960095

Torous J, Roberts LW: The ethical use of mobile health technology in clinical psychiatry. J Nerv Ment Dis 205(1):4–8, 2017 28005647

Trautmann S, Rehm J, Wittchen HU: The economic costs of mental disorders: do our societies react appropriately to the burden of mental disorders? EMBO Rep 17(9):1245–1249, 2016 27491723

Umpierrez GE, Klonoff DC: Diabetes technology update: use of insulin pumps and continuous glucose monitoring in the hospital. Diabetes Care 41(8):1579–1589, 2018 29936424

Van Ameringen M, Turna J, Khalesi Z, et al: There is an app for that! The current state of mobile applications (apps) for DSM-5 obsessive-compulsive disorder, posttraumatic stress disorder, anxiety and mood disorders. Depress Anxiety 34(6):526–539, 2017 28569409

Vigo D, Thornicroft G, Atun R: Estimating the true global burden of mental illness. Lancet Psychiatry 3(2):171–178, 2016 26851330

Vigo DV, Kestel D, Pendakur K, et al: Disease burden and government spending on mental, neurological, and substance use disorders, and self-harm: cross-sectional, ecological study of health system response in the Americas. Lancet Public Health 4(2):e89–e96, 2019 30446416

Vilches S, Tuson M, Vieta E, et al: Effectiveness of a pharmacogenetic tool at improving treatment efficacy in major depressive disorder: a meta-analysis of three clinical studies. Pharmaceutics 11(9):E453, 2019 31480800

Vu MT, Adalı T, Ba D, et al: A shared vision for machine learning in neuroscience. J Neurosci 38(7):1601–1607, 2018 29374138

Wang PS, Aguilar-Gaxiola S, Alonso J, et al: Use of mental health services for anxiety, mood, and substance disorders in 17 countries in the WHO world mental health surveys. Lancet 370(9590):841–850, 2007 17826169

Wendt J, Hamm AO, Pané-Farré CA, et al: Pretreatment cardiac vagal tone predicts dropout from and residual symptoms after exposure therapy in patients with panic disorder and agoraphobia. Psychother Psychosom 87(3):187–189, 2018 29533952

White House, Office of the Press Secretary: Fact sheet: President Obama's Precision Medicine Initiative. 2. 2015a. Available at: obamawhitehouse.archives.gov/the-press-office/2015/01/30/fact-sheet-president-obama-s-precision-medicine-initiative. Accessed February 19, 2021.

White House, Office of the Press Secretary: Remarks by the President on precision medicine. 2015b. Available at: obamawhitehouse.archives.gov/the-press-office/2015/01/30/remarks-president-precision-medicine. Accessed February 19, 2021.

World Federation for Mental Health: Depression: A Global Crisis. World Mental Health Day, October 10, 2012. Available at: www.who.int/mental_health/management/depression/wfmh_paper_depression_wmhd_2012.pdf. Accessed February 19, 2021.

World Health Organization: Basic Documents: 49th edition. 2020. Available at: www.who.int/mental_health/management/depression/wfmh_paper_depression_wmhd_2012.pdf. Accessed February 19, 2021.

Xing M, Fitzgerald JM, Klumpp H: Classification of social anxiety disorder with support vector machine analysis using neural correlates of social signals of threat. Front Psychiatry 11:144, 2020 32231598

Xu S, Zhang Y, Jia L, et al: Soft microfluidic assemblies of sensors, circuits, and radios for the skin. Science 344(6179):70–74, 2014 24700852

Zeier Z, Carpenter LL, Kalin NH, et al: Clinical implementation of pharmacogenetic decision support tools for antidepressant drug prescribing. Am J Psychiatry 175(9):873–886, 2018 29690793

Ziegler C, Grundner-Culemann F, Schiele MA, et al: The DNA methylome in panic disorder: a case-control and longitudinal psychotherapy-epigenetic study. Transl Psychiatry 9(1):314, 2019 31754096

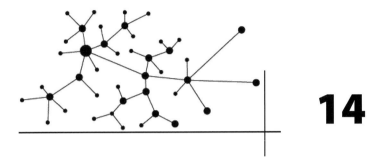

14

Preparing for the Future of Precision Psychiatry

The Critical Role of Neuroscience Education

David A. Ross, M.D., Ph.D.
Joseph J. Cooper, M.D.
Melissa R. Arbuckle, M.D., Ph.D.
Ashley E. Walker, M.D.
Michael J. Travis, M.D.

History

In the beginning, there was darkness. For thousands of years, psychiatric illness was treated as "madness." People were tried as witches and burned at the stake. They were shackled and forgotten. Some religious traditions inculcated a moral model in which symptoms were conceptualized as a choice, a personal failure, or divine punishment. Treatments, when they existed, may have been worse than the illnesses: bloodletting, to bring balance to the four body humors; trepanation, to let out evil spirits; exorcism, to remove the spirits forcefully. For most of history, psychiatric illness has been lumped together as a single, toxic entity, and those suffering from it were profoundly stigmatized, shunned from society, and exiled to the asylum.

The 1800s saw the first serious attempts to bring order and reason to the understanding of historical "madness." At the turn of the 19th century, Franz Joseph Gall was the first in recorded history to posit that specific regions of the brain were the centers for specific faculties (Zola-Morgan 1995). Although this work evolved into the carnival pseudoscience of phrenology, it marked an important shift away from Cartesian dualism. By the mid-century, support for the localization of higher-order behavioral functions emerged from the seminal case of Phineas Gage, who experienced disinhibition and personality change following injury to his prefrontal cortex (Macmillan 2000). The second half of the nineteenth century saw Broca's first precise localization of a higher cognitive function: the seat of spoken language on the inferior frontal gyrus (Broca 1861; Kann 1950). With efforts such as these, neuropsychiatric syndromes began to emerge from ancient concepts of "madness" and "lunacy." Researchers were so successful that some syndromes—for example, epilepsy through the work of Jackson (Reynolds 1988) and dementia through the work of Pick (Spatt 2003)—were no longer considered psychiatric disorders.

Other conditions were more elusive. Toward the late 1800s, a group of physicians turned their attention to some of the disorders that remained unexplained and dedicated themselves to the crucial task of psychiatric nosology. They sought to carve out categories that reflected discrete disease entities using meticulous observations of symptoms, phenomenology, and course of progression over time. Most famous is the work of Kraepelin on individuals with psychotic symptoms, in which he tried to differentiate those whom he felt to have a progressive decline from those with a more cyclical course. He ultimately settled on two broad entities: "dementia praecox" and "manic-depressive insanity." Though Kraepelin later appreciated that this was an oversimplification, the basic distinction still stands (Kendler and Engstrom 2018).

Through the early 1900s, new tools gradually emerged that enabled the measurement of brain activity. The advent of the lumbar puncture, electroencephalography, and advances in neuropathology furthered the growing schism between neurology and psychiatry—diseases of the nervous system versus diseases of the mind—with echoes of Cartesian dualism reverberating once more (Price et al. 2000). While these new developments helped to advance the field of neurology, psychiatry slipped backward. Leading psychiatric treatments of the era (e.g., cold sheet compresses, insulin coma, malarial fever, frontal lobotomy, hysterectomies) remained crude and imprecise. The burgeoning psychodynamic movement continued to push psychiatry further away from a medical model.

In the mid-1950s, widespread change overtook the field. Lithium's utility for acute mania had been rediscovered by John Cade, and the development of a blood test to monitor lithium levels helped to manage the safety profile of this markedly efficacious pharmacotherapy (Shorter 2009). At the same time, chlorpromazine offered a huge step forward in the treatment of chronic psychotic disorders (Carpenter and Davis 2012). Significant reduction in positive psychotic symptoms and agitation were seen, setting the stage for understanding the role of the brain's dopamine systems in perceptual disturbances, salience processing, and self-inferential reasoning.

Chlorpromazine's success prompted the development of derivative compounds, which included the tricyclic antidepressants and their descendants, the selective serotonin reuptake inhibitors. Meanwhile, happenstance during the treatment of tuberculosis with isoniazid led to the monoamine oxidase inhibitors (Carpenter and Davis 2012). The treatments themselves were hardly precise, but the sequential development of these drug classes was an important step toward precision. Psychiatric diseases were finally being conceptualized as biological entities.

In the 1960s, at the same time as the psychiatric world was widely expanding the use of these new pharmacotherapies, neurology was also about to change. Most of the field was focused on peripheral nerves, neuromuscular junctions, and movement syndromes. Moreover, psychodynamic models to explain higher-order functioning were just as accepted among neurologists as they were in psychiatric circles. But a subset of the community, led by Norman Geschwind, became interested in the serious study of behavior. Their approach derived from the neurology of the 1800s: observe patients with specific lesions (like Phineas Gage) and connect their disrupted neuroanatomy to circumscribed deficits of behavior or cognition. This work set the stage for a modern understanding of cortical networks that are involved in language, praxis, attention, visuospatial abilities, memory, and semantics (Mesulam 2015). The implications for understanding emotional processing, disorders of thought, consciousness, and behavior—the neurobiology of psychiatric illness—were not far behind. Sadly, though, the culture gap was so vast that this pioneering work went largely unnoticed by the field of psychiatry.

Meanwhile, in psychiatry, the challenges of nosology continued. By the 1970s, most fields of medicine had been able to describe their major disease processes, identify underlying pathophysiology, and develop corresponding treatments that could be evaluated via systematic clinical trials. But psychiatry was stuck. Much of the field persisted with older models of mental illness that conceptualized causality from a psychodynamic framework: from penis envy causing neuroses (Schafer 1974) to masturbatory impulses causing tics (Martin 2002). Psychiatry was decidedly lacking in both precision and reliability and was therefore incompatible with a modern medical approach. In 1980, DSM was revised specifically to address this problem: in the absence of biological data, the goal was to create a diagnostic system that would be based on observable behavioral features (DSM-III; American Psychiatric Association 1980). Though agnostic to causality, this system would at least enable inter-rater reliability as well as more valid and reproducible clinical trials.

While it was a critical step forward at the time, over the ensuing years the unintended consequences of DSM have become increasingly problematic. Since all major clinical trials are built around a DSM schema, the diagnostic criteria have become cemented as a foundation of clinical practice. Though DSM was intended as a tool for reliable categorization, over time clinicians have come to treat the DSM categories as if they reflect discrete diseases.

Similarly, while the discoveries of effective medications were an important step forward, they led to reductive disease models (e.g., schizophrenia as a hyperdopaminergic process or depression as a hyposerotonergic state) that have lingered beyond their utility. We have even designed animal models of psychiatric illness around these same oversimplifications. For example, we consider an animal model of depression to be valid if it is reversed by antidepressant medications.

Current Knowledge and Approaches

The dawn of the current century saw the beginning of the neuroscience revolution and the creation of a broad range of new tools that could finally bring light to psychiatry. As described in the previous chapters, modern approaches (including genetics, imaging, and interventional techniques) could enable us to achieve the holy grail of precision medicine: to make precise, pathophysiologically defined diagnoses for individual patients and use them as a basis for implementing specific custom treatments. Myriad examples are emerging that, while still limited in their scope, point the way to the future.

Yet even when these tools are ready, the field will still face a major obstacle. The successful implementation of precision psychiatry will require a skilled and ready workforce. Unfortunately, that workforce does not yet exist in the field of psychiatry. Sadly, our field remains defined by our history rather than our future.

Preparing for a future of precision psychiatry will require addressing several core challenges. First and foremost is the fact that major advances in our understanding of the brain are relatively new. This means that many— if not most—practicing clinicians were trained in an era when an understanding of neuroscience had relatively little impact on their day-to-day clinical practice. In fact, despite new hypothesis-driven treatments, much of neuroscience research has remained within the confines of academic institutions and leading research journals. The relevance of neuroscience to the practice of psychiatry today may not be readily apparent to most clinicians in the community.

As for those clinicians who do recognize the value of integrating a neuroscience perspective into clinical practice, where do they begin? The field is vast, and much of the scientific literature is intended to communicate with other researchers. The content is inherently intricate and is often inaccessible to a clinical audience. In addition, the relevance of these data and their potential translation to clinical practice are often unclear. The increasingly complex landscape of medicine has driven specialization, with clinicians and researchers each working within smaller and smaller niches. As a result, opportunities for dialogue between researchers and clinicians are limited, and this is further complicated by the fact that each group fundamentally speaks a different language. Thus, a major challenge is facilitating communication across these distinct communities (Arbuckle et al. 2017; Cooper et al. 2019).

Conclusion and Future Directions: Medical Education for Precision Psychiatry

Preparing the field for precision psychiatry will require major changes in medical education and how psychiatry residents are trained. Although most psychiatric residency training directors appreciate the importance of integrating neuroscience into training, a lack of appropriate faculty and the unavailability of curricula are major barriers (Benjamin et al. 2014). Few programs have faculty with sufficient expertise in neuroscience. For those that do, the same challenges described above apply (i.e., expertise in neuroscience may be independent of the skills necessary to teach a clinical audience). These barriers underscore the importance of collaborating across institutions to develop resources that can be implemented by non-experts. In addition, resources must be adaptable to cover a broad range of topics and keep pace with new discoveries (Ross et al. 2015).

To this end, the National Neuroscience Curriculum Initiative (NNCI) was developed in 2013 with the goal of creating a set of shared, open-access materials that could be used by residency training programs to help learners incorporate a robust neuroscience presence into their clinical work. The guiding principles were as follows: 1) all materials should maintain an integrative, patient-centered approach to care; rather than teaching neuroscience in isolation, it should be brought alongside the other rich traditions of our field; 2) in recognition of limitations of traditional medical education (including overreliance on a lecture format), all resources would be designed according to principles of adult learning (e.g., clear learning objectives for each session; embracing experiential learning methods); and 3) focusing on dissemination, sessions must be easy to implement regardless of the content expertise of the facilitator. From the beginning, it was clear that no single program would be able to do this on its own. Rather, a core belief of the NNCI team was that *in the same way that cutting-edge science requires teamwork and collaboration, so too does cutting-edge education.*

Over the first several years, the NNCI focused on creating classroom teaching and learning resources that embody these principles. These included more than a dozen different modules, each reflecting a unique pedagogical approach, with multiple sessions designed around each approach. To assist with implementation, the NNCI ensured that each session was accompanied by a facilitator's guide with detailed descriptions of how to run the session, answers to all of the exercises, and additional background materials. Recognizing that many instructors may not feel comfortable with the content, the NNCI also focused heavily on faculty development by providing training sessions at the annual meetings of many professional organizations.

At the same time, it quickly became clear that these efforts were intrinsically limited. Even if programs were able to successfully implement the most radical of classroom curricula (perhaps 50–100 hours), it would still be only a small fraction of a resident's total educational experience (approximately 10,000 hours). If faculty were not reinforcing core neuroscience concepts in clinical settings, a hidden curriculum might emerge: that neuroscience is an academic topic intended for classroom discussion only and is not important to clinical practice. To address this challenge, the NNCI began developing a set of resources that could be easily implemented within a clinical setting while highlighting the relevance of neuroscience to patient care. For example, a team could treat a patient with borderline personality disorder and then watch together a brief video of an expert demonstrating how to speak with a patient about the neurobiology of borderline personality disorder, or a different video illustrating how adverse childhood experiences could cause lasting changes to hypothalamic-pituitary-adrenal axis regulation through epigenetic mechanisms.

Another limitation of this approach became apparent: the majority of these materials were aimed at residency programs. In order to effect meaningful change in our field, the scope of this effort needed to expand to engage individuals throughout levels of training and across disciplines, including medical students, practicing psychiatrists, other physicians, psychologists, social workers, nurses, and even patients and families. To this end, the NNCI began investing effort into a set of resources that were designed to engage a wider audience. These resources include TED-style talks, a series of narrative clinical commentaries in the journal *Biological Psychiatry*, and a new podcast. Each of these pieces is designed to take one core concept in neuroscience and make it clear, relevant, and accessible.

Since its inception, the NNCI has compiled over 200 teaching resources. These include materials that are designed for classroom settings and those designed for clinical supervision, as well as a collection of videos and narrative-style commentaries that are designed to engage a broader audience. Recognizing the challenges of implementation and dissemination, the NNCI has run more than 50 faculty development workshops at the annual meetings of national organizations and in other venues. As a reflection of the demand for such resources, as of March 2021, more than 200 training programs have implemented NNCI teaching materials within their curricula, and the NNCI website has registered more than 90,000 unique users from 164 countries. Even more encouragingly, regulatory agencies have begun to embrace neuroscience in psychiatric training standards. The Accreditation Council for Graduate Medical Education has included neuroscience in the Psychiatry Milestones benchmarks for resident competence, and the Royal College of Psychiatrists in the United Kingdom has changed both its curriculum and its assessment process to incorporate modern neuroscience.

Psychiatry is on the cusp of a revolution. Modern neuroscience is already enabling us to move from broad syndromes to more focused diagnostic entities. Over a century ago, Kraepelin's dementia praecox laid the groundwork for today's broad categorization of psychosis. Since then, we have been able to carve a few actual diseases from this category. Psychosis that presents with progressive paresis, sensory ataxia, and pupils that accommodate but do not react to light is a disease caused by a spirochete and requires treatment with penicillin. Delusions and hallucinations following a cluster of seizures require improved seizure control rather than treatment with antipsychotic medications. The occurrence of isolated visual hallucinations in the setting of blindness requires only psychoeducation to inform that this is normal. More recently, catatonia in first-episode psychosis should prompt testing for autoimmune causes (Pollak et al. 2020). Each of these more precise diagnoses (neurosyphilis, postictal psychosis, Charles Bonnet syndrome, and autoimmune encephalitis, respectively) enables targeted treatment planning at the *disease* level.

The promise of precision medicine is that we can leverage modern tools to continue this work, not only for psychosis but also across all of psychiatric illness. Other examples are just around the corner: from the identification of novel autoimmune antibodies to appreciating the impact of the microbiome; from applying complex machine learning algorithms to functional imaging–based diagnostics. However, advances in precision psychiatry will also require precision education to ensure that clinicians have the knowledge, skills, and attitudes that will enable them to embrace new approaches as they emerge.

As Joshua Gordon, director of the National Institute of Mental Health, described: "It's incredibly important that our psychiatrists training for tomorrow understand that they too are neuroscientists. They're studying the brain. They're studying the brain in a very different way, in a very patient-focused way....If they don't understand that, one of two things will happen, and maybe both: they will be left behind, they won't be able to do the psychiatry of tomorrow; or the psychiatry of tomorrow won't be" (Ross 2019).

KEY POINTS

- The field of psychiatry has progressed a long way from the conceptualization of psychiatric illness as "madness" to the neuroscience revolution in which modern approaches described in previous chapters are paving the way for the precision psychiatry revolution.

- Preparing the field for precision psychiatry will require major changes in medical education and how psychiatry residents are trained.

- The National Neuroscience Curriculum Initiative (NNCI) was developed in 2013 with the goal of creating a set of shared, open-access materials that could be used by psychiatry residency training programs to help learners incorporate a robust neuroscience presence into their clinical work.

- Initially focused on creating classroom resources that embody principles of adult learning, the NNCI has adapted over the years to now developing resources implementable in clinical settings and that are designed to engage individuals throughout levels of training and across disciplines.

- The vital importance of incorporating modern neuroscience into psychiatric training is clearly reflected in the high demand for the NNCI's materials, its adoption by regulatory agencies into psychiatric training standards, and recognition by the past two directors of the National Institute of Mental Health that psychiatrists must incorporate neuroscience into their clinical practice.

References

American Psychiatric Association: Diagnostic and Statistical Manual of Mental Disorders, 3rd Edition. Washington, DC, American Psychiatric Association, 1980

Arbuckle MR, Travis MJ, Ross DA: Integrating a neuroscience perspective into clinical psychiatry today. JAMA Psychiatry 74(4):313–314, 2017 28273288

Benjamin S, Travis MJ, Cooper JJ, et al: Neuropsychiatry and neuroscience education of psychiatry trainees: attitudes and barriers. Acad Psychiatry 38(2):135–140, 2014 24643397

Broca P: Remarks on the seat of the faculty of articulated language, following an observation of aphemia (loss of speech). Bulletin de la Société Anatomique 6:330–357, 1861

Carpenter WT Jr, Davis JM: Another view of the history of antipsychotic drug discovery and development. Mol Psychiatry 17(12):1168–1173, 2012 22889923

Cooper JJ, Korb AS, Akil M: Bringing neuroscience to the bedside. Focus Am Psychiatr Publ 17(1):2–7, 2019 31975952

Kann J: A translation of Broca's original article on the location of the speech center. J Speech Hear Disord 15(1):16–20, 1950

Kendler KS, Engstrom EJ: Criticisms of Kraepelin's psychiatric nosology: 1896–1927. Am J Psychiatry 175(4):316–326, 2018 29241358

Macmillan M: Restoring Phineas Gage: a 150th retrospective. J Hist Neurosci 9(1):46–66, 2000 11232349

Martin JB: The integration of neurology, psychiatry, and neuroscience in the 21st century. Am J Psychiatry 159(5):695–704, 2002 11986119

Mesulam MM: Fifty years of disconnexion syndromes and the Geschwind legacy. Brain 138 (Pt 9):2791–2799, 2015 26163663

Pollak TA, Lennox BR, Müller S, et al: Autoimmune psychosis: an international consensus on an approach to the diagnosis and management of psychosis of suspected autoimmune origin. Lancet Psychiatry 7(1):93–108, 2020 31669058

Price BH, Adams RD, Coyle JT: Neurology and psychiatry: closing the great divide. Neurology 54(1):8–14, 2000 10636118

Reynolds EH: Hughlings Jackson. A Yorkshireman's contribution to epilepsy. Arch Neurol 45(6):675–678, 1988 3285819

Ross DA: Episode 1: What's in a name? [podcast]. Ten to the Fifteenth. National Neuroscience Curriculum Initiative, September 3, 2019. Available at: www.nncionline.org/course/episode-1-whats-in-a-name/. Accessed May 29, 2020.

Ross DA, Travis MJ, Arbuckle MR: The future of psychiatry as clinical neuroscience: why not now? JAMA Psychiatry 72(5):413–414, 2015 25760896

Schafer R: Problems in Freud's psychology of women. J Am Psychoanal Assoc 22(3):459–485, 1974 4616980

Shorter E: The history of lithium therapy. Bipolar Disord 11 (suppl 2):4–9, 2009 19538681

Spatt J: Arnold Pick's concept of dementia. Cortex 39(3):525–531, 2003 12870825

Zola-Morgan S: Localization of brain function: the legacy of Franz Joseph Gall (1758–1828). Annu Rev Neurosci 18:359–383, 1995 7605066

INDEX

Page numbers printed in **boldface** *type refer to tables or figures.*